NEUROPATHIC PAIN

NEUROPATHIC PAIN

A Case-Based Approach to Practical Management

EDITED BY

JIANGUO CHENG, MD, PHD

Professor of Anesthesiology
Cleveland Clinic Lerner College of Medicine
Case Western Reserve University
Director, Cleveland Clinic Multidisciplinary
Pain Fellowship Program
Departments of Pain Management and Neurosciences

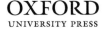

OXFORD
UNIVERSITY PRESS

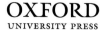

Oxford University Press is a department of the University of Oxford. It furthers
the University's objective of excellence in research, scholarship, and education
by publishing worldwide. Oxford is a registered trade mark of Oxford University
Press in the UK and certain other countries.

Published in the United States of America by Oxford University Press
198 Madison Avenue, New York, NY 10016, United States of America.

CIP data is on file at the Library of Congress
ISBN 978–0–19–029835–7

1 3 5 7 9 8 6 4 2

Printed by Sheridan Books, Inc., United States of America

CONTENTS

CONTRIBUTORS

Magdalena Anitescu, MD, PhD
Associate Professor, Director, Pain Medicine
Fellowship Program
Section Chief, Division of Pain Management,
Department of Anesthesia and Critical
Care, University of Chicago Medical Center,
Chicago, IL

Sailesh Arulkumar, MD
Interventional Pain Medicine Specialist,
Tulsa, OK

Justin F. Averna, DO
Interventional Pain Medicine,
New Mexico Pain and Spine Institute,
Albuquerque, NM

Hersimren Basi, MD
Staff, Department of Pain Management,
Cleveland Clinic, Cleveland, OH

Alexander Bautista, MD
Assistant Professor, Department of
Anesthesiology, University of Oklahoma
Health Sciences Center, Oklahoma City, OK

Timothy Bednar, MD
Pain Medicine Specialist, Greater Austin Pain
Center, Kyle, TX

John Blackburn, MD
Pain Fellow, Department of Anesthesiology,
University of Oklahoma Health Sciences
Center, Oklahoma City, OK

Whit Braddy, MD, MBA
Interventional Pain Medicine, National Spine
and Pain, Cary, NC and Henderson, NC

Randall P. Brewer, MD
Attending Physician, River Cities
Interventional Pain Specialists, Shreveport, LA
Clinical Assistant Professor, Departments of
Anesthesiology and Neurology, Louisiana
State University Health Science Center in
Shreveport, LA
Assistant Consulting Professor, Department
of Anesthesiology, Duke University Medixal
Center, Durham, NC

Harold J. Campbell, MD, MPH
Resident, Department of Surgery, Mountain
Area Health Education Center, Asheville, NC

Martin J. Carney, MD
Resident, Division of Plastic Surgery,
Yale School of Medicine, New Haven, CT

Elizabeth Casserly, PharmD
Pain Pharmacy Specialist, Department of
Pain Management, Cleveland Clinic,
Cleveland, OH

George C. Chang Chien, DO
Director of Pain Management, Ventura
County Medical Center, Ventura, CA
Director, GCC Institute, Arcadia, CA

Jianguo Cheng, MD, PhD
Professor of Anesthesiology, Cleveland Clinic
Lerner College of Medicine, Case Western
Reserve University
Director, Cleveland Clinic Multidisciplinary
Pain Fellowship Program, Departments
of Pain Management and Neurosciences,
Cleveland, OH

Armin Deroee, MD
Interventional Pain Physician, Pacific Pain and Spine Center, Visalia, CA

Jagan Devarajan, MD, EMBA
Medical Director, Department of Anesthesiology, Medina Hospital, Cleveland Clinic, Westlake, OH

Gulshan Doulatram, MD
Professor of Anesthesiology, University of Texas Medical Branch at Galveston, Galveston, TX

Theodore G. Eckman, MD
Interventional Pain Physician, The Center for Pain Management at Saint Vincent, Erie, PA

Dalia Elmofty, MD
Assistant Professor, Pain Medicine Division, Department of Anesthesia & Critical Care, University of Chicago, Chicago, IL

Jonathan P. Eskander, MD, MBA
Senior Resident, Department of Anesthesiology, Tulane Medical Center, New Orleans, LA

Victor Foorsov, MD
Marianjoy Rehabilitation Hospital/ Northwestern Medicine, Chicago, IL

Joshua Frenkel, MD
Attending Physician, Department of Anesthesiology, Staten Island University Hospital, New York, NY

Timothy Furnish, MD
Associate Clinical Professor of Anesthesiology, Center for Pain Medicine
Pain Fellowship Program Director, UC San Diego Medical Center, San Diego, CA

Radhika Grandhe, MD
Assistant Professor, Department of Anesthesiology, University of New Mexico, Albuquerque, NM

Eli Johnson Harris, MD
Resident, Department of Anesthesiology, University of New Mexico, Albuquerque, NM

Maximilian Hsia-Kiung, MD
Instructor, Harvard Medical School, Department of Anesthesiology, Critical Care, and Pain Medicine, Massachusetts General Hospital, Boston, MA

Erik C. Hustak, MD
Associate Professor, Pain Medicine Fellowship Director, Department of Anesthesiology, The University of Texas Medical Branch, Galveston, TX

Eduardo E. Icaza, MD
Interventional Pain Physician, Mendelson Kornblum Orthopedics and Spine Specialists, Livonia, MI

Preya K. Jhita, MD
Resident, Department of Anesthesiology, Stanford Medical School, Palo Alto, CA

Mark R. Jones, MD
Senior Resident, Department of Anesthesiology, Beth Israel Deaconess Medical Center, Harvard Medical School, Boston, MA

Abdullah Kandil, MD
Pain Medicine Fellow, Dartmouth Hitchcock Medical Center, Lebanon, NH

Alan D. Kaye, MD, PhD
Professor and Chairman, Department of Anesthesiology, Louisiana State University School of Medicine, New Orleans, LA

John P. Kenny IV, MD
Fellow, Pain Medicine Division, Department of Anesthesia & Critical Care, University of Chicago, Chicago, IL

Brian A. Kim, MD
Pain Specialist, Center for Interdisciplinary Spine, Sacramento, CA

Eugene Koshkin, MD
Associate Professor, Department of Anesthesiology, University of New Mexico, Albuquerque, NM

Aliza Kumpinsky, MD
Resident, Department of Neurology, Emory University, Atlanta, GA

Zeeshan Malik, DO
Interventional Pain Physician, Arizona Pain Specialists, Gilbert, AZ

Beth H. Minzter, MD, MS
Staff, Medical Director, Department of Pain Management, Anesthesiology Institute, Cleveland Clinic, Cleveland, OH

Ravi Mirpuri, DO
Chief Resident, Physical Medicine and
Rehabilitation, UC Irvine Medical Center,
Orange, CA

Mark Motejunas, MD
Senior Resident, Department of
Anesthesiology, Louisiana State University
School of Medicine, New Orleans, LA

Sai Munjampalli, MD
Attending Physician, River Cities
Interventional Pain Specialists, Shreveport, LA

Sarah M. Pastoriza, DO
Fellow, Interventional Pain Medicine,
University of Alabama-Birmingham,
Birmingham, AB

Shilpadevi Patil, MD
Associate Professor, Program Director,
Director of PACU, Louisiana State University
Health Sciences Center-Shreveport,
Shreveport, LA

Danielle Perret, MD
Associate Dean for Graduate Medical
Education, Associate Clinical Professor,
Departments of Physical Medicine &
Rehabilitation;
Anesthesiology & Perioperative Care and
Neurological Surgery, The University of
California, Irvine, CA

Varun Rimmalapudi, MD
Fellow, Department of Anesthesiology,
University of New Mexico, Albuquerque, NM

Samuel W. Samuel, MD
Associate Program Director, Pain Medicine
Fellowship, Cleveland Clinic, Cleveland, OH

Michael Saulino, MD, PhD
Director of Neuromodulation, MossRehab,
Associate Professor, Rehabilitation Medicine,
Thomas Jefferson University, Philadelphia, PA

Rinoo V. Shah, MD, MBA
Professor, Director of Chronic Pain, Pain
Fellowship Director, Louisiana State
University Health Sciences Center-Shreveport,
Shreveport, LA

Bradley A. Silva, MD, JD
Multidisciplinary Pain Medicine Fellow,
Department of Anesthesia and Critical Care,
The University of Chicago Medicine,
Chicago, IL

Michelle St. Romain, BS
Senior Medical Student, Louisiana State
University School of Medicine, New
Orleans, LA

Agnes R. Stogicza, MD
St. Paul's Hospital, University of British
Columbia, Vancouver, Canada

Andrea M. Trescot, MD
Pain and Headache Center, Wasilla, AK

Trevor Van Oostrom, MD
Interventional Pain Physician & Clinical
Instructor, Nanaimo Regional Gen. Hospital,
Vancouver, British Columbia, Canada

Ashwin Varma, MD
University of Texas Medical Branch at
Galveston, Galveston, TX

Wenbao Wang, MD
Attending Physician, Department of Physical
Medicine and Rehabilitation, Baylor Scott &
White, Dallas, TX

Jiang Wu, MD
Assistance Professor, Department of
Anesthesiology and Pain Medicine, University
of Washington Medical Center, University of
Washington, Seattle, WA

PART I

Overview of Neuropathic Pain

Concept and Overview of Neuropathic Pain

JIANGUO CHENG

DEFINING NEUROPATHIC PAIN

Our understanding and management of pain as a familiar part of life or as a symptom of various diseases have improved tremendously over the past century. Neuropathic pain, however, remains a significant challenge in patients' lives and in clinical practice. Defined by the International Association for the Study of Pain (IASP) "*neuropathic pain* refers to pain arising as a direct consequence of a lesion or disease affecting the somatosensory system."[1] It is noteworthy that *neuropathic pain* is a clinical description, not a diagnosis, which requires a demonstrable lesion or a disease that satisfies established neurological diagnostic criteria. Postherpetic neuralgia, diabetic neuropathy, and post-stroke central pain syndrome are prominent examples of neuropathic pain, as there are demonstrable lesions or diseases in these cases that clearly fulfill the established neurological diagnostic criteria. Neuropathic pain is commonly associated with other sensory abnormalities.

Peripheral neuropathic pain is caused by a lesion or a disease of the peripheral nervous system (PNS). Painful diabetic neuropathy, complex regional pain syndrome type II (causalgia), postherpetic neuralgia, various nerve entrapments, and radicular pain are examples of this category of neuropathic pain. The pain is often described as "burning," "tingling," "electrical," "stabbing," or "pins and needles." Central neuropathic pain is caused by a primary lesion or disease in the central nervous system (CNS) and is usually associated with abnormal sensibility to temperature and noxious stimulation. Common examples include post-stroke pain, pain related to spinal cord injury, and pain due to multiple sclerosis. Phantom pain (pain felt in a part of the body that has been lost or from which the brain no longer receives signals) may also be considered in this category.

The current definition of neuropathic pain was developed with considerations of a number of important factors that render intricacy and nuances to the differentiation of neuropathic from non-neuropathic pain. Taking into account these factors, the new definition represents the current consensus among experts in the field.[2]

1. Our current understanding of the neural pathophysiology is limited even for the most common neuropathic pain conditions, such as postherpetic neuralgia, painful diabetic neuropathy, and spinal cord injury.
2. Some of the clinical features of neuropathic pain, such as allodynia and hyperalgesia, can also occur in normal nociceptors. The specificity of these clinical features for diagnosis or mechanistic understanding of neuropathic pain is limited.
3. Such conditions as cervical and lumbar radicular pain are likely results of physiological function of nociceptors that reside in the connective tissue sheaths and respond to inflammatory processes around the nerve root due to mechanical compression or chemical irritation.
4. Several pain conditions, such as migraine and cluster headaches, are clearly associated with dysfunction of the nervous system but not commonly considered neuropathic pain.
5. Some clinical conditions of unknown etiology, such as fibromyalgia, share certain clinical features with syndromes that are clearly neuropathic.
6. Under the new definition, complex regional pain syndrome (CRPS), which has been traditionally considered a type of neuropathic pain, may no longer be

classified as neuropathic pain. It is more likely autoimmune related instead.

EPIDEMIOLOGY

Neuropathic pain is one of the most common forms of chronic pain. The first systematic review of epidemiological studies of neuropathic pain in the general population concluded that a best estimate of population prevalence of pain with neuropathic characteristics is likely to lie between 6.9% and 10%.[3] A telephone survey based on a random sampling of both urban and rural households of the general population in Canada employed the Douleur Neuropathique en 4 questionnaire (DN4Q) to identify neuropathic pain symptoms in those patients with chronic pain and found that chronic pain was present in 35.0% of the surveyed population, with neuropathic pain symptoms present in 17.9%.[4]

A cross-sectional study of 1,857 patients recruited from 137 US medical institutions nationwide revealed high prevalence of neuropathic pain in patients with chronic pain associated with spinal disorders.[5] The overall prevalence of neuropathic pain was 53.3%. It was particularly high in patients with cervical spondylotic myelopathy (77.3%) and ligament ossification (75.7%) and relatively low in those with low back pain (29.4%) and spondylolysis (40.4%). Similarly, the prevalence of neuropathic pain characteristics in patients with painful knee osteoarthritis (OA) was also as high as 33.3%.[6] A recent systematic review concluded that neuropathic pain prevalence in people with knee or hip OA is 23% and may be higher after other potential causes of neuropathic pain are excluded.[7] In cancer patients, 54.2% suffered from pain, and 20.4% had a clinical diagnosis of pure neuropathic or mixed pain.[8]

The methodological means used to identify patients with neuropathic pain, such as the Leeds Assessment of Neuropathic Symptoms and Signs (LANSS) pain scale and the DN4Q, may account for some of the variations between different studies.[9,10] Regardless, it is evident that neuropathic pain has high prevalence both in the general population and among patients with specific medical conditions. The 2016 revision of the IASP Special Interest Group on Neuropathic Pain (NeuPSIG) grading system[11] uses information from patient history, physical examination, and confirmatory diagnostic test as clinical classification criteria for the diagnosis of unlikely, possible, probable, and definite neuropathic pain (Figure 1.1). This system is recommended for consistent use in clinical practice and research.[12]

IMPACT

Neuropathic pain has enormous impact on patients' quality of life and cost of care. A review of 52 high-quality studies examined the association between neuropathic pain and health-related quality of life (HRQoL) in patients with six neuropathic pain conditions associated with lesions of either the CNS (post-stroke pain, spinal cord injury pain, multiple sclerosis pain) or the PNS (postsurgical neuropathic pain associated with breast and amputation surgery, postherpetic neuralgia, and painful diabetic neuropathy).[13] The results provide strong evidence that the presence and severity of neuropathic pain are associated with greater impairments in a number of important HRQoL domains.

Patients with neuropathic pain experience substantially lower HRQoL than the general population. A systematic review and meta-analysis included 24 studies and examined the level of health utility in patients with neuropathic pain.[14] The use of a single-index health utility measure is a common way to assess HRQoL.[15] Health utility measures evaluate patients' subjective preferences on a scale where 0 represents death and 1 represents full health. Utility scores are frequently used to quantify the cost-effectiveness of therapies and are therefore often required by health policymakers. Utility measures combine many different health domains into a single number, weigh the different domains with the values people have for the particular health states, and reflect the preferences of groups of persons for particular treatment outcomes and disease states.[15] A significant relationship between increasing neuropathic pain severity and a reduction in utility and HRQoL was identified.[14] Neuropathic pain severity emerged as a primary predictor of the negative health impact.

A study using a large US health insurance claims database demonstrated that the total calendar-year healthcare charges were threefold higher for patients with painful neuropathic pain disorders (PNDs) than for matched control subjects.[16] Patients with PNDs are generally in poorer health and have higher healthcare costs than their peers without these conditions. There were a total of 55,686 patients with PNDs in the study database, and the most frequently noted PNDs were back and neck pain with neuropathic involvement (62.3% of PND patients),

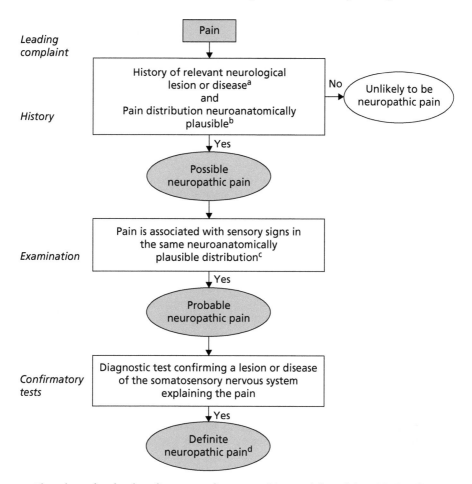

FIGURE 1.1. Flow chart of updated grading system for neuropathic pain (adopted from NeuPSIG). **a**. History, including pain descriptors, the presence of nonpainful sensory symptoms, and aggravating and alleviating factors, suggestive of pain being related to a neurological lesion and not other causes such as inflammation or non-neural tissue damage. The suspected lesion or disease is reported to be associated with neuropathic pain, including a temporal and spatial relationship representative of the condition; includes paroxysmal pain in trigeminal neuralgia. **b**. The pain distribution reported by the patient is consistent with the suspected lesion or disease. **c**. The area of sensory changes may extend beyond, be within, or overlap with the area of pain. Sensory loss is generally required but touch-evoked or thermal allodynia may be the only finding at bedside examination. Trigger phenomena in trigeminal neuralgia may be counted as sensory signs. In some cases, sensory signs may be difficult to demonstrate, although the nature of the lesion or disease is confirmed; for these cases the level "probable" continues to be appropriate, if a diagnostic test confirms the lesion or disease of the somatosensory nervous system. **d**. The term "definite" in this context means "probable neuropathic pain with confirmatory tests" because the location and nature of the lesion or disease have been confirmed to be able to explain the pain. "Definite" neuropathic pain is a pain that is fully compatible with neuropathic pain, but it does not necessarily establish causality.

causalgia (12.1%), and diabetic neuropathy (10.8%). Compared to matched control subjects, PND patients were more likely to have other pain-related conditions, including fibromyalgia (6.0% vs. 0.6% for control subjects), OA (13.6% vs. 3.6%), and other chronic comorbidities, such as coronary heart disease (13.6% vs. 6.5%) and depression (6.4% vs. 2.3%).

A number of different diseases or injuries can damage the CNS or PNS and produce neuropathic pain, which seems to be more difficult to treat than many other types of chronic pain.[17] As a group, patients with neuropathic pain have greater medical comorbidity burden than age- and sex-adjusted controls, which makes determining the humanistic and economic burden attributable to neuropathic pain challenging. Patients with neuropathic pain describe pain-related interference in multiple HRQoL and functional domains, as well as reduced ability to work and reduced mobility due to their pain. In addition, the spouses of neuropathic pain patients have been shown to experience adverse social consequences related to neuropathic pain. Several medications have been shown to improve various measures of HRQoL in randomized controlled trials. Changes in HRQoL appear to be tightly linked to pain relief. However, cross-sectional studies showed that many patients continue to have moderate or severe pain and markedly impaired HRQoL, despite taking medications prescribed for neuropathic pain.

The substantial costs of neuropathic pain to society derive from direct medical costs, loss of the ability to work, loss of caregivers' ability to work, and possibly greater need for institutionalization or other living assistance.[17] So far, no single study has measured all of these costs to society for chronic neuropathic pain. Cost-effectiveness of various interventions for the treatment or prevention of different types of neuropathic pain has been assessed in several different studies. The most-studied diseases are postherpetic neuralgia and painful diabetic neuropathy, for which tricyclic antidepressants (both amitriptyline and desipramine) have been found to be cost-effective compared to other strategies. Increasing the use of cost-effective therapies such as tricyclic antidepressants for postherpetic neuralgia and painful diabetic neuropathy may improve the HRQoL of patients and decrease societal costs. Comparative effectiveness clinical trials using HRQoL and health utility measures are needed to help assess the relative clinical efficacy of neuropathic pain therapies. Improved relative efficacy, utility, and cost estimates would facilitate future cost-effectiveness research in neuropathic pain.

CHALLENGES AND OPPORTUNITIES

There are enormous challenges in understanding and managing neuropathic pain given the diversity of causes, pathology, mechanisms, and clinical presentations of neuropathic pain conditions.[18] Our understanding is limited regarding how an injury or disease of the peripheral nerves leads to molecular, cellular, and histological changes in the CNS. We know even less about how a lesion or a disease of the CNS can cause central neuropathic pain. Likewise, our tools to investigate neuropathic pain are also limited. Most of the clinical neuropathic pain conditions don't have suitable animal models to study. Even for those for which animal models do exist, such as animal models of peripheral nerve injury induced neuropathic pain, diabetic neuropathy, and chemotherapy-induced neuropathy, the translation of laboratory findings to humans is often challenging and can be misleading, for various reasons. One of the reasons, for example, is that most of the animals used for this purpose (rats and mice) have life expectancies of about 2 years. This makes it difficult to study chronic pain states due to neurological injury or disorders. A second reason is that we don't have reliable objective measures of neuropathic pain in animals, or in humans for that matter. This lack of objectivity often compromises the quality of experimental investigations. Third, biological differences between species also complicate the interpretation of findings in animal models of neuropathic pain and the translation to humans. Because of our very limited mechanistic understanding of most of the neuropathic pain conditions, our ability to design and develop new and effective treatment is significantly hindered.

It has been a daunting challenge to manage most of the neuropathic pain conditions in clinical practice. The challenges of neuropathic pain are not limited to the research arena but also extend to clinical practice. Many treatment modalities, ranging from physical/cognitive, pharmacological, interventional, to surgical therapies, have been or are being used in clinical practice with limited efficacy in the majority of cases. Clearly, there are unmet needs in the treatment of neuropathic pain.

Along with these challenges are enormous opportunities for advancement.[18] In the last couple of decades, particularly in the last few years, the field of neuropathic pain has witnessed exciting progress in exploring the molecular and cellular mechanisms of neuropathic pain. In recent years, technologies such as transgenesis, optogenetics, and RNA-sequencing have been developed, which alongside the more traditional use of animal neuropathic pain models and insights from genetic variations in humans have enabled significant advances in the mechanistic understanding of neuropathic pain.[19] The roles of cytokines, chemokines, and other inflammatory factors in the development and maintenance OF chronic neuropathic pain are also being recognized.[20] The significant contributions from glial cells and immune cells (microglia in the CNS and other immune cells in the PNS) are being established.[21-24] It is now recognized that during chronic neuropathic pain, maladaptation occurs in the peripheral and central nervous systems, including a shift in microglial phenotype from a surveillance state to an activated state.[25,26] Microglial activation may lead to altered expression of cell surface proteins and release of growth factors and other intracellular signaling molecules that contribute to development of neuroinflammation and chronic pain sensitization.[25,27] Specific targeting of these cellular and molecular mechanisms may provide the key to development of effective neuropathic pain therapies with minimal side effects.

Rapid technological advances are being made in clinical diagnostics.[28] Magnetic resonance neurography, diffusion tensor imaging, and nerve ultrasonography are increasingly entering the diagnostic workup of peripheral neuropathies. These tools complement neurophysiology and enable investigation of proximal structures, such as plexuses and roots. The improved design of magnetic resonance scanners and sequences and the development of high-frequency ultrasound probes make it possible to have high-resolution peripheral nerve imaging, allowing detailed examination of nerve size, morphology, and internal fascicular structure that can integrate nerve conduction studies into clinical practice. Skin biopsy has become a reliable tool for diagnosis of small-fiber neuropathy, for which traditional nerve conduction studies are of little or no use.[28] Corneal confocal microscopy, nociceptive evoked potentials, and microneurography are emerging techniques that are not only critical in clinical research settings but also increasingly relevant to clinical practice.

New, promising therapeutic strategies are emerging in pharmacotherapy,[29] stem cell therapy,[30-33] and neuromodulation. For example, monoclonal antibodies antagonizing the calcitonin gene-related peptide (CGRP) pathway represent a novel approach to migraine prevention and mechanism-specific migraine-targeted therapy.[34-37] Monoclonal antibodies against CGRP or the CGRP receptor have shown efficacy in preventing or aborting migraine headaches in high-profile controlled trials. No safety issues have arisen to date. EMA401, an orally administered highly selective angiotensin II type 2 receptor antagonist, has shown promise as a novel treatment for postherpetic neuralgia in a randomized trial.[38] Acetyl-L-carnitine (ALC) and alpha-lipoic-acid (ALA) were effective for painful diabetic neuropathy in randomized controlled trials.[29] Cannabinoids were shown to be effective for HIV neuropathy in randomized trials. Experimental data and preliminary clinical investigations have demonstrated enormous promise of stem cell therapy for neuropathic pain.[30-33,39-41] Furthermore, new modalities in neuromodulation, such as high-frequency spinal cord stimulation, burst stimulation, dorsal root ganglion stimulation, closed-loop stimulation, transcranial direct current stimulation, and many others, have yielded exciting results.[42]

Inspired by these emerging therapeutic strategies and advances, the authors of this textbook strive to provide the readers with the current understanding of the mechanisms of the common neuropathic pain disorders, state-of-the art management strategies of neuropathic pain, and future directions in research and clinical practice.

REFERENCES

1. Treede RD, Jensen TS, Campbell JN, et al. Neuropathic pain: redefinition and a grading system for clinical and research purposes. *Neurology.* 2008;70;1630–1635. doi:10.1212/01.wnl.0000282763.29778.59.

2. Treede RD. Chapter 2, Peripheral and central mechanisms of neuropathic pain. In: Simpson DM, McArthur JC, Dworkin RH, eds. *Neuropathic Pain, Mechanisms, Diagnosis and Treatment.* New York: Oxford University Press; 2012: 14–24.

3. van Hecke O, Austin SK, Khan RA, Smith BH, Torrance N. Neuropathic pain in the general population: a systematic review of epidemiological studies. *Pain.* 2014;155:654–662. doi:10.1016/j.pain.2013.11.013.

4. Toth C, Lander J, Wiebe S. The prevalence and impact of chronic pain with neuropathic pain symptoms in the general population. *Pain Med.* 2009;10:918–929. doi:10.1111/j.1526-4637.2009.00655.x.

5. Yamashita T, Takahashi K, Yonenobu K, Kikuchi S. Prevalence of neuropathic pain in cases with chronic pain related to spinal disorders. *J Orthopaed Sci.* 2014;19:15–21. doi:10.1007/s00776-013-0496-9.

6. Oteo-Álvaro Á, Ruiz-Ibán MA, Miguens X, Stern A, Villoria J, Sánchez-Magro I. High prevalence of neuropathic pain features in patients with knee osteoarthritis: a cross-sectional study. *Pain Pract.* 2015;15:618–626. doi:10.1111/papr.12220.

7. French HP, Smart KM, Doyle F. Prevalence of neuropathic pain in knee or hip osteoarthritis: a systematic review and meta-analysis. *Semin Arthritis Rheum.* 2017;47:1–8. doi:10.1016/j.semarthrit.2017.02.008.

8. Pérez C, Sánchez-Martínez N, Ballesteros A, et al. Prevalence of pain and relative diagnostic performance of screening tools for neuropathic pain in cancer patients: a cross-sectional study. *Eur J Pain.* 2015;19:752–761. doi:10.1002/ejp.598.

9. Hamdan A, Luna JD, Del Pozo E, Galvez R. Diagnostic accuracy of two questionnaires for the detection of neuropathic pain in the Spanish population. *Eur J Pain.* 2014;18:101–109. doi:10.1002/j.1532-2149.2013.00350.x.

10. Vaegter HB, Andersen PG, Madsen MF, Handberg G. Enggaard TP. Prevalence of neuropathic pain according to the IASP grading system in patients with chronic non-malignant pain. *Pain Med.* 2014;15:120–127. doi:10.1111/pme.12273.

11. Finnerup NB., Haroutounian S, Kamerman P, et al. Neuropathic pain: an updated grading system for research and clinical practice. *Pain.* 2016;157:1599–1606, doi:10.1097/j.pain.0000000000000492.

12. Hasvik, E, Haugen, AJ, Gjerstad, J. Grovle, L. Assessing neuropathic pain in patients with low back-related leg pain: comparing the painDETECT Questionnaire with the 2016 NeuPSIG grading system. *Eur J Pain.* 2018;22(6):1160–1169. doi:10.1002/ejp.1204.

13. Jensen, MP, Chodroff, MJ. Dworkin, RH. The impact of neuropathic pain on health-related quality of life: review and implications. *Neurology.* 2007;68:1178–1182. doi:10.1212/01.wnl.0000259085.61898.9e.

14. Doth, AH, Hansson, PT, Jensen, MP. Taylor, RS. The burden of neuropathic pain: a systematic review and meta-analysis of health utilities. *Pain.* 2010;149:338–344. doi:10.1016/j.pain.2010.02.034.

15. Cramer JA. *Quality of life and pharmacoeconomics: an introduction.* Philadelphia: Lippincott-Raven Publishers; 1998.

16. Berger A, Dukes EM. Oster G. Clinical characteristics and economic costs of patients with painful neuropathic disorders. *J Pain.* 2004;5:143–149. doi:10.1016/j.jpain.2003.12.004.

17. O'Connor AB. Neuropathic pain: quality-of-life impact, costs and cost effectiveness of therapy. *Pharmacoeconomics.* 2009;27:95–112. doi:10.2165/00019053-200927020-00002.

18. Cheng J. State of the art, challenges, and opportunities for pain medicine. *Pain Med.* 2018. doi: 10.1093/pm/pny073.

19. St John Smith, E. Advances in understanding nociception and neuropathic pain. *J. Neurol.* 2018;265:231–238. doi:10.1007/s00415-017-8641-6.

20. Basbaum AI, Bautista DM, Scherrer G. Julius D. Cellular and molecular mechanisms of pain. *Cell.* 2009;139:267–284. doi:10.1016/j.cell.2009.09.028.

21. Ji RR, Chamessian A, Zhang YQ. Pain regulation by non-neuronal cells and inflammation. *Science.* 2016;354:572–577. doi:10.1126/science.aaf8924.

22. Colombo E. Farina C. Astrocytes: key regulators of neuroinflammation. *Trends Immunol.* 2016;37:608–620. doi:10.1016/j.it.2016.06.006.

23. Ren K. Dubner R. Interactions between the immune and nervous systems in pain. *Nat Med.* 2010;16:1267–1276, doi:10.1038/nm.2234.

24. Scholz J. Woolf CJ. The neuropathic pain triad: neurons, immune cells and glia. *Nat Neurosci.* 2007;10:1361–1368. doi:10.1038/nn1992.

25. Fernandes V, Sharma D, Vaidya S, et al. Cellular and molecular mechanisms driving neuropathic pain: recent advancements and challenges. *Expert Opin Ther Targets.* 2018;22:131–142. doi:10.1080/14728222.2018.1420781.

26. von Hehn CA, Baron R. Woolf CJ. Deconstructing the neuropathic pain phenotype to reveal neural mechanisms. *Neuron.* 2012;73:638–652. doi:10.1016/j.neuron.2012.02.008.

27. Tsuda M. P2 receptors, microglial cytokines and chemokines, and neuropathic pain. *J Neurosci Res.* 2017;95:1319–1329. doi:10.1002/jnr.23816.

28. Gasparotti R, Padua L, Briani C. Lauria G. New technologies for the assessment of neuropathies. *Nat Rev Neurol.* 2017;13:203–216. doi:10.1038/nrneurol.2017.31.

29. Pessoa BL, Escudeiro G. Nascimento OJ. Emerging treatments for neuropathic pain. *Curr Pain Headache Rep.* 2015;19:56. doi:10.1007/s11916-015-0530-z.

30. Chen G, Park CK, Xie RG. Ji RR. Intrathecal bone marrow stromal cells inhibit neuropathic pain via TGF-beta secretion. *J Clin Invest.* 2015;125:3226–3240. doi:10.1172/jci80883.

31. Li F, Liu L, Cheng K, Chen Z. Cheng J. The use of stem cell therapy to reverse opioid tolerance. *Clin Pharmacol Ther,* 2018;103(6):971–974. doi:10.1002/cpt.959.

32. Hua Z, Liu L, Shen J, et al. Mesenchymal stem cells reversed morphine tolerance and opioid-induced hyperalgesia. *Sci Rep.* 2016;6:32096. doi:10.1038/srep32096.

33. Liu L, Hua Z, Shen J, et al. Comparative efficacy of multiple variables of mesenchymal stem cell transplantation for the treatment of neuropathic pain

in rats. *Mil Med.* 2017;182:175–184. doi:10.7205/milmed-d-16-00096.

34. Tso AR. Goadsby PJ. Anti-CGRP monoclonal antibodies: the next era of migraine prevention? *Curr Treat Options Neurol.* 2017;19:27. doi:10.1007/s11940-017-0463-4.

35. Goadsby PJ, Reuter U, Hallström Y, et al. A controlled trial of erenumab for episodic migraine. *N Engl J Med.* 2017;377:2123–2132. doi:10.1056/NEJMoa1705848.

36. Silberstein SD, Dodick DW, Bigal ME, et al. Fremanezumab for the preventive treatment of chronic migraine. *N Engl J Med.* 2017;377:2113–2122. doi:10.1056/NEJMoa1709038.

37. Tepper S, Ashina M, Reuter U, et al. Safety and efficacy of erenumab for preventive treatment of chronic migraine: a randomised, double-blind, placebo-controlled phase 2 trial. *Lancet Neurol.* 2017;16:425–434. doi:10.1016/s1474-4422(17)30083-2.

38. Rice ASC, Dworkin RH, McCarthy TD, et al. EMA401, an orally administered highly selective angiotensin II type 2 receptor antagonist, as a novel treatment for postherpetic neuralgia: a randomised, double-blind, placebo-controlled phase 2 clinical trial. *Lancet.* 2014;383:1637–1647. doi:10.1016/s0140-6736(13)62337-5.

39. Vickers ER, Karsten E, Flood J. Lilischkis R. A preliminary report on stem cell therapy for neuropathic pain in humans. *J Pain Res.* 2014;7:255–263. doi:10.2147/jpr.s63361.

40. Vaquero J, Zurita M, Rico MA, et al. Intrathecal administration of autologous bone marrow stromal cells improves neuropathic pain in patients with spinal cord injury. *Neurosci Lett.* 2018;670:14–18. doi:10.1016/j.neulet.2018.01.035.

41. Venturi M, Boccasanta P, Lombardi B, et al. Pudendal neuralgia: a new option for treatment? Preliminary results on feasibility and efficacy. *Pain Med.* 2015;16:1475–1481. doi:10.1111/pme.12693.

42. Xu J, Liu A. Cheng J. New advancements in spinal cord stimulation for chronic pain management. *Curr Opin Anaesthesiol.* 2017;30:710–717. doi:10.1097/aco.0000000000000531.

2

Classification of Neuropathic Pain

ABDULLAH KANDIL AND DANIELLE PERRET

BACKGROUND

Pain can be considered physiological and adaptive when nociceptors are activated by a stimulant, alerting the individual of impending harm or injury. By contrast, neuropathic pain results from disease or lesions of the somatosensory nervous system and can be present from absent or very minimal stimulation.[1] *Neuropathy* refers to a pathological change, injury, or a disease process affecting the nervous system.[2] Sensory abnormalities are commonly associated with neuropathic pain.[1]

Classification of neuropathic pain can be central, peripheral, or mixed. Central neuropathic pain results from involvement of the brain or spinal cord. Peripheral neuropathic pain results from involvement of the peripheral nerve, plexus, dorsal root ganglion/cranial nerve ganglion, or nerve root.[3] Further categorization of neuropathic pain can be made on the basis of etiology of the pain, chronicity, anatomical location, and treatment.[3] Additionally, some have advocated for the classification of neuropathic pain based on the underlying cellular and molecular biology following neuropathic injury.[4] In this book, we will classify neuropathic pain based on the anatomical location (central, peripheral, or mixed) and the causes of neuropathic pain wherever possible. In this chapter, we provide a few examples from each category of neuropathic pain (see Table 2.1). More detailed discussion and management strategies will be provided in subsequent chapters.

CENTRAL NEUROPATHIC PAIN

Pain can be generated within the brain and spinal cord owing to vascular disease, traumatic injury, autoimmune disease, degenerative changes, and other causes.

Post-Stroke Pain

First described in 1906 as thalamic pain syndrome, central post-stroke pain (CPSP) is the most common cause of central pain originating in the brain.[1] Occurring in up to 35% of patients after stroke, it is commonly diagnosed but difficult to treat.[15] Considered a diagnosis of exclusion, CPSP can be diagnosed after peripheral neuropathy and psychological and other causes of pain have been ruled out after stroke. Some studies hypothesize that damage to central inhibitory pathways, hyperexcitation of the sensory pathways, or some combination is responsible.[16] It is characterized by spontaneous and/or evoked pain, which can be continuous or paroxysmal.[15] It is often associated with allodynia, dysesthesia, or hyperalgesia.[15] It should be differentiated from pain generated from the periphery, such as the shoulder, due to immobility and contraction following paresis.[16]

Spinal Cord Injury Pain

Pain after spinal cord injury (SCI) is very common and can be present in as many as 80% of patients.[5] SCI pain incidence varies widely.[17] Studies have shown that SCI pain is not correlated with completeness or injury level, but may be associated with age at the time of injury.[17] The reasons for this association remain unexplained, but the association with age seems to have been replicated in multiple studies and is adjusted for increased prevalence of pain in SCI with time.[17] SCI pain can have aspects of nociceptive as well as neuropathic pain. Unlike persons with incomplete SCI, those with complete SCI will not experience nociceptive pain below the level of injury. SCI pain is often chronic, recalcitrant to treatment, and associated with depression and anxiety.[17,18]

TABLE 2.1. CLASSIFICATION
OF NEUROPATHIC PAIN AND EXAMPLES

Classification	Examples
Central	Post-stroke pain[1]
	SCI pain[5]
	Spinal infarction
	Syringomyelia
	Multiple sclerosis
	Phantom limb pain[6]
	Parkinson's pain[7]
	Fibromyalgia[1]
Peripheral	Postherpetic neuralgia[8]
	Post-amputation stump pain[9]
	Chronic pelvic pain[10]
	Entrapment neuropathies[1]
	Neuromas
	Radiculopathies[1]
	Diabetic neuropathy
	HIV-related neuropathy
	Immune-related neuropathy
	Hereditary sensory neuropathies
	Metabolic, endocrine, and other toxic neuropathies
Mixed	Spinal stenosis[11]
	Complex regional pain syndrome (CRPS)[12]
	Charcot-Marie-Tooth[13]
	Cancer pain[14]

Phantom Limb Pain

Phantom limb pain (PLP) is a type of neuropathic pain that is felt in the same distribution of a previously present body part after amputation of the body part. PLP is very common (40–80% prevalence) and varies in time of onset from days to years post-amputation.[6] The leading predictor of PLP is pain in the extremity prior to amputation.[6] The character of PLP is also variable and has been described as sharp, dull, aching, throbbing, burning, cramping, or shooting in nature.

Multiple Sclerosis/Parkinson's Pain

Multiple sclerosis (MS) pain due to demyelination of nerve fibers in the central nervous system (CNS) is a type of central pain that is often refractory to treatment.[1] Pain in Parkinson's disease is common and was mentioned in James Parkinson's earliest descriptions of the disease.[7] Prevalence is high, noted to be up to 83%.[19] The mechanism is unclear but is thought to involve a combination of musculoskeletal, radicular, dystonic, and central pain.[7]

Fibromyalgia

Fibromyalgia is a condition with aspects of chronic generalized as well as localized pain, fatigue, insomnia, cognitive and memory problems, psychological issues, stiffness, oral and ocular involvement, sexual dysfunction, and headaches.[1] Many of these symptoms may be present at a particular point in time but the symptoms may not overlap. There is a diminished quality of life due to multifocal pain and psychological symptoms that do not occur with a clear pathological cause.[20] Although the etiology is unclear, fibromyalgia is considered by some as a central type of neuropathic pain.[21] Diagnosis traditionally required a history of multifocal pain as well as assessment of 11 out of 18 tender points on physical examination.[22] In 2011, the American College of Rheumatology revised the criteria for the diagnosis of fibromyalgia. This criteria includes widespread myofascial pain and generalized pain in at least 7 of 19 areas with cognitive, fatigue and sleep disturbances; symptoms must be present for at least 3 months and no other disorder can explain these findings.

PERIPHERAL NEUROPATHIC PAIN

Postherpetic Neuralgia

Varicella-zoster virus lies latent in the dorsal root ganglia after chicken pox infection, sometimes for decades. However, occasionally it can reemerge and cause a localized cutaneous eruption along a characteristic dermatomal distribution; this is called herpes zoster, or shingles.[8] Pain (typically described as burning in nature) frequently accompanies herpes zoster along the dermatomal distribution and may persist for weeks and sometimes years.[23] When the acute pain of herpes zoster lasts for longer than 30 days, it is termed postherpetic neuralgia (PHN). The most predictive risk factors for PHN are pain during acute rash, age, and intensity of infection.[23] Allodynia is common and dominates as the main feature of PHN.[24]

Post-Amputation Stump Pain

Stump pain is pain that is felt at the site of the residual limb after an amputation. Outside of the universal immediate postoperative pain, stump pain is less common than phantom limb pain (approximately 20% prevalence).[9] Stump pain can have multiple etiologies, including infection, soft tissue or bone lesions (pain from an ill-fitting prosthesis), or ischemia.[1] Types of pain vary and include both nociceptive and neuropathic types.

Chronic Pelvic Pain

Chronic pelvic pain (CPP) can be debilitating for patients and difficult to diagnose and treat for the practitioner. It is defined as nonmenstrual pelvic pain (in females or males) that lasts for more than 6 months. Prevalence among females is approximately 5%.[10] CPP can have both nociceptive and neuropathic etiology that includes pathology in the reproductive tract, urological, gastrointestinal, musculoskeletal, and psychological systems.[25] Males with CPP typically have a history of chronic prostatitis.[25]

Entrapment Neuropathies

Entrapment neuropathies are caused by anatomical compression. There are many well-described entrapment neuropathies and most of them are painful. They include carpal tunnel syndrome, tarsal tunnel syndrome, thoracic outlet syndrome, and meralgia paresthetica. Sensory loss in the distribution of the affected nerve, in addition to weakness, and special physical examination tests help in the diagnosis of entrapment neuropathies. Electrodiagnostic studies may help confirm the diagnosis.[1]

Radiculopathies

A *radiculopathy* refers to a lesion or injury to a nerve root exiting the spinal cord. Symptoms include pain along the distribution of the nerve root, and often sensory changes and/or weakness. Compression is the most common cause of radiculopathy, but other causes may include tumors, fracture, or infection.[1] Disk herniations are the most common type of compression, with the L5–S1 disk being most common.[1]

MIXED NEUROPATHIC PAIN

Spinal Stenosis

Spinal stenosis is a narrowing of the spinal canal. This may lead to impingement on the spinal cord leading to pain, numbness, and loss of sensory or motor function. Claudication is often described, which includes leg pain bilaterally with walking, standing, and walking downhill, with the resolving of symptoms with walking uphill or leaning forward on a shopping cart. It is one of the most commonly diagnosed and treated conditions of the spine.[11] Pain is caused not only from mechanical compression but also from venous congestion and arterial insufficiency that results because of stenosis. Causes of spinal stenosis include congenital, acquired, and traumatic causes.

Complex Regional Pain Syndrome (CRPS)

Complex regional pain syndrome (CRPS) is a term that was developed by the International Association for the Study of Pain (IASP) at a meeting in 1994. CRPS is divided into to types: type 1, formerly known as reflex sympathetic dystrophy (RSD), and type 2, formerly known as causalgia. CRPS-I is usually caused by injury, immobilization, or trauma to an extremity which leads to allodynia, hyperalgesia, sudomotor and vasomotor changes, and motor dysfunction or trophic changes. CRPS-I is not considered neuropathic pain under the new IASP definition of neuropathic pain, whereas CRPS-II is, because it is triggered by nerve injury or lesion and leads to burning pain, allodynia, and hyperalgesia not necessarily limited to a particular nerve's distribution.[12] It may also be characterized by sudomotor, vasomotor, and motor dysfunction or trophic changes. CRPS has peripheral, central, and sympathetic mediated factors that influence its symptoms.[1]

Charcot-Marie-Tooth

Charcot-Marie-Tooth (CMT), also known as hereditary motor and sensory neuropathy (HMSN), is a commonly inherited neuromuscular disorder. Caused by a genetic mutation in one of multiple myelin genes, it leads to defects in myelin structure and integrity and axonal degeneration.[13] Symptoms begin distally in the lower extremities. There is a stereotypical phenotype that accompanies CMT, which includes muscle wasting, sensory loss, hyporeflexia, weakness, hammer toes, and high arches.[13] Pain results from peripheral polyneuropathic causes as well as musculoskeletal causes.

Cancer Pain

Cancer pain varies drastically among cancer patients, based on type, stage, and location of the cancer.[14] Like SCI pain, cancer pain can have aspects of nociceptive, neuropathic, or mixed pain. Etiology of the pain differs and can be caused by tumor growth in bone, nerves, viscera, or skin or may be due to adverse effects of chemotherapy or radiation therapy. A recent meta-analysis of cancer-prevalence literature showed that an average of 64% of patients with metastatic or terminal cancer, 59% of patients on anticancer treatment, and 33% of patients cured of cancer had cancer pain.[26] Clinical practice has emphasized actively treating cancer pain, especially in terminal cancers.[14]

TAXONOMY

All taxonomy definitions are from the *Classification of Chronic Pain*, second edition, IASP Task Force on Taxonomy, 1994.[27]

Pain: An unpleasant sensory and emotional experience associated with actual or potential tissue damage

Allodynia: Pain due to a stimulus that does not normally produce pain

Analgesia: Absence of pain in response to stimulation, which would normally be painful

Dysesthesia: An unpleasant, abnormal sensation, whether spontaneous or evoked

Hyperalgesia: Increased pain from a stimulus that normally provokes pain

Hyperesthesia: Increased sensitivity to stimulation, excluding the special senses

Hyperpathia: A painful syndrome characterized by an abnormally painful reaction to a stimulus, especially a repetitive stimulus, as well as an increased threshold

Hypoalgesia: Diminished pain in response to a normally painful stimulus

Hypoasthesia: Decreased sensitivity to stimulation, excluding the special senses

Neuralgia: Pain in the distribution of a nerve or nerves

Neuritis: Inflammation of a nerve or nerves

Neuropathic pain: Pain caused by a lesion or disease of the somatosensory nervous system

Central neuropathic pain: Neuropathic pain resulting from a lesion or disease of the brain or spinal cord

Peripheral neuropathic pain: Neuropathic pain resulting from a lesion or disease of the peripheral nerve, plexus, dorsal root ganglion or root

Neuropathy: A disturbance of function or pathological change in a nerve: in one nerve, mononeuropathy; in several nerves, mononeuropathy multiplex; if diffuse and bilateral, polyneuropathy

Nociceptive pain: Pain that arises from actual or threatened damage to non-neural tissue and is due to the activation of nociceptors

Paresthesia: An abnormal sensation, whether spontaneous or evoked

Central sensitization: Increased responsiveness of nociceptive neurons in the central nervous system to their normal or subthreshold afferent input

Peripheral sensitization: Increased responsiveness and reduced threshold of nociceptive neurons in the periphery to the stimulation of their receptive fields

REFERENCES

1. McCartney CJL. *Essentials of Pain Medicine.* 3rd ed. Philadelphia, PA: Saunders Elsevier; 2011. doi:10.1016/B978-1-4377-2242-0.00044-4.
2. Nijs J, Apeldoorn A, Hallegraeff H, et al. Low back pain: guidelines for the clinical classification of predominant neuropathic, nociceptive, or central sensitization pain. *Pain Phys.* 2015;18:E333–E346. http://www.scopus.com/inward/record.url?eid=2-s2.0-84929455261&partnerID=40&md5=71800674f0f5edd40883bb31c3a91732.
3. Haanpää M. Treede R-D. Diagnosis and classification of neuropathic pain epidemiology and impact of neuropathic pain. *Pain Clin Updates.* 2010;XVIII(7):1–6.
4. Baron R. Mechanisms of disease: neuropathic pain—a clinical perspective. *Nat Clin Pract Neurol.* 2006;2(2):95–106. doi:10.1038/ncpneuro0113.
5. Cardenas DD, Jensen MP. Treatments for chronic pain in persons with spinal cord injury: a survey study. *J Spinal Cord Med.* 2006;29(2):109–117.
6. Postone N. Phantom limb pain. A review. *Int J Psychiatry Med.* 1987;17(1):57–70.
7. Kubo S, Hamada S, Maeda T, et al. A Japanese multicenter survey characterizing pain in Parkinson's disease. *J Neurol Sci.* 2016;365:162–166. doi:10.1016/j.jns.2016.04.015.
8. Maltha J, Jacobs J. Herpes zoster clinical practice. *Eur J Pediatr.* 2011;170(7):821–829.
9. Ehde DM, Czerniecki JM, Smith DG, et al. Chronic phantom sensations, phantom pain, residual limb pain, and other regional pain after lower limb amputation. *Arch Phys Med Rehabil.* 2000;81(8):1039–1044. doi:10.1053/apmr.2000.7583.
10. Howard F. Chronic pelvic pain. *Obstet Gynecol.* 2003;101(3):594–611. doi:10.1016/S0029-7844(02)02723-0.

11. Kalichman L, Cole R, Kim DH, et al. Spinal stenosis prevalence and association with symptoms: the Framingham Study. *Spine J.* 2009;9(7):545–550. doi:10.1016/j.spinee.2009.03.005.

12. Raja SN, Grabow TS. Complex regional pain syndrome I (reflex sympathetic dystrophy). *Anesthesiology.* 2002;96:1254–1260.

13. Pareyson D, Marchesi C. Diagnosis, natural history, and management of Charcot-Marie-Tooth disease. *Lancet Neurol.* 2009;8(7):654–667. doi:10.1016/S1474-4422(09)70110-3.

14. Ripamonti CI, Santini D, Maranzano E, Berti M, Roila F. Management of cancer pain: ESMO clinical practice guidelines. *Ann Oncol.* 2012;23(Suppl. 7): vii139–vii154. doi:10.1093/annonc/mds233.

15. Kumar B, Kalita J, Kumar G, Misra UK. Central poststroke pain: a review of pathophysiology and treatment. *Anesth Analg.* 2009;108(5):1645–1657. doi:10.1213/ane.0b013e31819d644c.

16. Kim JS. Post-stroke pain. *Exp Rev Neurother.* 2009;9(5):711–721.

17. Werhagen L, Budh CN, Hultling C, Molander C. Neuropathic pain after traumatic spinal cord injury—relations to gender, spinal level, completeness, and age at the time of injury. *Spinal Cord.* 2004;42(12):665–673. doi:10.1038/sj.sc.3101641.

18. Nicholson Perry K, Nicholas MK, Middleton J. Spinal cord injury-related pain in rehabilitation: a cross-sectional study of relationships with cognitions, mood and physical function. *Eur J Pain.* 2009;13(5):511–517. doi:10.1016/j.ejpain.2008.06.003.

19. Beiske AG, Loge JH, Ronningen A, Svensson E. Pain in Parkinson's disease: prevalence and characteristics. *Pain.* 2009;141(1–2):173–177. doi:10.1016/j.pain.2008.12.004.

20. Walitt B, Nahin RL, Katz RS, Bergman MJ, Wolfe F. The prevalence and characteristics of fibromyalgia in the 2012 National Health Interview Survey. *PLoS One.* 2015;10(9):1–16. doi:10.1371/journal.pone.0138024.

21. Doppler K, Rittner HL, Deckart M, Sommer C. Reduced dermal nerve fiber diameter in skin biopsies of patients with fibromyalgia. *Pain.* 2015;156(11):1. doi:10.1097/j.pain.0000000000000285.

22. Wolfe F, Clauw DJ, Fitzcharles MA, et al. The American College of Rheumatology preliminary diagnostic criteria for fibromyalgia and measurement of symptom severity. *Arthritis Care Res.* 2010;62(5):600–610. doi:10.1002/acr.20140.

23. Hope-Simpson RE. Postherpetic neuralgia. *J R Coll Gen Pract.* 1975;25(157):571–575.

24. Haanpää M, Laippala P, Nurmikko T. Allodynia and pinprick hypesthesia in acute herpes zoster, and the development of postherpetic neuralgia. *J Pain Symptom Manage.* 2000;20(1):50–58. doi:10.1016/S0885-3924(00)00149-4.

25. Vercellini P, Somigliana E, Viganò P, Abbiati A, Barbara G, Fedele L. Chronic pelvic pain in women: etiology, pathogenesis and diagnostic approach. *Gynecol Endocrinol.* 2009;25(3):149–158. doi:10.1080/09513590802549858.

26. van den Beuken-van Everdingen MHJ, de Rijke JM, Kessels AG, Schouten HC, van Kleef M, Patijn J. Prevalence of pain in patients with cancer: a systematic review of the past 40 years. *Ann Oncol.* 2007;18(9):1437–1449. doi:10.1093/annonc/mdm056.

27. Merskey H, Bogduk N. *Classification of Chronic Pain: Description of Chronic Pain Syndromes and Definitions of Pain Terms.* 2nd ed. Seattle: IASP Press; 1994. doi:10.1002/ana.20394.

3

Mechanisms of Neuropathic Pain

JIANGUO CHENG

INTRODUCTION

Patients with neuropathic pain often experience spontaneous burning or electrical-like shouting pain, heightened pain in response to stimuli applied to their skin (hyperalgesia), or pain upon light touch (allodynia). These symptoms are typically accompanied by evidence of sensory deficit. Neuropathic pain is almost always pathological as it is, by definition, a result of a lesion or disease of the somatosensory nervous system. Pain is pathological when it has no physiological, protective function, as in the case of neuropathic pain, or when it outlives its usefulness as an acute warning system and instead becomes chronic and debilitating.[1]

There are enormous challenges in understanding the mechanisms of neuropathic pain, given the diversity in cause, pathology, and clinical presentation of neuropathic pain conditions.[2] We know little about how an injury or a disease of the peripheral nerve leads to molecular, cellular, and histological changes in the central nervous system (CNS). We know even less about how a lesion or a disease of the CNS can cause central neuropathic pain. This is in part due to limitations in the ways to investigate neuropathic pain. For most clinical neuropathic pain conditions there are no suitable animal models that can be used to study such conditions. Even for those for which animal models do exist, such as peripheral nerve injury–induced neuropathic pain, diabetic neuropathy, and chemotherapy-induced neuropathy, the translation of laboratory findings to humans is often challenging. First, we don't have reliable objective measures of neuropathic pain in animals, or in humans for that matter. This lack of objectivity often compromises the quality of experimental investigations. Second, it is almost impossible to create animal models that match the diversity of clinical presentations of various neuropathic pain disorders in humans. Human experiences are often dramatically different even for the same neuropathic pain condition. What appears to be the same lesion may induce no pain in one person but severe pain in another. Third, most of the animals used for this purpose (rats and mice) have life expectancies of about 2 years. This makes it difficult to study chronic pain states due to neurological injury or disorders. Fourth, biological differences between species also complicate the interpretation of findings in animal models of neuropathic pain and the translation of findings to humans.

Despite these challenges and limitations, intensive efforts from the pain and neuroscience research community have yielded significant insights into molecular and cellular mechanisms of neuropathic pain.[3,4] It is commonly believed that various neuropathic pain conditions may share common peripheral and central mechanisms.[4,5]

PERIPHERAL MECHANISMS

A lesion or a disease of the peripheral nerve due to trauma, mechanical compression, chemical irritation, degeneration, infection, toxicity, autoimmune reaction, cancer, or genetic disorders can cause neuropathic pain in many patients. Common examples include post-trauma/surgery neuropathic pain, painful diabetic neuropathy, postherpetic neuralgia, various nerve entrapment syndromes, and cancer-related pain due to tumor invasion, surgery, chemotherapy, or radiation therapy. Although not completely understood, diverse causes may lead to pathological changes that directly compromise the integrity of somatosensory nerve fibers or cause dysfunction of the nerve fibers indirectly, owing to inflammatory, ischemic, or metabolic changes surrounding the nerves. Structural or functional changes of the nerve fibers may lead to abnormally high-intensity injury discharge, ectopic discharge, or loss of somatosensory input to the second-order neurons in the spinal cord or brainstem.

Evidence for the role of primary afferent inputs in the pathogenesis of neuropathic pain comes from several pharmacological experiments. Selective blockade of CB2 cannabinoid receptor, which is not expressed in the CNS, reversed mechanical and thermal hyperalgesia following a lesion from spinal nerve ligation.[6] Anti-sense oligodeoxynucleotides directed against Nav1.8, a sodium channel primarily expressed in small-diameter primary afferent neurons, reversed signs of mechanical hyperalgesia.[7] These results suggest that primary afferent neurons contribute to the development of neuropathic pain.

Nociceptors or other somatosensory neurons can develop hypersensitivity or spontaneous activity at the receptive field (nerve endings) due to peripheral sensitization, which is defined as increased responsiveness and/or reduced threshold for firing action potentials of nociceptive neurons upon stimulation of their receptive fields (Figure 3.1). After a peripheral nerve lesion, change of function or aberrant regeneration of the nociceptors may occur. These neurons

become abnormally sensitive and may develop spontaneous pathological activity, unusual excitability, and increased sensitivity to chemical, thermal, and mechanical stimuli. Peripheral sensitization usually involves activation of several types of cells, such as macrophages, mast cells, platelets, endothelial cells, fibroblasts, and other immune cells, in reaction to tissue injury or inflammation.[3,8–10] These cells release a milieu of inflammatory factors, which in turn bind to specific receptors of the nerve endings. These factors include cytokines (interleukin-1β [IL-1β], interleukin 6 [IL-6], tumor necrosis factor-α [TNF-α], leukemia inhibiting factor [LIF]), nerve growth factor (NGF), histamine, bradykinin, prostaglandin E2 (PGE2), adenosine triphosphate (ATP), adenosine, and proton. These factors act on specific receptors or channels such as receptor tyrosine kinases (RTK), two-pore potassium (K2P) channels, G protein–coupled receptors (GPCR), transient receptor potential (TRP) channels, acid-sensitive ion channels (ASIC), and purinergic receptors (e.g., P2X) in the sensory nerve endings and lead to increased excitability of the peripheral sensory neurons.

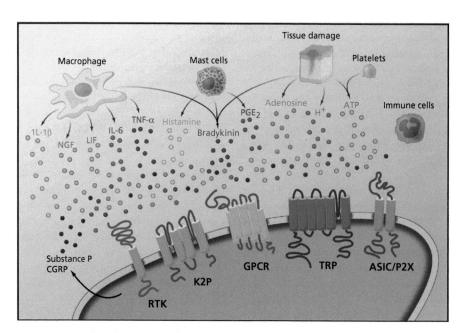

FIGURE 3.1. Factors contributing to peripheral sensitization

ASIC, acid-sensitive ion channels; ATP, adenosine triphosphate; CGRP, calcitonin gene-related peptide; GPCR, G protein–coupled receptor; IL-1β, interleukin 1β; IL-6, interleukin 6; K2P, two-pore potassium; LIF, leukemia inhibiting factor; NGF, nerve growth factor; PGE₂, prostaglandin E2; RTK, receptor tyrosine kinases; TRP, transient receptor potential.

From Basbaum AI, Bautista DM, Scherrer G, Julius D. Cellular and molecular mechanisms of pain. *Cell.* 2009;139(2):267–284.

In addition, nerve endings of the nociceptors may release substance P (acting on neurokinin-1 receptor) and calcitonin gene-related peptide (CGRP), both of which have been associated with neurogenic inflammation and possibly peripheral sensitization. Nociceptors are thus often referred to as "bidirectional signaling machine" because they not only release neurotransmitters and neuromodulators at the central ends in the spinal cord but also release active agents from nerve endings in the periphery.

Sensitization of nociceptors may be achieved either by enhancing the transduction channel to generate bigger generator potential to a given stimulus or by reducing the threshold of the sodium channels responsible for spike initiation. NGF, for example, can regulate TRPV1 expression and enhance its transduction-channel function.[11] Abnormal transduction, at least in part, underlies the pathophysiology of the sensitized "intact nociceptors." Another example of abnormal transduction is that intact nociceptors acquire sensitivity to norepinephrine and transduction capacity for stimuli that ordinarily do not activate nociceptors. An additional example is that abnormal expression of transduction channels such as TRPA1, or TRPM8 in nociceptors likely accounts for cooling hyperalgesia, which is prominent in neuropathic pain.[4] In addition to influencing the amplitude of generator potentials, many inflammatory factors can modulate the threshold of action potential initiation. Inflammatory factors, such as IL-1β or a mixture of bradykinin, ATP, histamine, PGE2, and noradrenaline, increased the current density (a measure that reflects the number of active channels) of NaV1.9, enhanced the excitability of these neurons by lowering the threshold for action potential generation, and increased the number of action potentials in response to injected depolarizing stimulus.[12]

Apart from increased nociceptive input from sensitized afferent fibers, damaged nociceptors may also fire ectopic discharge at the site of axonal damage (neuroma), at the soma of the damaged neurons (dorsal root ganglion), or even from adjacent uninjured fibers. All of these phenomena have been well documented.[13–15] Displacement of transduction from nerve endings to these pathological sites has been linked to the "Tinel sign," a clinical finding that, when the area over the nerve injury is tapped, patients experience paresthesias (tingling sensation) or dysesthesia (an unpleasant or painful sensation). The Tinel sign

may be present at a point of entrapment where continuity of the axon has not necessarily been interrupted. Presumably, a disturbance of fast axonal transport leads to ectopic expression of the transduction channels. Alternatively, axotomy may lead to neuroma, an entangled mass formed by budding regenerative nerve sprouts devoid of growth guidance from denervated Schwann cells. Areas of nerve injury may be tethered to adjacent structures so that otherwise normal movements evoke an increase in pain, presumably by activating mechanoreceptive transduction channels. Not all neuromas are painful, for reasons that are largely unknown.

Ectopic discharge has also been linked to spontaneous pain and may be related to expression of heterotopic sodium channels, such as Nav1.3, Nav1.7, and Nav1.8, and calcium channels such as the α2δ subunit of voltage-gated calcium channels at the site of neuroma or in the soma of injured nociceptors.[16] It is a common clinical observation that local-anesthetic blockade of an injured nerve in patients relieves pain for the duration of the nerve blockade or beyond.[17–19] Additionally, anesthetics or tetrodotoxin applied to the L5 dorsal root ganglia reversed the neuropathic pain behavior induced by L5 spinal nerve ligation in rats.[20] These findings favor the "injured afferent hypothesis" and support the notion that ectopic discharge plays a role in the genesis or maintenance of neuropathic pain. It is worth noting, however, that neuropathic pain may still develop in the absence of neural input from the injured nerve. For example, neuropathic pain behavior is observed after an L5 ganglionectomy, where the injured afferents are removed altogether, indicating other mechanisms are likely at play in the development of neuropathic pain.[21]

The "intact nociceptor hypothesis" postulates that intact nociceptors, innervating the region affected by the injured nerve fibers, sensitize and generate spontaneous activity. The changes in the intact nociceptors may cause spontaneous, ongoing neuropathic pain. This hypothesis is supported by several lines of evidence. First, spontaneous activity was found to develop in the uninjured, unmyelinated nociceptors as well as in the uninjured, myelinated fibers in the same innervation territory of the transected fibers in monkeys and rats.[22–25] Second, the intact L4 dorsal root ganglion underwent significant phenotype changes after injury to the adjacent L5 spinal nerve (L5 spinal nerve ligation [SNL]), including increased expression of TRPV1 and TRPA1, mRNA for CGRP,[26] brain-derived neurotrophic factor (BDNF),[27] and P2X3 mRNA.[28] Third, in a primate model of neuropathic pain, an L6 SNL led to loss of about one-half of the afferents to the top of the foot. The other half reached the foot from the adjoining and putatively uninjured spinal nerves.[22] More than 60% of the intact nociceptors had spontaneous activity (rarely seen in normal controls), and more than 50% had sensitivity to the select α-adrenergic agonist phenylephrine, indicating that these adjacent uninjured afferent fibers are sensitive to influence from sympathetic nerves and likely responsible for sympathetically maintained neuropathic pain. Fourth, low-frequency electrical stimulation of intact C fibers led to hyperalgesia in humans and behavioral signs of hyperalgesia in rats.[29,30] Fifth, local treatment with capsaicin, the effects of which are specific to nociceptors, may significantly relieve ongoing pain in patients. Thus the uninjured sensory nerve fibers may contribute to the pathogenesis of neuropathic pain. In addition, motor nerve fibers may also contribute, since ventral root rhizotomy induced long-lasting neuropathic pain behavior.[21,31,32] Taken together, it is highly plausible that interactions between degenerating motor and sensory fibers of the injured nerve and intact afferent fibers of neighboring nerves play a critical role for both the initiation and maintenance of neuropathic pain.[21]

Damaged nociceptors may also lead to loss of somatosensory input and negative sensory symptoms and signs. This helps explain patients' experiences of numbness, insensitivity to touch and pressure, loss of proprioception, and abnormal nociception to mechanical, thermal, or visceral stimulation.

CENTRAL MECHANISMS

The changes in the peripheral nerves do not occur in isolation but often lead to changes in the CNS, characterized by central sensitization, cortical reorganization, and changes in thalamic activities and the descending control pathways. These central mechanisms play a key role in the pathogenesis of neuropathic pain and may underlie many clinical phenomena such as expansion of nociceptive field, hyperalgesia, allodynia, deafferentation pain, and phantom limb pain.

Central Sensitization

The term *central sensitization* refers to the augmented response of central signaling neurons.[33]

The dorsal horn of the spinal cord serves as an interface with afferent input in pain processing. An increased volley of afferent input from nociceptors can trigger a prolonged but reversible increase in the excitability and synaptic efficacy of neurons in nociceptive pathways. Central sensitization is not unique to neuropathic pain but has been linked to the pain phenotype in patients with fibromyalgia, osteoarthritis, musculoskeletal disorders with generalized pain hypersensitivity, and visceral pain hypersensitivity disorders. Development of or increase in spontaneous activity is one of the hallmarks of central sensitization.[34,35]

Pain wind-up is the perceived increase in pain intensity over time when a given painful stimulus is delivered repeatedly above a critical rate. It is caused by repeated stimulation of group C peripheral nerve fibers, leading to progressively increasing electrical response in output neurons in lamina I of the superficial dorsal horn. In the spinal cord, wind-up results in dramatic increase in neuron firing, from 0.3 Hz up to 50 Hz. Wind-up lasts tens of seconds and represents a short-term form of sensitization. Nociceptive inputs also alter synaptic efficacy such that A-β mechanoreceptors acquire the capacity to evoke pain responses. This form of sensitization, called *heterosynaptic sensitization*, presumably accounts for allodynia. Electrophysiological evidence for heterosynaptic sensitization has been shown in primate studies of dorsal horn cells where the response to light stroking of the skin was enhanced after capsaicin injection.[36] At least five interrelated mechanisms have been proposed to explain central sensitization.

Presynaptically, nerve injury leads to an upregulation of the α-2-δ subunit of voltage-gated calcium channels in the dorsal root ganglion and spinal cord,[37] a downregulation of μ-opioid receptors,[38] and a phenotypic switch of A-β fibers such that they begin to express substance P.[39] These changes synergistically enhance the release of transmitters (glutamate, ATP, substance P, and CGRP) onto the dorsal horn neurons. Postsynaptically, fast depolarization induced by glutamate leads to opening of the calcium-permeable AMPA receptor,[40] while slow depolarization induced by substance P and other peptides leads to an opening of the NMDA receptor, which in turn leads to calcium entry[41] and a multitude of calcium-dependent intracellular events that lead to sensitization. Inhibitory neurons reduce the sensitivity of dorsal horn neurons,[40] but this function is compromised after nerve injury. Evidence exists that nerve injury leads to a decreased expression of inhibitory receptors on primary afferent terminals and postsynaptic neurons,[38] a downregulation of the potassium-chloride transporter KCC2 on superficial dorsal horn cells,[42] and a selective apoptosis of inhibitory γ-aminobutyric acid (GABA)-ergic interneurons.[43] These changes contribute to sensitization of the spinothalamic projection neurons. Descending modulatory pathways also influence dorsal horn sensitization in neuropathic pain. Cortical, thalamic, parabrachial, and periaqueductal inputs converge on the rostroventromedial medulla (RVM), which gives rise to both inhibitory and excitatory inputs to the dorsal horn via an ipsilateral pathway in the dorsolateral funiculus. Many of the cells in the RVM express μ-opioid receptors and form serotonergic pathways (inhibitory through 5HT1 receptor and facilitatory via 5HT3 receptor) and noradrenergic pathways (predominantly inhibitory via α2 receptor). Lidocaine microinjection[44] or selective ablation[45] of these cells either before or after establishment of the SNL model can eliminate hyperalgesia.

Central sensitization is summarized here and illustrated in Figures 3.2 and 3.3. Three mechanisms are emphasized:

(1) *Glutamate/NMDA receptor–mediated sensitization.* Increased nociceptive afferent input leads to a massive release from nociceptor central endings of several neurotransmitters and/or neuromodulators, including glutamate (Glu), substance P (SP), CGRP, and ATP, onto the output neurons in lamina I of the superficial dorsal horn. Consequently, an increased release of glutamate activates NMDA receptors, in addition to non-NMDA receptors (kainate receptors and AMPA receptors) located in the postsynaptic neuron, by displacing magnesium ions that normally keep NMDA receptors silent. Activation of NMDA receptor allows calcium influx through its open pores. Intracellular calcium in turn triggers a cascade of intracellular signaling processes through enzymatic amplifications that involves a host of calcium-dependent signaling pathways and second messengers, including mitogen-activated protein kinase (MAPK), protein kinase C (PKC), protein kinase A (PKA), phosphatidylinositol 3-kinase (PI3K), and proto-oncogene tyrosine-protein kinase Src (Src). These cascades of events

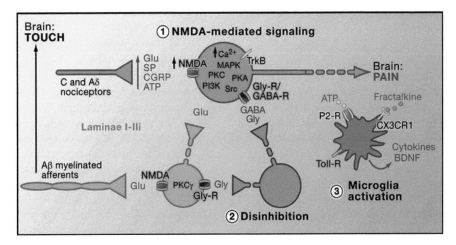

FIGURE 3.2. Factors contributing to central sensitization

Glutamate/NMDA receptor–mediated sensitization. ATP, adenosine triphosphate; BDNF, brain-derived neurotrophic factor; CGRP, calcitonin gene-related peptide; CX3CR1, CX3CL1 (Fractalkine) receptor; GABA-R, γ-aminobutyric acid receptor; Glu, glutamate; Gly, glycine; MAPK, mitogen-activated protein kinase; NMDA, N-methyl-D-aspartate; P2-R, P2 receptor; PI3K, phosphatidylinositol 3-kinase; PKA, protein kinase A; PKC, protein kinase C; Src, proto-oncogene tyrosine-protein kinase Src; SP, substance P; TrkB, tropomyosin receptor kinase B.

From Basbaum AI, Bautista DM, Scherrer G, Julius D. Cellular and molecular mechanisms of pain. *Cell.* 2009;139(2):267–284.

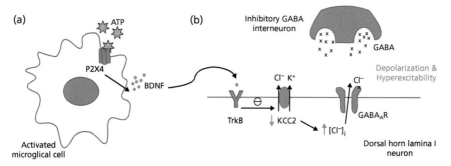

FIGURE 3.3. Molecular mechanism for the reversal of GABAergic response from inhibition to excitation

ATP, adenosine triphosphate; BDNF, brain-derived neurotrophic factor; GABA, γ-aminobutyric acid; KCC2, potassium-chloride cotransporter 2; TrkB, tropomyosin receptor kinase B.

Modified from Mifflin KA, Kerr BJ. The transition from acute to chronic pain: understanding how different biological systems interact. *Can J Anaesth.* 2014;61(2):112–122.

eventually lead to phosphorylation and/or upregulation of expression of relevant ion channels and receptors of the output neurons, increase their excitability, and facilitate the transmission of nociceptive signals to the brain.

(2) *Disinhibition.* Spinal cord inhibitory interneurons, under normal circumstances, keep an inhibitory tone on lamina I output neurons by continuously releasing GABA and/or glycine (Gly). However, this inhibition can be lost in the case of inhibitory interneuronal cell death in the setting of injury. The inhibition can also be lost when the property of the inhibitory neurons changes from inhibitory to excitatory in the setting of increased release of BDNF from activated microglia (Figure 3.3). Upon activation by a number of mechanisms, microglial cells in the spinal cord release BDNF and cytokines. BDNF acts on tropomyosin receptor kinase B (TrkB) receptor of lamina I output neurons and leads to inhibition of potassium-chloride cotransporter 2 (KCC2) of these neurons. Consequently, intracellular chloride concentration rises and exceeds the extracellular concentration. When GABAₐ receptors are activated by GABA released by the inhibitory interneurons, an outflux of chloride ions occurs, leading to depolarization and excitation of lamina I output neurons.

In addition, disinhibition is believed to contribute to allodynia through activation of the PKCγ expressing interneurons in inner lamina II. These neurons receive synaptic input from non-nociceptive myelinated Aβ primary afferents and project to excitatory synaptic output to the lamina I output neurons. However, under normal circumstances, this group of neurons is silent owing to strong input from inhibitory interneurons. This pathway can be activated by disinhibition, allowing non-nociceptive myelinated Aβ primary afferents to engage in the pain transmission circuitry. Consequently, normally innocuous stimuli are perceived as painful (allodynia).

(3) *Microglial activation and glial–neuron interactions.* In addition to Glu, SP, and CGRP, peripheral nerve injury promotes release of ATP and the chemokine fractalkine that can stimulate microglial cells. Specifically, activation of purinergic P2-R receptors, CX3CR1, and Toll-like receptors on microglia results in the release of BDNF, which through activation of TrkB receptor and inhibition of KCC2, both expressed by lamina I output neurons, promotes increased excitability and enhanced pain in response to both noxious and innocuous stimulation. Activated microglia also release a host of cytokines, such as TNF-α, IL-1β, IL-6, and other factors that contribute to central sensitization, by

mechanisms similar to sensitization of nociceptors in the periphery.

Besides changes in the dorsal horn of the spinal cord, neuroplasticity also occurs in other areas of the CNS. Cortical reorganization, measured by topographical shifts in peak activity in the brain through functional magnetic resonance imaging (fMRI), has been linked specifically to neuropathic pain in patients with spinal cord injury,[47,48] complex regional pain syndrome,[49–51] and amputation.[52–54] Spontaneous burst activity in the thalamus has been observed in patients with central neuropathic pain[55] and in animal models of neuropathic pain after spinal cord injury.[56,57] In addition, a disease or a lesion may directly take place in the CNS. Examples include stroke, multiple sclerosis, and spinal cord injury. These conditions may directly or indirectly affect CNS structures that are critical for pain processing and perception.

In recent years, technologies such as transgenesis, optogenetics, and RNA sequencing have been developed, which alongside the more traditional use of animal neuropathic pain models and insights from genetic variations in humans have enabled significant advances to be made in the mechanistic understanding of neuropathic pain.[58] The roles of cytokines, chemokines, and other inflammatory factors in the development and maintenance chronic neuropathic pain are being recognized.[3] The significant contributions from glial cells and immune cells (microglia in the CNS and other immune cells in the peripheral nervous system) are being established.[8–10,59] It is now recognized that, in neuropathic pain conditions, maladaptation occurs in the peripheral and central nervous systems, including a shift in microglial phenotype from a surveillance state to an activated state.[60,61] Microglial activation may lead to altered expression of cell surface proteins and release of growth factors and other intracellular signaling molecules that contribute to development of neuroinflammation and central sensitization.[60,62] Specific targeting of these cellular and molecular mechanisms may provide the key to development of effective neuropathic pain therapies with minimal side effects.

REFERENCES

1. Cheng J. Mechanisms of pathological pain. In: Cheng J, Rosenquist RW, eds. *Fundamentals of Pain Medicine*. Cham, Switzerland: Springer-Nature; 2018:21–25.

2. Cheng J. State of the art, challenges, and opportunities for pain medicine. *Pain Med.* 2018;19(6):1109–1111. http://www.painmed.org/membercenter/presidents-message/.

3. Basbaum AI, Bautista DM, Scherrer G, Julius D. Cellular and molecular mechanisms of pain. *Cell.* 2009;139(2):267–284.

4. Campbell JN, Meyer RA. Mechanisms of neuropathic pain. *Neuron.* 2006;52(1):77–92.

5. Treede RD. Peripheral and cental mechanimsms of neuropathic pain. In: Simpson DM, McArthur JC, Dworkin RH, eds. *Neuropathic Pain, Mechanisms, Diagnosis and Treatment.* New York: Oxford University Press; 2012:14–24.

6. Ibrahim MM, Deng H, Zvonok A, et al. Activation of CB2 cannabinoid receptors by AM1241 inhibits experimental neuropathic pain: pain inhibition by receptors not present in the CNS. *Proc Natl Acad Sci U S A.* 2003;100(18):10529–10533.

7. Porreca F, Lai J, Bian D, et al. A comparison of the potential role of the tetrodotoxin-insensitive sodium channels, PN3/SNS and NaN/SNS2, in rat models of chronic pain. *Proc Natl Acad Sci U S A.* 1999;96(14):7640–7644.

8. Ji RR, Chamessian A, Zhang YQ. Pain regulation by non-neuronal cells and inflammation. *Science.* 2016;354(6312):572–577.

9. Ren K, Dubner R. Interactions between the immune and nervous systems in pain. *Nat Med.* 2010;16(11):1267–1276.

10. Scholz J, Woolf CJ. The neuropathic pain triad: neurons, immune cells and glia. *Nat Neurosci.* 2007;10(11):1361–1368.

11. Cortright DN, Szallasi A. Biochemical pharmacology of the vanilloid receptor TRPV1. An update. *Eur J Biochem.* 2004;271(10):1814–1819.

12. Dib-Hajj SD, Black JA, Waxman SG. NaV1.9: a sodium channel linked to human pain. *Nat Rev Neurosci.* 2015;16(9):511–519.

13. Blumberg H, Janig W. Discharge pattern of afferent fibers from a neuroma. *Pain.* 1984;20(4):335–353.

14. Devor M. *Response of Nerves to Injury in Relation to Neuropathic Pain.* London: Elsevier; 2006.

15. Wall PD, Devor M. Sensory afferent impulses originate from dorsal root ganglia as well as from the periphery in normal and nerve injured rats. *Pain.* 1983;17(4):321–339.

16. Cohen SP, Mao J. Neuropathic pain: mechanisms and their clinical implications. *BMJ (Clin Res Ed).* 2014;348:f7656.

17. Arner S, Lindblom U, Meyerson BA, Molander C. Prolonged relief of neuralgia after regional anesthetic blocks. A call for further experimental and systematic clinical studies. *Pain.* 1990;43(3):287–297.

18. Burchiel KJ, Johans TJ, Ochoa J. The surgical treatment of painful traumatic neuromas. *J Neurosurg.* 1993;78(5):714–719.

19. Gracely RH, Lynch SA, Bennett GJ. Painful neuropathy: altered central processing maintained dynamically by peripheral input. *Pain.* 1992;51(2):175–194.

20. Lyu YS, Park SK, Chung K, Chung JM. Low dose of tetrodotoxin reduces neuropathic pain behaviors in an animal model. *Brain Res.* 2000;871(1):98–103.

21. Sheth RN, Dorsi MJ, Li Y, et al. Mechanical hyperalgesia after an L5 ventral rhizotomy or an L5 ganglionectomy in the rat. *Pain.* 2002;96(1–2):63–72.

22. Ali Z, Ringkamp M, Hartke TV, et al. Uninjured C-fiber nociceptors develop spontaneous activity and alpha-adrenergic sensitivity following L6 spinal nerve ligation in monkey. *J Neurophysiol.* 1999;81(2):455–466.

23. Djouhri L, Koutsikou S, Fang X, McMullan S, Lawson SN. Spontaneous pain, both neuropathic and inflammatory, is related to frequency of spontaneous firing in intact C-fiber nociceptors. *J Neurosci.* 2006;26(4):1281–1292.

24. Wu G, Ringkamp M, Hartke TV, et al. Early onset of spontaneous activity in uninjured C-fiber nociceptors after injury to neighboring nerve fibers. *J Neurosci.* 2001;21(8):Rc140.

25. Boucher TJ, Okuse K, Bennett DL, Munson JB, Wood JN, McMahon SB. Potent analgesic effects of GDNF in neuropathic pain states. *Science.* 2000;290(5489):124–127.

26. Fukuoka T, Tokunaga A, Kondo E, Miki K, Tachibana T, Noguchi K. Change in mRNAs for neuropeptides and the GABA(A) receptor in dorsal root ganglion neurons in a rat experimental neuropathic pain model. *Pain.* 1998;78(1):13–26.

27. Fukuoka T, Kondo E, Dai Y, Hashimoto N, Noguchi K. Brain-derived neurotrophic factor increases in the uninjured dorsal root ganglion neurons in selective spinal nerve ligation model. *J Neurosci.* 2001;21(13):4891–4900.

28. Tsuzuki K, Kondo E, Fukuoka T, et al. Differential regulation of P2X(3) mRNA expression by peripheral nerve injury in intact and injured neurons in the rat sensory ganglia. *Pain.* 2001;91(3):351–360.

29. Klede M, Handwerker HO, Schmelz M. Central origin of secondary mechanical hyperalgesia. *J Neurophysiol.* 2003;90(1):353–359.

30. Wu G, Ringkamp M, Murinson BB, et al. Degeneration of myelinated efferent fibers induces spontaneous activity in uninjured C-fiber afferents. *J Neurosci.* 2002;22(17):7746–7753.

31. Xiao L, Cheng J, Zhuang Y, et al. Botulinum toxin type A reduces hyperalgesia and TRPV1 expression in rats with neuropathic pain. *Pain Med.* 2013;14(2):276–286.

32. Xie X, Cheng J, Liu Z, Shen L. Changes of the immunological parameters in patients with epilepsy. *Chin J Neurol Psychiatry.* 1990;23(3):182–184.

33. Woolf CJ. Central sensitization: implications for the diagnosis and treatment of pain. *Pain.* 2011;152(3 Suppl):S2–S15.

34. Latremoliere A, Woolf CJ. Central sensitization: a generator of pain hypersensitivity by central neural plasticity. *J Pain.* 2009;10(9):895–926.

35. Costigan M, Scholz J, Woolf CJ. Neuropathic pain: a maladaptive response of the nervous system to damage. *Annu Rev Neurosci.* 2009;32:1–32.

36. Simone DA, Sorkin LS, Oh U, et al. Neurogenic hyperalgesia: central neural correlates in responses of spinothalamic tract neurons. *J Neurophysiol.* 1991;66(1):228–246.

37. Li CY, Song YH, Higuera ES, Luo ZD. Spinal dorsal horn calcium channel alpha2delta-1 subunit upregulation contributes to peripheral nerve injury-induced tactile allodynia. *J Neurosci.* 2004;24(39):8494–8499.

38. Kohno T, Ji RR, Ito N, et al. Peripheral axonal injury results in reduced mu opioid receptor pre- and post-synaptic action in the spinal cord. *Pain.* 2005;117(1–2):77–87.

39. Noguchi K, Dubner R, De Leon M, Senba E, Ruda MA. Axotomy induces preprotachykinin gene expression in a subpopulation of dorsal root ganglion neurons. *J Neurosci Res.* 1994;37(5):596–603.

40. Gu JG, Albuquerque C, Lee CJ, MacDermott AB. Synaptic strengthening through activation of Ca2+-permeable AMPA receptors. *Nature.* 1996;381(6585):793–796.

41. Yoshimura M, Yonehara N. Alteration in sensitivity of ionotropic glutamate receptors and tachykinin receptors in spinal cord contribute to development and maintenance of nerve injury-evoked neuropathic pain. *Neurosci Res.* 2006;56(1):21–28.

42. Coull JA, Boudreau D, Bachand K, et al. Trans-synaptic shift in anion gradient in spinal lamina I neurons as a mechanism of neuropathic pain. *Nature.* 2003;424(6951):938–942.

43. Moore KA, Kohno T, Karchewski LA, Scholz J, Baba H, Woolf CJ. Partial peripheral nerve injury promotes a selective loss of GABAergic inhibition in the superficial dorsal horn of the spinal cord. *J Neurosci.* 2002;22(15):6724–6731.

44. Burgess SE, Gardell LR, Ossipov MH, et al. Time-dependent descending facilitation from the rostral ventromedial medulla maintains, but does not initiate, neuropathic pain. *J Neurosci.* 2002;22(12):5129–5136.

45. Porreca F, Burgess SE, Gardell LR, et al. Inhibition of neuropathic pain by selective ablation of brainstem medullary cells expressing the mu-opioid receptor. *J Neurosci.* 2001;21(14):5281–5288.

46. Mifflin KA, Kerr BJ. The transition from acute to chronic pain: understanding how different biological systems interact. *Can J Anaesth.* 2014;61(2):112–122.

47. Wrigley PJ, Press SR, Gustin SM, et al. Neuropathic pain and primary somatosensory cortex reorganization following spinal cord injury. *Pain.* 2009;141(1–2):52–59.

48. Jutzeler CR, Freund P, Huber E, Curt A, Kramer JLK. Neuropathic pain and functional reorganization in the primary sensorimotor cortex after spinal cord injury. *J Pain.* 2015;16(12):1256–1267.

49. Maihofner C, Handwerker HO, Neundorfer B, Birklein F. Patterns of cortical reorganization in complex regional pain syndrome. *Neurology.* 2003;61(12):1707–1715.

50. Geha PY, Baliki MN, Harden RN, Bauer WR, Parrish TB, Apkarian AV. The brain in chronic CRPS pain: abnormal gray-white matter interactions in emotional and autonomic regions. *Neuron.* 2008;60(4):570–581.

51. Barad MJ, Ueno T, Younger J, Chatterjee N, Mackey S. Complex regional pain syndrome is associated with structural abnormalities in pain-related regions of the human brain. *J Pain.* 2014;15(2):197–203.

52. MacIver K, Lloyd DM, Kelly S, Roberts N, Nurmikko T. Phantom limb pain, cortical reorganization and the therapeutic effect of mental imagery. *Brain.* 2008;131(Pt 8):2181–2191.

53. Raffin E, Richard N, Giraux P, Reilly KT. Primary motor cortex changes after amputation correlate with phantom limb pain and the ability to move the phantom limb. *NeuroImage.* 2016;130:134–144.

54. Makin TR, Scholz J, Henderson Slater D, Johansen-Berg H, Tracey I. Reassessing cortical reorganization in the primary sensorimotor cortex following arm amputation. *Brain.* 2015;138(Pt 8):2140–2146.

55. Lenz FA, Kwan HC, Dostrovsky JO, Tasker RR. Characteristics of the bursting pattern of action potentials that occurs in the thalamus of patients with central pain. *Brain Res.* 1989;496(1–2):357–360.

56. Gerke MB, Duggan AW, Xu L, Siddall PJ. Thalamic neuronal activity in rats with mechanical allodynia following contusive spinal cord injury. *Neuroscience.* 2003;117(3):715–722.

57. Klit H, Finnerup NB, Jensen TS. Central poststroke pain: clinical characteristics, pathophysiology, and management. *Lancet Neurol.* 2009;8(9):857–868.

58. St John Smith E. Advances in understanding nociception and neuropathic pain. *J Neurol.* 2018;265(2):231–238.

59. Colombo E, Farina C. Astrocytes: key regulators of neuroinflammation. *Trends Immunol.* 2016;37(9):608–620.

60. Fernandes V, Sharma D, Vaidya S, et al. Cellular and molecular mechanisms driving neuropathic pain: recent advancements and challenges. *Expert Opin Ther Targets.* 2018;22(2):131–142.

61. von Hehn CA, Baron R, Woolf CJ. Deconstructing the neuropathic pain phenotype to reveal neural mechanisms. *Neuron.* 2012;73(4):638–652.

62. Tsuda M. P2 receptors, microglial cytokines and chemokines, and neuropathic pain. *J Neurosci Res.* 2017;95(6):1319–1329.

4

Assessment and Diagnosis of Neuropathic Pain

ERIK C. HUSTAK

INTRODUCTION

The assessment and diagnosis of neuropathic pain are important in order to develop a better understanding of the complex mechanisms responsible for this syndrome. Also, there is a tremendous need for the development of more effective targeted drug delivery strategies for neuropathic pain.[1] In this chapter, the evolving definition of neuropathic pain will be reviewed along with a standardized approach utilizing history, physical exam, and applicable confirmatory tests. An exploration of screening tool development along with validated questionnaires specific to neuropathic pain is important to gaining a better appreciation of high-yield neuropathic pain descriptors. Finally, a brief review of some confirmatory tests is provided. Hopefully this information, along with the key resources referenced in this chapter, will promote progress in the accurate assessment and diagnosis of this complex syndrome.

THE EVOLVING DEFINITION OF NEUROPATHIC PAIN

Before analyzing large publications from various neuropathic pain interest societies, it is informative to look at the evolving definition of neuropathic pain over the last 25 years to highlight its complexity and impact on society. The semantics of this definition are important because they influence the accurate assessment and diagnosis of this multifaceted syndrome as well as the development of research protocols and treatment paradigms. In 1994, the International Association for the Study of Pain (IASP) defined neuropathic pain as "pain initiated or caused by a primary lesion or dysfunction in the nervous system."[2] Discussion regarding the 1994 term "dysfunction" served as part of the impetus that led to a re-evaluation of the 1994 IASP definition of neuropathic pain, because some

"found it difficult to accept conditions in which symptoms and signs were not reflected in abnormal neuropathophysiology."[3] Subsequently, in 2008, an IASP special interest group on neuropathic pain (NeuPSIG) published a paper in which neuropathic pain was defined as "pain arising as a direct consequence of a lesion or disease affecting the somatosensory system."[4] Ultimately, in 2011, the IASP Taxonomy Committee simplified NeuPSIG's language, defining neuropathic pain as "pain caused by a lesion or disease of the somatosensory nervous system."[3,5]

The subtle insertion of "disease" and "somatosensory nervous system" into the neuropathic pain definition deserves special attention. A normally functioning nociceptive system with abundant afferent traffic can lead to plasticity changes that do not represent neuropathic pain, and the word "disease" attempts to address this issue.[6,7] "Somatosensory nervous system" specifically narrows the focus of the neuropathic pain diagnosis, to exclude motor system diseases which can cause neuropathic pain symptoms indirectly.[7] For example, muscle spasticity is not considered neuropathic pain.[8]

The 2008 NeuPSIG document also introduced a flow chart culminating in a grading system paradigm that categorizes the diagnostician's neuropathic pain diagnosis as unlikely, possible, probable, or definite. This degree of certainty is obtained from a directed history, physical exam, and confirmatory tests, if applicable.

Over the last 8 years, the NeuPSIG's 2008 neuropathic pain definition has been widely referenced. However, an in-depth citation analysis showed limited implementation of the grading system, although slightly improving with time, as it was used in only 25% of clinically based studies.[9] In an effort to improve the clinical application of the neuropathic pain diagnosis algorithm in the clinical and research setting, a modification to the flow chart was made that provides a more practical approach when dealing with a potential neuropathic pain patient. The revised grading system categorizes "possible neuropathic pain" if a history of a relevant neurological lesion or disease is obtained along with a pain distribution that is "neuroanatomically plausible." In a stepwise fashion, "probable neuropathic pain" classification is appropriate if the clinical exam supports the clinician's history with a range of positive and negative signs, as discussed later in the chapter. Finally, "definite neuropathic pain" is applicable when an objective diagnostic test and/or direct anatomical verification (by a surgeon in an operating room, for example) confirms a lesion or disease of the somatosensory nervous system (see Figure 4.1).

Important points regarding the revised guidelines, as introduced by Finnerup et al.'s[9] article, deserve special mention:

1. A classification of probable neuropathic pain should direct the clinician to consider empiric treatment, as discussed in subsequent chapters.
2. Definite neuropathic pain classification, as defined by the algorithm, does not explain causality and multiple pain generators are possible, including concomitant nociceptive or inflammatory components to one's pain syndrome. In other words, an astute clinician should consider the possibility of multifactorial etiologies, which may dictate multifactorial treatment strategies.
3. The guidelines were intended neither for disease classification nor for medicolegal purposes.

The final point, though not necessarily within the scope of this chapter, deserves a brief comment. The clinical diagnoses of many chronic pain conditions are not necessarily reflected accurately in the International Classification of Diseases (ICD) of the World Health Organization (WHO). This lack of available accurate classification can subsequently confound accurate coding required by various payers. This problem also presents a barrier to conducting accurately inclusive research studies, which ultimately impedes the development of novel targeted therapy. A task force is currently developing the ICD-11 chronic pain glossary that will hopefully address some of these systematic shortcomings.[10,11]

RELEVANT NEUROLOGICAL LESIONS OR DISEASES

Lesions or diseases affecting the somatosensory nervous system can occur on a macroscopic or microscopic scale and have been classified in the literature according to disease-based and anatomy-based classification schemes.[12,13] Many of these entities will be reviewed in depth elsewhere in this book, but one needs to have a generalized understanding of some of the common pathological states affecting the nervous system. Categorization of lesions in the literature is often anatomy based and disease based.

Anatomically, lesions are often broken down into central and peripheral classification schemes. Peripheral lesions include post-traumatic injuries, such as surgical trauma, entrapment syndromes, postherpetic neuralgia (PHN), and ischemic neuropathies among other entities. Central lesions include, but are not limited to, infarctions of the brain and spinal cord, spinal cord injuries, and multiple sclerosis. Regional classifications include neuropathic pain entities specific to the head and neck, including trigeminal, glossopharyngeal, and occipital neuralgias. Radicular pain complaints in the cervical, thoracic, and lumbar spine are often considered a separate category of syndromes. In addition, generalized polyneuropathies can also result from nutritional deficiencies, metabolic derangements including diabetes, toxin-related diseases like chemotherapy-induced neuropathies, immune system derangements secondary to infectious or post-infectious states, and hereditary syndromes like Charcot-Marie-Tooth disease. Finally, complex disorders, including complex regional pain syndrome (CRPS) types 1 and 2, are generally categorized separately. Inclusive lists should be referenced regularly to expand one's differential diagnosis.[12]

The European Federation of Neurological Societies (EFNS) 2004 publication[14] along with the 2009 revision[15] and the NeuPSIG 2011 publication[7] serve as a comprehensive review of guidelines for neuropathic pain assessment. After understanding some of the major neuropathic pain–causing lesions and diseases, clinicians are advised to follow a systematic approach (like that referenced here), starting with a focused history and followed by an effective physical exam, and then utilize applicable confirmatory tests in an economically reasonable fashion.

Questionnaires	10 Pain	NPQ	PainDETECT	LANSS	DN4	StEP
Symptoms reported						
Ongoing pain						–
Pricking, tingling pins, needles (any dysesthesia)	+	+	+	+	+	+
Electric shocks or shooting	+	+	+	+	+	
Hot or burning	+	+	+	+	+	
Numbness	+	+	+		+	
Pain evoked by light touching	+	+	+	+		
Painful cold or freezing pain		+			+	–
Pain evoked by mild pressure			+			
Pain evoked by heat or cold			+			
Pain evoked by changes in weather		+				
Pain limited to joints	–					
Itching					+	–
Temporal patterns or temporal summation			+			
Radiation of pain			+			
Autonomic changes	+					
Physical examination						
Abnormal response to cold temperature (decrease or allodynia)						+
Hyperalgesia						+
Abnormal response to blunt pressure (decreased or evoked pain)						+
Decreased response to vibration						+
Brush allodynia				+	+	–
Raised soft touch threshold					+	–
Raised pinprick threshold				+	+	+
Straight-leg-raising test						+
Skin changes						–

The minus sign (–) indicates items that reduce the score.
doi:10.1371/journal.pmed.1000045.t002

FIGURE 4.1. Symptoms reported and physical examination required in six questionnaires for assessing neuropathic pain.

CLINICAL HISTORY IDENTIFIES POSSIBLE NEUROPATHIC PAIN

When the chief complaint is reported as, "It's numb . . . but it hurts," one should implement one's neuropathic pain assessment algorithm. Often these paradoxical descriptors coexist when a lesion or disease affects the somatosensory nervous system. Numbness can indicate lack of normal sensory input, but neuropathic pain mechanisms, reviewed in Chapter 3, are thought to reflect spontaneous ectopic discharges and hypersensitivity of afferent input into the dorsal horn and transmitted to higher centers of the brain.[16] Clinically, this may explain patients' apparently contradictory complaint of "shooting sensations" in the "numb" area. Mechanistically and clinically, neuropathic pain is different from nociceptive pain, and one needs to be able to differentiate between the two.

Clinicians first need to explore the chronology, onset, duration, and intensity of pain and exacerbating and remitting factors surrounding the chief complaint. In clinical practice, this is generally achieved during the medical interview. Verbal rating scales (VRS), 100-millimeter visual analog scales (VAS), and 11-point numerical rating scales (NRS) are used in the attempt to quantify the complex experience of pain symptoms in a one-dimensional fashion.[17] In contrast, the aim of multidimensional pain assessment tools, including the McGill Pain Questionnaire (MPQ) and Brief Pain Inventory (BPI), is to quantify the complex and dynamic pain experience in a more comprehensive fashion.[18]

However, tools and questionnaires that have been developed specifically for neuropathic pain are now being implemented. Although pain perception is influenced by cultural attitudes and psychiatric health (among other factors), certain universal patterns of neuropathic pain emerge that clinicians need to understand.[19] The clinician should be familiar with basic pain terminology that can be reviewed in various pain texts or online[5]; some of those key points will be reviewed here. "Negative" symptoms and signs include hypoesthesia defined as a *reduced* sensation of various stimuli, which is described commonly as "numb." Subclasses of hypoesthesia include pall-hypoesthesia (vibration), and therm-hypoesthesia (cold/warm). "Positive" symptoms, on the other hand, can be spontaneous or evoked. They can be described as paroxysmal "shooting

electric shock–like attacks." Furthermore, paresthesias, described as abnormal sensations, and dysesthesias, described as abnormal *and unpleasant* sensations, are commonly found. Hyperalgesia, described as increased pain from a stimulus that normally provokes pain, is often present, although this is sometimes difficult to quantify because of the subjective nature of pain. Furthermore, allodynia, described as painful sensation to a normally nonpainful stimulus, can result from cold, heat, or mechanical stimuli.[13] As one conducts an interview, certain patterns of neuropathic pain descriptors emerge that are statistically distinct from other pain syndromes. Fortunately, there are several published reports attempting to clarify some of these patterns, as discussed next.

QUANTIFYING TREATMENT OUTCOMES UTILIZING NEUROPATHIC DESCRIPTORS

The Neuropathic Pain Scale (NPS) was introduced in 1996. This scale includes two global pain scales (intensity and unpleasantness), one temporal sequence assessment (background pain versus flare-ups), and eight specific neuropathic pain descriptors (sharp, hot, dull, cold, sensitive, itchy, deep pain, and surface pain).[20] Two points regarding the NPS deserve mention. The first is that the NPS was developed using patients with PHN and, as a result, found that PHN patients characteristically described their pain as less cold but more sharp, sensitive, and itchy than other neuropathic pain syndromes. Perhaps more useful, however, is that, relative to other simple global pain assessments (like the 11-point NRS), the NPS provides more neuropathic descriptors, which may better quantify responsiveness to a particular intervention. Providing documentation of improved efficacy is of particular importance when trying to justify implementation of a therapy.

The Neuropathic Pain Symptom Inventory (NPSI) questionnaire, with 10 descriptors and 2 temporal items, was introduced in 2004. Like the NPS, the NPSI provided a more detailed analysis of one's pain syndrome. In addition, the NPSI attempts to quantify five distinct dimensions of neuropathic pain expression: pain which is evoked, paroxysmal, superficially spontaneous, deep spontaneous, and/or associated with paresthesias or dysesthesias.[21] Interestingly, the NPSI has been studied to confirm the "universality of core neuropathic pain descriptors" across multiple cultures, including Brazil, Japan, China, Finland, Spain, and the United States.[19]

Ultimately, however, the clinically relevant inference of the NPS and NPSI development is that certain descriptors and "dimensions" of the NPS and NPSI may reflect specific pathological mechanisms. Furthermore, they have been validated for neuropathic pain and are sensitive to changes in treatment, which can be used clinically to document treatment effects. As a result, the NPS and NPSI are recommended to evaluate treatment outcomes for neuropathic pain clinically instead of relying on unidimensional global pain assessments.[7] This has been the trend in the literature over the last two decades.[22]

After quantifying discriminant neuropathic pain descriptors, one needs to ascertain if there is a "neuroanatomically plausible" lesion or disease somewhere in the somatosensory nervous system explaining the symptoms. Following Finnerup's flow chart application of the NeuPSIG's definition, if the patient's history confirms a "possible" neuropathic diagnosis, a directed physical examination is needed to advance into the "probable" category.[9] Some of the tools and questionnaires discussed next incorporate physical exam findings in order to take this step.

NEUROPATHIC PAIN QUESTIONNAIRES AND HELPFUL OBJECTIVE ASSESSMENTS

Many questionnaires are available to aid in assessment of neuropathic pain, including the Leeds Assessment of Neuropathic Symptoms and Signs (LANSS) and the simplified self-LANSS (S-LANSS), the Neuropathic Pain Questionnaire (NPQ) and the simplified short-NPQ (S-NPQ), the Douleur Neuropathique en 4 (DN4), PainDETECT (PD-Q), ID-Pain, and the Standardized Evaluation of Pain (StEP). The recent trend in the literature highlights the beneficial utilization of some of these validated tools in providing support for the diagnosis. Each tool is reviewed in the sections that follow.[7,9,23,24]

Leeds Assessment of Neuropathic Symptoms and Signs (LANSS)

The LANSS was introduced in 2001, followed in 2005 by a simplified version that can be self-administered (self-LANSS, or S-LANSS).[25,26] Both the LANNS and the S-LANSS are useful tools when trying to distinguish nociceptive from neuropathic pain. This has implications for treatment. Furthermore, the LANNS and S-LANSS were the first tools introduced for this purpose.

The LANNS is a five-item questionnaire reflecting potential dysesthesias, autonomic, evoked, paroxysmal, and thermal pain symptoms. In addition, two physical exam items reflecting allodynia and altered pinprick thresholds were introduced. Different predictive values of neuropathic pain were assigned a numeric value. A scoring system out of 24 was created, with any number greater than 12 indicative of a syndrome encompassing likely involvement of neuropathic mechanisms.

The S-LANSS was subsequently introduced to clarify some of the descriptive vocabulary of the LANSS and to address the physical-exam difficulties faced in the reality of clinical practice. The pinprick threshold assessments were replaced with self-evaluation by the patient subjectively pressing his or her fingertip into affected and unaffected areas and making a comparison. Finally, an anatomical diagram was also added, to help subjects illustrate the location of their pain characteristics, which helps the examiner determine if the pain distribution is neuroanatomically plausible, based on one's understanding of neuroanatomy.

Several points deserve special mention regarding the LANSS and S-LANSS. First, symptoms related to dysesthesias, autonomic phenomenon, and evoked discomfort were found to be more associated with neuropathic mechanisms and, as a result, carry a point value of 5, 5, and 3, respectively. By contrast, paroxysmal "electric shock" and thermal changes including "hot and burning" descriptors carry a score of 2 and 1, respectfully. The S-LANSS is a self-report instrument, but when the S-LANSS is given in interview format, the sensitivity of the assessment does increase by 5%, perhaps not surprisingly. However, describing a subjective pain experience has its inherent challenges. The author hypothesized that the discriminate ability of certain descriptors may also depend on the context in which it was obtained. This suggests that an open interview may carry more weight than priming the patient with descriptive terminology choices in a questionnaire format.[25,26] Either approach is probably acceptable, but an understanding of which descriptors carry more meaning may increase one's diagnostic acumen and illustrates the importance of understanding the development of some of these neuropathic pain tools and questionnaires.

Neuropathic Pain Questionnaire (NPQ)

The NPQ and the NPQ–Short Form (NPQ-S) were introduced in 2003[22,27] and, like the LANSS/S-LANSS, can help differentiate neuropathic from nociceptive pain. The NPQ consists of 12 items with an NRS of 1–100 for each item. A discriminate analysis was conducted by the authors that led to the assignment of statistical coefficients to each pain descriptor. Each score is multiplied by the discriminant coefficient and the 12 results are summed together. After conducting the arithmetic and subtracting a constant, a discriminant function score is observed which "at or greater than zero" predicts neuropathic pain. The sensitivity and specificity is quoted at 66% and 74%, respectively, compared to the clinical diagnosis in the validated sample and represents the lowest reported accuracy among the tests discussed in this chapter. Furthermore, the arithmetic required for each patient encounter might be viewed as more labor intensive than desired. Alternatively, the NPQ-S utilized the three most important descriptors—numbness (hypoesthesia), tingling pain (dysesthesia), and increased pain due to touch (allodynia)—which, when trying to distinguish between neuropathic and nociceptive pain, resulted in a comparable sensitivity and specificity of 64.5% and 78.6%, respectively. However, just understanding the high-yield symptoms used in the NPQ-S provides clinically meaningful information, irrespective of NPQ or NPQ-S utilization.

Douleur Neuropathique 4 (DN4)

In 2005, the French Neuropathic Pain Group introduced a simple, clinically administered questionnaire, the Douleur Neuropathique 4 (DN4).[28] The DN4 comprises four questions, the first two of which relate to seven characteristics or associated symptoms (burning, painful cold, electric shocks, tingling, pins and needles, numbness, and itching). The final two relate to three physical exam findings (hypoesthesia to touch, hypoesthesia to pinprick, increased pain following brush stimulus) to comprise 10 total data points. A score of 4 or greater is suggestive of neuropathic pain. The authors quote the sensitivity and specificity of the DN4 at 82.9 and 89.9%, respectively, compared to clinical diagnosis in the development study. The DN4 is easy to administer and score and has been used to characterize treatment effects as well.[29]

ID Pain

In 2006, the ID Pain screening tool was developed to differentiate nociceptive from neuropathic pain.[30] The validation of this tool suggests that a formal pain specialist would label the patient with probable neuropathic mechanisms when scores were 3 or more, indicating that this tool is perhaps best used in a primary care setting. ID Pain is simple to use and can be self-administered with no need for examination. It is a six-question tool, which assigns points to the descriptors (paresthesias, numbness, allodynia, dysesthesia, and burning) and subtracts a point if the pain is limited to the joints. Neuropathic pain patients scored 3 or greater (the recommended cut-off for neuropathic pain) 58% of the time, compared to only 22% of nociceptive pain patients in the validation studies mentioned.

PainDETECT

Developed in 2004 and published in 2006, PainDETECT was introduced as a screening questionnaire in back pain patients to assess for neuropathic components.[31] Since its inception, PainDETECT has been translated and validated in multiple languages, applied to multiple neuropathic pain conditions, and utilized to follow pain symptom response to treatment course.[32] PainDETECT has seven pain descriptor questions (categorized verbally and scored 0 to 5), along with temporal assessment (scored -1 to 2) and assessment of radiating patterns (scored 0 to 2) for a total point range from -1 to 38. Cut-off point values suggest unlikely (if -1 to 12), ambiguous (if 13 to 18), and likely patterns of neuropathic pain (if 19 to 38). The sensitivity was reported at 84%–85%.

Standardized Evaluation of Pain (StEP)

In 2009, the Standardized Evaluation of Pain (StEP) was introduced, which combined 6 interview questions with 10 physical exam tests to differentiate axial low back pain (aLBP) from radicular low back pain (rLBP), and also to identify different pain subtypes possibly reflecting different mechanisms.[16] The authors report a validation of the StEP at 92% sensitivity and 97% specificity with respect to the discriminate ability of differentiating axial versus radicular back pain. The most significant indicators for radicular pain on physical exam included a positive straight-leg raise, deficit in cold detection, and decreased response to pinprick. The gold standard comparison was an interdisciplinary team of at least two attending physicians and a spinal physiotherapist along with any available diagnostic studies including imaging. The StEP authors also applied the 10-item DN4 (which comprises two physical exam questions yielding three parameters, as discussed previously) for comparison purposes to differentiate rLBP from aLBP and found the DN4 to yield a sensitivity and specificity of only 61% and 73%, respectively. In addition to aLBP versus rLBP discriminatory ability, the StEP also found pain subtypes reflected in the diagnostic categories of the patient population studied, including those with diabetic polyneuropathy (DPN), PHN, rLBP, and aLBP. Important clusters distinguishing between the diagnoses were cited, but a few points deserve special mention:

1. Altered response to pinprick was the most sensitive and specific test distinguishing DPN, rLBP, and PHN (95%) from aLBP (7%).
2. A positive straight-leg raise was 100% specific when distinguishing rLBP from DPN and PHN.
3. Decreased response to vibration distinguished DPN from PHN.

ROLE OF PHYSICAL EXAM FINDINGS

Three of the six tools just discussed (LANSS, DN4, and StEP) utilize physical exam findings and thus are administered by a clinician, providing the support for a "probable neuropathic pain" diagnosis. A comparison of the strengths and weaknesses of the aforementioned six tools has been discussed in the literature, and various charts (see Figure 4.1) citing similarities and differences are helpful to explore.[23,24,29,33,34]

It is important to note that the "gold standard" used in validation of many these tools is the expert clinical evaluation with physical examination. The EFNS 2004 publication[14] along with the 2009 revision[15] and the NeuPSIG 2011 publication[7] serve as a comprehensive review of guidelines for neuropathic pain assessment. Both groups strongly endorse clinical examination as a necessary step in the diagnosis of neuropathic pain. As taught in medical school, the standardized approach to the physical exam, including inspection, palpation, percussion, and auscultation, should not be disregarded, as the physician needs to avoid examination bias despite his or her clinical interests. However, when dealing with the potential neuropathic pain patient, one needs to focus on the neurological exam with an emphasis on the somatosensory nervous system, including the evaluation of autonomic signs, reflexes, motor response, and, most importantly, sensory testing.

Anatomical diagrams mapping patient signs and symptoms as well as quantification of response to various stimuli are important. The NeuPSIG stresses the importance of sensory testing, including touch (cotton wool), vibration (128 Hz tuning fork), pinprick (broken tongue blade), cold, and warmth (metal thermorollers).[7] The examiner needs to differentiate the locations of allodynia (mechanical, brush, cold, and heat), hyperalgesia, blunt-pressure responses, soft-touch threshold comparisons, and pinprick thresholds and note any skin changes. As previously discussed, some of the assessment tools contain various portions of the aforementioned physical exam findings (see Figure 4.1). Nerve distribution borders as well as contralateral assessment and comparison are key. If the sensory signs are "neuroanatomically plausible," then the diagnostician may conclude that the patient has "probable neuropathic pain." Common neuropathic pain conditions with plausible distributions of signs and symptoms are helpful to reference in the clinical setting.[9] A straight-leg raise has particular diagnostic implications as reflected in the StEP scoring system[16] for radicular back pain. In addition, use of von Frey filaments for discriminative testing may help provide more information on physical exam and is included in tools like StEP as well as in research studies. Resources available might dictate the depth of the physical examination, but a basic somatosensory exam with the tools described here should be part of every clinician's practice.

CONFIRMATORY TESTS IDENTIFY DEFINITE NEUROPATHIC PAIN

Confirmatory tests categorizing definitive neuropathic pain are used in research publications for the evaluation of pain in human subjects. However, the reality of clinical practice often precludes performance of such testing secondary to time, cost, reimbursement, and the availability of specialty centers with resources capable of such testing.[16] Quantitative sensory testing (QST), somatosensory-evoked potentials (SEP), nerve conduction studies (NCS), A-delta laser-evoked potentials (LEP), and skin biopsies are occasionally performed and are discussed briefly in the next sections. Functional magnetic resonance imaging (fMRI), positron emission tomography (PET), and microneurography are interesting tools in evaluation of neuropathic pain but not routinely recommended. Readers are directed to literature for further review, if desired.[7,14,15]

Quantitative Sensory Testing

QST is a helpful adjunct to the clinical exam to objectively document the sensory exam; an abnormality would provide evidence needed for a definite neuropathic pain diagnosis. QST is useful to evaluate evoked pain response and possible treatment response. However, QST abnormalities exist in non-neuropathic pain conditions as well; therefore, QST by itself does not make for a definitive diagnosis and should be interpreted with caution. QST may be helpful in documenting responses to subtypes of pain (discriminate characteristics). Unfortunately, QST is not readily available and not frequently used in a non-research setting.

Neurophysiological Testing

SEP and NCS are readily available and recommended for objectively locating and quantifying abnormalities in the large, non-nociceptive afferent tracts like the dorsal column lemniscal system. This information is helpful to objectively delineate topographical mapping of peripheral or central lesions.[35] However, to specifically assess the nociceptive pathway, laser stimulators to superficial skin layers (LEPs) selectively excite nociceptive pathways (A-delta and C) and can further provide diagnostic information. Specialized centers are needed for this evaluation, which limits its routine use in clinical practice.[7,23,35]

Skin Biopsy

Intraepidermal nerve fiber density (IENFD) and clues for possible dysfunction can be assessed by visualization of immunostaining of punch skin biopsies.[7,15] This information can also be correlated with other objective assessments, including evoked potentials, QST findings, and NPS/NPSI, to provide objective confirmation of definite neuropathic pain. The use of skin biopsy is recommended if patients show clinical signs of small fiber dysfunction in order to document IENFD, but experienced centers are needed with application of standardized assessment.

CONCLUSION AND KEY POINTS

The refinement in our ability to accurately assess and diagnose neuropathic pain conditions will ultimately lead to potential treatment targets to alleviate suffering in our patients. The preceding discussion explored some important aspects that the clinician needs to understand when dealing with this challenging patient population. Some key points are summarized as follows.

- Neuropathic pain is defined as "pain arising as a direct consequence of a lesion or disease affecting the somatosensory system."
- A grading system categorizing possible, probable, and definite neuropathic pain, based on the clinician's history, physical exam, and confirmatory tests, should be used.
- The NPS and NPSI are tools specific to neuropathic pain, which can be repeatedly followed to assess treatment outcomes and provide more meaningful data relative to one-dimensional global pain assessments.
- The use of questionnaires and screening tools (LANSS, NPQ, DN4, PainDETECT, ID PAIN, StEP) may aid in the accurate assessment of neuropathic pain, and understanding their development is insightful.
- Physical examination (part of LANSS, DN4, and StEP) focusing on the neurological exam is recommended and can be performed with basic instruments.
- Surgical confirmation or imaging confirming a somatosensory lesion, as well as confirmatory tests such as QST, SEP, LEP, NCS, and skin biopsy (among other tests) can help categorize definitive neuropathic pain.

REFERENCES

1. Dworkin RH. Introduction: recommendations for the diagnosis, assessment, and treatment of neuropathic pain. *Am J Med.* 2009;122(10 Suppl):S1–S2.
2. Merskey H, Bogduk N. *Classification of Chronic Pain.* 2nd ed. Seattle: IASP Press; 1994.
3. Jensen TS, Baron R, Haanpaa M, et al. A new definition of neuropathic pain. *Pain.* 2011;152(10):2204–2205.
4. Treede RD, Jensen TS, Campbell JN, et al. Neuropathic pain: redefinition and a grading system for clinical and research purposes. *Neurology.* 2008;70(18):1630–1635.

5. IASP Task Force on Taxonomy; Merskey H, Bogduk N (eds.). IASP taxonomy. https://www.scribd.com/document/257946411/IASP-Taxonomy. Accessed July 7, 2018.

6. May S, Serpell M. Diagnosis and assessment of neuropathic pain. *F1000 Med Rep.* 2009;1.

7. Haanpaa M, Attal N, Backonja M, et al. NeuPSIG guidelines on neuropathic pain assessment. *Pain.* 2011;152(1):14–27.

8. Geber C, Baumgartner U, Schwab R, et al. Revised definition of neuropathic pain and its grading system: an open case series illustrating its use in clinical practice. *Am J Med.* 2009;122(10 Suppl):S3–S12.

9. Finnerup NB, Haroutounian S, Kamerman P, et al. Neuropathic pain: an updated grading system for research and clinical practice. *Pain.* 2016;157(8):1599–1606.

10. Finnerup NB, Scholz J, Attal N et al. Neuropathic pain needs systematic classification. *Eur J Pain.* 2013;17(7):953–956.

11. Treede RD, Rief W, Barke A, et al. A classification of chronic pain for ICD-11. *Pain.* 2015;156(6):1003–1007.

12. Baron R, Binder A, Wasner G. Neuropathic pain: diagnosis, pathophysiological mechanisms, and treatment. *Lancet Neurol.* 2010;9(8):807–819.

13. Baron R, Tolle TR. Assessment and diagnosis of neuropathic pain. *Curr Opin Support Palliat Care.* 2008;2(1):1–8.

14. Cruccu G, Anand P, Attal N, et al. EFNS guidelines on neuropathic pain assessment. *Eur J Neurol.* 2004;11(3):153–162.

15. Cruccu G, Sommer C, Anand P, et al. EFNS guidelines on neuropathic pain assessment: revised 2009. *Eur J Neurol.* 2010;17(8):1010–1018.

16. Scholz J, Mannion RJ, Hord DE, et al. A novel tool for the assessment of pain: validation in low back pain. *PLoS Med.* 2009;6(4):e1000047.

17. Breivik EK, Bjornsson GA, Skovlund E. A comparison of pain rating scales by sampling from clinical trial data. *Clin J Pain.* 2000;16(1):22–28.

18. Katz J, Melzack R. Measurement of pain. *Surg Clin North Am.* 1999;79(2):231–252.

19. Crawford B, Bouhassira D, Wong A, Dukes E. Conceptual adequacy of the neuropathic pain symptom inventory in six countries. *Health Qual Life Outcomes.* 2008;6:62.

20. Galer BS, Jensen MP. Development and preliminary validation of a pain measure specific to neuropathic pain: the Neuropathic Pain Scale. *Neurology.* 1997;48(2):332–338.

21. Bouhassira D, Attal N, Fermanian J, et al. Development and validation of the Neuropathic Pain Symptom Inventory. *Pain.* 2004;108(3):248–257.

22. Krause SJ, Backonja MM. Development of a neuropathic pain questionnaire. *Clin J Pain.* 2003;19(5):306–314.

23. Cruccu G, Truini A. Tools for assessing neuropathic pain. *PLoS Med.* 2009;6(4):e1000045.

24. Bennett MI, Attal N, Backonja MM, et al. Using screening tools to identify neuropathic pain. *Pain.* 2007;127(3):199–203.

25. Bennett M. The LANSS Pain Scale: the Leeds assessment of neuropathic symptoms and signs. *Pain.* 2001;92(1–2):147–157.

26. Bennett MI, Smith BH, Torrance N, Potter J. The S-LANSS score for identifying pain of predominantly neuropathic origin: validation for use in clinical and postal research. *J Pain.* 2005;6(3):149–158.

27. Backonja MM, Krause SJ. Neuropathic pain questionnaire—short form. *Clin J Pain.* 2003;19(5):315–316.

28. Bouhassira D, Attal N, Alchaar H, et al. Comparison of pain syndromes associated with nervous or somatic lesions and development of a new neuropathic pain diagnostic questionnaire (DN4). *Pain.* 2005;114(1–2):29–36.

29. Jones RC, III, Backonja MM. Review of neuropathic pain screening and assessment tools. *Curr Pain Headache Rep.* 2013;17(9):363.

30. Portenoy R. Development and testing of a neuropathic pain screening questionnaire: ID Pain. *Curr Med Res Opin.* 2006;22(8):1555–1565.

31. Freynhagen R, Baron R, Gockel U, Tolle TR. painDETECT: a new screening questionnaire to identify neuropathic components in patients with back pain. *Curr Med Res Opin.* 2006;22(10):1911–1920.

32. Freynhagen R, Tolle TR, Gockel U, Baron R. The painDETECT project—far more than a screening tool on neuropathic pain. *Curr Med Res Opin.* 2016;32(6):1033–1057.

33. Hallstrom H, Norrbrink C. Screening tools for neuropathic pain: can they be of use in individuals with spinal cord injury? *Pain.* 2011;152(4):772–779.

34. Bouhassira D, Attal N. Diagnosis and assessment of neuropathic pain: the saga of clinical tools. *Pain.* 2011;152(3 Suppl):S74–S83.

35. Garcia-Larrea L. Objective pain diagnostics: clinical neurophysiology. *Neurophysiol Clin.* 2012;42(4):187–197.

5

Nonpharmacological Treatment of Neuropathic Pain

RAVI MIRPURI AND DANIELLE PERRET

INTRODUCTION

Nonpharmacological management of neuropathic pain can offer patient-centered treatment options with various modalities, which typically have better safety profiles, reduce pain intensity, and improve overall function. They can be applied on an as-needed basis to a wide range of patients of varying ages and are accepted in many ethnic and cultural settings. Limitations include few randomized controlled trials to provide evidence for treatment efficacy, lack of provider education and comfort, incomplete patient access to services, and difficult patient compliance with treatment. Although many of the modalities described here can complement or serve as stand-alone treatments, it should be noted that non-pharmacotherapy typically provides better outcomes in combination with a comprehensive multimodal pain management plan that also includes pharmacological agents and interventional modalities.[1] A summary of the classification and types of nonpharmacological treatment can be found in Table 5.1.

EXERCISE AND PHYSIOTHERAPY

A variety of exercise and training techniques can be used by physicians, physical therapists, and occupational therapists. Since neuropathic pain can be accompanied by sensory and motor deficits, any individual exercise plan must be tailored to each patient on the basis of his or her deficits. Additionally, it is important to note that kinesiophobia, or "fear of movement," can be a common maladaptive behavior in patients with neuropathic pain and should be addressed in all the treatments. Following are some types of exercise and physiotherapy programs that may be useful in treating neuropathic pain.

- *Balance, sensory, and proprioceptive training.* Poor balance and proprioception can result from sensory neuropathy. As a result, treatment may focus on balance, gait, and spatial reorientation retraining. Depending on the severity of deficits, evaluation of ambulation equipment (e.g., cane, walker, or wheelchair) may be appropriate during this training.[2]

- *Aquatic therapy.* This treatment strategy is typically employed in patients unable to tolerate land-based therapy because of pain limitations. It is proposed that water buoyancy may act on thermal and mechanoreceptors to block nociception and thus improve treatment tolerance. Additionally, warm water may enhance blood flow and facilitate flexibility, muscle relaxation, and general analgesia.[2]

- *Strength and postural training.* Impairments of muscle weakness, poor activity tolerance, posture, and decreased range of motion can develop over time as with many chronic conditions. Treatments, depending on the deconditioned sites, may include stretching, aerobic training, and strengthening. One popular technique commonly used for sciatic pain is the McKenzie program, which places emphasis on core strengthening to reduce pain.[3]

- *Ergonomics.* This treatment focuses on the biomechanics and efficiency of an individual in a particular work environment. If improper, adjusting body mechanics during sitting or lifting to the most biologically advantageous position can help reduce pain. Another consideration in ergonomics is energy conservation techniques. Chronic neuropathic pain can be associated with quick fatigue; the treatment for preventing early fatigue is focused on modifying work tasks to eliminate steps, pace activity, and

TABLE 5.1. CLASSIFICATION OF NONPHARMACOLOGICAL TREATMENTS
FOR NEUROPATHIC PAIN

Movement/ Biomechanical*	Peripheral System[†]	Central System[‡]
• Physiotherapy • Tai chi** • Yoga** • Orthotics	• Structured graded desensitization • Heat/cold modalities • Transcutaneous electrical nerve stimulation (TENS) • Acupuncture	• Mirror therapy • Psychotherapy • Transcranial magnetic stimulation (TMS) • Tai chi** • Yoga**

* Movement/Biomechanical: treatments focus more on movement, exercise, and correcting underlying biomechanics to treat pain.
[†] Peripheral System: treatments focus on stimulating the peripheral nervous system, which may also then affect the central nervous system.
[‡] Central System: treatments focus on treating the brain or central nervous system to influence the peripheral system.
** These modalities have roles that apply in more than one category.

adding environmental modifications for simplicity.[2]

- *Work hardening.* Typically the work hardening program is performed under the supervision of an occupational therapist who will design a work circuit specific to the targeted job, such as climbing ladders, heavy lifting, or performing overhead activities. Programs typically range from 2 to 5 days per week for 2–8 hours per day, all depending on the tolerance of the patient. Eventually, most patients progress to transitional work programming, where job duties are performed at the actual employment site.[2]

MIRROR THERAPY

Mirror therapy was originally invented by Vilayanur Ramachandran to treat phantom limb pain. Mirror therapy has also been shown to have some benefit in treating stroke effects and complex regional pain syndrome (CRPS). The

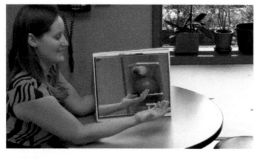

FIGURE 5.1. Mirror box therapy being used to treat hand or wrist pain.

principal is to exploit the brain's preference in prioritizing visual feedback over somatosensory feedback. A mirror is used to create a reflective illusion of an affected limb moving without pain, thus creating false feedback.[2,4]

Treatment is performed by placing the sound limb in front of the mirror box and the affected limb behind the mirror. This creates a reflection of the sound limb so that it appears in place of the affected hidden limb (see Figure 5.1). Once limbs are in the appropriate place, the patient then looks into the mirror on the sound side and makes "mirror symmetric" movements, such as clapping hands or circular movements. This artificial feedback sometimes makes it possible for patients to unclench themselves from potentially painful positions.[4]

STRUCTURED GRADED DESENSITIZATION PROGRAM

Desensitization is a useful strategy specifically for patients with allodynia or hyperalgesia. The goal is to normalize sensitivity in a progressive manner. Three primary methods of desensitization include tactile, thermal, and pressure.

Thermal—This approach usually occurs in either form, using temperature changes:
1. *Contrast bath therapy.* In this treatment the affected limb is immersed in ice water first, followed by immediate immersion of the same limb in warm water. This is repeated several times for multiple sessions.

2. *Gradual thermal desensitization.* This therapy is used primarily to treat symptoms of cold intolerance. A hot bath is warmed to approximately 96° F and the limb is immersed for 2 minutes, rested for 5 minutes, and then the sequence repeated multiple times. For each new session the temperature of the water is lowered a few degrees until the goal is reached; this usually requires several weeks of treatment.

Tactile—A typical protocol for this approach involves massaging the skin with soft fabrics, such as silk, and progressing toward more irritating textures, such as Velcro.[2,5]

Pressure—Light pressure forces are applied to the affected limb; initially this may include rolling a soft ball over the region. This protocol is then progressed by rolling increasingly firmer balls over the area until the goal is met.[5]

Desensitization techniques can be performed directly at the painful site or also in remote areas with anatomical nerve relation. For example, a patient who complains of hypersensitivity of the palmar thumb (median nerve innervated) can be desensitized in the skin over the thenar eminence (also median nerve innervated). All desensitization techniques require multiple sessions with a total duration of 1 to 4 months.[6]

HEAT/COLD MODALITIES

Physical modalities have both observational and limited hypothesis-driven research to support their use as adjunct analgesics. Little research is available on heat/cold modalities for the specific treatment of neuropathic pain. Heat has been shown to increase nerve conduction velocity, increase arterial blood flood flow by vasodilation, and increase tendon extensibility.[7] Generally speaking, deep heat approaches, such as ultrasound and short-wave diathermy, should be avoided in the neuropathic pain setting as these approaches could potentially exacerbate pain with increased nerve activity. Additionally, since neuropathy may present with decreased temperature sensation, prolonged heat exposure is contraindicated. Superficial heating modalities, including hot packs, hydrocollator packs, and heating pads, may play an important role in reducing pain by increasing the flexibility of connective tissue prior to stretching deconditioned muscles, joint contractures, or adhesions.[8]

Cold therapy has been shown to slow nerve conduction velocity, which can diminish the neurotransmission of pain, decrease arterial blood flood flow by vasoconstriction, and decrease tendon extensibility. Cold packs or ice massage can be trialed for analgesia. Although there is plenty of observational short-term benefit, there is little evidence to show any significant long-term efficacy.[7,8]

PAIN PSYCHOTHERAPY

Pain psychology is typically focused more toward treatment of chronic pain among a variety of domains including physical functioning, pain medication consumption, mood, cognitive patterns, and quality of life. Once these domains are addressed, pain intensity is believed to be decreased as a secondary effect. Thus, like other nonpharmacological treatments, pain psychotherapy is better suited as a treatment complementary to other medical approaches.

There are multiple psychological interventions with different theoretical approaches, therapeutic targets, and areas of efficacy. All approaches are intended to address behavioral, cognitive, and social contributions to pain. In this chapter, we will focus on four primary approaches: cognitive-behavioral therapy, operant-behavioral therapy, mindfulness-based stress reduction, and acceptance and commitment therapy, summarized next.[9] It is also important to note that chronic pain can significantly affect mental health with multiple psychological comorbidities. Some studies at tertiary-care pain clinics have shown that 33% of chronic-pain patients have anxiety and 40%–60% have a depressive disorder.[2]

- *Cognitive-behavioral therapy (CBT).* CBT is one of the most commonly used behavior approaches for pain and focuses on developing coping skills to manage pain. CBT also addresses maladaptive patient views on pain through cognitive restructuring where unrealistic or helpless thoughts about pain are oriented towards adaptation and improved functioning. Activity pacing, mood strategies, stress management, assertive communication, problem solving, goal setting, and relaxation are usually incorporated into the approach.[9]

- *Operant-behavioral therapy.* This theory treats underlying maladaptive behaviors of pain avoidance that can lead to deconditioning, depression, and worsening chronicity. The goal of this therapy is to use reinforcement and punishment to foster more adaptive behaviors. Kinesiophobia and fear of pain are targeted for extinction through progressive exposure to painful behaviors without catastrophic consequences causing the patient to realize unrealistic pain expectations of doing certain activities.[9]
- *Mindfulness-based stress reduction (MBSR).* This approach attempts to separate the sensory and physical components of pain from the emotional aspect. Acceptance and awareness of physical pain as something familiar could potentially eliminate the emotionally maladaptive behavioral responses to pain. Meditation is a significant component of this treatment to promote a mindful awareness of the body's physical sensations, breathing, and other aspects occurring in the present moment. This technique teaches acceptance of the present instead of judgement.[9]
- *Acceptance and commitment therapy (ACT).* ACT teaches a nonjudgmental approach of accepting all thoughts and emotions while trying to modify the negative responses that may be produced. Individuals are instructed to react in way consistent with their goals and values instead of focusing on immediate relief of pain. ACT and MBSR share a similar concept in acceptance of pain, but ACT is notable for not incorporating meditation and for placing more emphasis on goal directed behavior.[9]

Common psychological techniques include supportive counseling, hypnosis, relaxation, biofeedback, and meditation. In particular biofeedback is popularly used in CBT where an individual's bodily functions are noninvasively measured (e.g., blood pressure, muscle tension, heart rate, skin temperature, sweat gland output, and electroencephalography). The goal is to increase patient's awareness and conscious control of unconscious physiologic activities that may exacerbate pain.[10]

Overall, psychotherapy can be a valuable adjunctive tool in the treatment of pain. One study showed that multidisciplinary cognitive behavior programs had statistical improvements in pain intensity, pain-related disability, and anxiety for those with chronic neuropathic spinal cord pain. Other evidence for potential uses of psychotherapies for neuropathic pain includes CRPS, chronic migraines, fibromyalgia, multiple sclerosis, and spinal cord injury.[9]

TRANSCUTANEOUS ELECTRICAL NERVE STIMULATION (TENS)

Transcutaneous electrical nerve stimulation (TENS) is carried out with a noninvasive device that emits small electrical currents to stimulate nerves. Although there are varying devices, a unit is normally connected to the skin with two adhesive electrodes and produces stimulation of a set pulse width, frequency, and intensity (Figure 5.2).[11] The mechanism of treatment is believed to occur, at least partially, via the "gate-theory of pain": large Aβ sensory fibers are stimulated and cause temporary interruption of smaller C and Aδ pain fibers. Analgesia may also occur through activation of μ-opioid receptors in the spinal cord and brainstem.[12]

Ideally, a TENS unit should be used immediately before or after activity, not at rest. Contraindications for TENS unit usage include patients with implantable electric devices (e.g., pacemaker, defibrillator, or peripheral stimulator), pregnant patients, placement over infected regions, patients with seizures, or patients with malignancy.[13]

Two randomized controlled trials have shown therapeutic benefit in the treatment of diabetic polyneuropathy. A meta-analysis showed efficacy for the management of central pain in multiple sclerosis. In terms of phantom limb

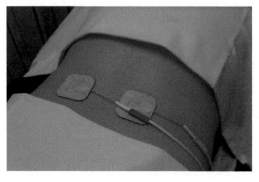

FIGURE 5.2. Transcutaneous electrical nerve stimulation (TENS) unit electrodes placed for treatment of back pain.

pain, only low-grade evidence has shown support of treatment efficacy. Nonetheless, given its relatively safe profile and low cost, TENS can be trialed across a variety of neuropathic conditions, typically during physical therapy sessions.[8,11] For musculoskeletal pain, a Cochrane review revealed conflicting data about the effectiveness of TENS.

TAI CHI AND YOGA

Both tai chi and yoga are methods of physical engagement that have been studied specifically for treatment of pain. Although these may be categorized under exercise and physiotherapy techniques, they are being discussed separately because they incorporate targeting a state of mental tranquility and provide exercise. The meditation component in both tai chi and yoga is intended to reduce pain by increasing self-awareness and cultivating the role of an impartial observer. Once this is achieved, patients may be able to detach themselves of subjective phenomena, including pain.

Tai Chi

Tai chi is a form of Chinese martial arts that includes slow, graceful movements, breathing exercises, and meditation. The slow movements are typically practiced in a semi-squat position where knee angle is adjusted to modify intensity. For example, elderly patients would use a high-squat posture and younger patients, if healthy, would typically use a more intense low-squat posture. All major muscle groups and joints are typically incorporated into the training to improve muscle strength, balance, range of motion, stamina, and coordination. Tai chi has been shown to have some benefit for a variety of chronic pain conditions, such as fibromyalgia, and in particular tai chi has been shown to improve hemoglobin A1C and plantar sensation in diabetic neuropathy.[14,15]

Yoga

Originating in India, yoga incorporates both exercise and philosophy. The goal is to treat the physical body and influence the mental state emotionally, intellectually, and spiritually. A yoga practitioner typically assumes a seated fixed posture called an "asana." There are a variety of asana positions with different purposes such as strengthening, stretching, improving balance, initiating relaxation, or placing one into a meditative state. Relaxation throughout the entire process is emphasized. Some studies have shown yoga to improve balance and reduce myofascial pain. Yoga has also been linked to increasing awareness of optimal joint positions that have been used to treat carpal tunnel syndrome.[16]

ACUPUNCTURE

Originating from traditional Chinese medicine (TCM), acupuncture typically involves placement of thin needles into various acupuncture points. There are many variations for treating different acupuncture points, as listed in Table 5.2.[17-20] Also, acupuncture treatments vary between Western medicine and TCM. In traditional acupuncture, qi, or "life force," circulates throughout the body in lines called meridians. Thus in TCM, a diagnosis is based on a TCM theory of disease, which can be philosophically different from a Western-medicine diagnosis.

TABLE 5.2. TYPES OF ACUPUNCTURE RELATED PRACTICES

Type	Technique
Acupressure	Noninvasive technique using pressure applied by hand or elbow to various locations
Cupping therapy	Localized suction is placed on the skin to increase blood flow to certain areas
Electroacupuncture	Acupuncture needles are connected to a device that produces electrical pulses
Sonopuncture	Uses sound instead of needles to stimulate different regions using either a tuning fork or ultrasound beam
Acupuncture point injection	Injection of various substances into different acupuncture points
Auriculotherapy	Needles are placed over various stimulation points on the outer ear
Bee venom acupuncture	Injection of bee venom into acupuncture points
Acupuncture with moxibustion	Involves burning of cone-shaped preparations of moxa on or near the skin

Sources: Patil et al. (2016),[17] Sur et al. (2016),[18] Wu et al. (2016),[19] and Yao et al. (2016).[20]

Nonetheless, Western medical acupuncture exists using adaptations to treat specific Western diagnoses.[17]

In theory, acupuncture may treat the body through biochemical changes to the body's homeostasis that improve physical and emotional well-being. Some studies have suggested that acupuncture can specifically treat neuropathic pain by affecting spinal opioid receptors, influencing the neurotrophic factor signaling system, increasing local microcirculation to muscles and joints, and increasing the release of adenosine, which has antinociceptive properties.[17]

Randomized controlled trials have been performed showing benefit for treatment of trigeminal neuralgia, peripheral neuropathy due to chemotherapy, and greater occipital neuralgia. Many other studies have been performed as well for a variety of chronic pain syndromes; these have shown mixed results.[17,21]

ORTHOTICS

An *orthotic* is defined as an external device that provides support or alignment to correct the function of any moveable part of the body. In general, the goal is to correct or support any deformity that may produce or cause pain. Thus, the appropriate orthotic is selected on the basis of specific pathology to be treated.

For example, someone with an entrapment neuropathy like carpal tunnel syndrome could benefit from a carpal tunnel wrist splint. This splint fixates the wrist in a neutral position where there is less pressure in the carpal tunnel and thus reduces pain.[22] Foot orthotics may be applied in a similar fashion. In the case of tarsal tunnel syndrome, where excessive eversion may provoke the entrapment, a custom orthotic could be fashioned to hold the hind foot in a neutral position.[23]

Some orthotics may be used to treat the underlying cause of neuropathic pain. If a patient has piriformis syndrome or sacroiliac joint pain caused by a leg-length discrepancy, then a heel lift applied to the shortened side could help resolve some of the symptoms. This same principal applies to any form of neuropathic pain secondary to myofascial restriction or biomechanical imbalance.

Finally, some orthotics are used for protective reasons. Diabetic shoes, for example, are designed with extra depth to accommodate custom shoe inserts to prevent skin breakdown in the insensate foot of those with peripheral neuropathy. This principal also applies to certain spinal braces which stabilize the spine to prevent

cord impingement after unstable fractures occur. In summary, orthotics can be used in the treatment, correction, or prevention of neuropathic pain.[24]

TRANSCRANIAL MAGNETIC STIMULATION (TMS)

Transcranial magnetic stimulation (TMS) is performed by inducing current through coils of wire inside a paddle (typically a figure-eight design) to produce a magnetic field. These paddles are then noninvasively placed over the head to stimulate select locations of the brain. It is theorized that the magnetic field will induce action potentials in axons and modulate activity of superficial and deep structures within the brain. The US Food and Drug Agency (FDA) approved TMS in 2008 for the treatment of major depression, but it is currently being investigated for treatment of neuropathic pain. In several studies, including randomized controlled trials, TMS showed some efficacy in treating neuropathic pain in thalamic stroke, brainstem strokes, spinal cord injury, brachial plexus injury, CRPS, diabetic polyneuropathy, and fibromyalgia.[25,26]

Repetitive TMS (rTMS), which is a series of pulses delivered in rapid succession within a single session, is more frequently used for pain treatment. Once the area of the motor cortex corresponding to the painful side is determined, the pulses are delivered with varying protocols of pulse frequency, stimulation intensity, number of stimuli, and pulse duration. Most studies have used a pulse frequency between 1 and 10 Hz. Frequencies of less than 5 Hz are believed to hyperpolarize axons and reduce firing rates, whereas frequencies greater than 5 Hz cause axon depolarization and trigger action potentials to nearby neurons. In the treatment of pain, higher frequencies (>5 Hz) and more stimuli per session (>500) are generally preferred for better efficacy.[26]

TMS requires multiple sessions, which can occur as frequent as daily, weekly, monthly, or a combination of all three. To date, there is limited evidence for sustained analgesia after treatments. One study documented continued benefit 4 weeks after treatment in patients with fibromyalgia.[27] Another study showed continued benefit 17 days after treatment in 70 patients with neuropathic pain. However, no cumulative effects were seen after each treatment session.[28]

Although TMS is noninvasive, there are multiple safety considerations. Absolute contraindications include patients with ferromagnetic implants or shrapnel in the head or neck, as magnetic fields might cause heating or movement of the metal. TMS is also contraindicated in patients with electronic implants, such as a deep brain stimulator or pacemaker, since magnetic pulses can cause these to malfunction. Relative contraindications apply to persons at high risk for seizure, including patients with epilepsy or those taking select medications that lower the seizure threshold (select antibiotics, antidepressants, psychiatric medications, or illicit drugs). It should be noted that a single seizure is an expected consequence in TMS. The most common adverse effect reported is headache, which occurs in 1 of 10 patients, and is usually responsive to acetaminophen.[26]

KEY POINTS

- Nonpharmacological modalities can complement or serve as stand-alone treatments. Typically, they provide better outcomes in combination with a comprehensive multimodal pain management plan that also includes pharmacological agents and interventional modalities.
- Exercise and physiotherapy treatments can include the following: balance, sensory, and proprioceptive training; aquatic therapy; strength and postural training; ergonomics; and work hardening.
- Mirror therapy has been shown to have benefits in treating neuropathic pain from stroke, phantom limb pain, and CRPS.
- Chronic pain clinics may have a significant percentage of patients with underlying psychological comorbidities—as high as 33% with anxiety and 40%–60% with a depressive disorder.
- There are multiple psychological approaches to treating neuropathic pain, including CBT, operant-behavioral therapy, MBSR, and ACT.
- Tai chi and yoga are two methods of physical engagement that have been studied specifically for the treatment of neuropathic pain; these incorporate a goal of reaching mental tranquility in addition to exercise.
- Some studies have suggested that acupuncture can specifically treat neuropathic pain by affecting spinal opioid receptors, influencing the neurotrophic factor signaling system, increasing local microcirculation to muscles and joints, and increasing the release of adenosine, which has antinociceptive properties.
- Repetitive TMS may have benefit in treating neuropathic pain in thalamic stroke, brainstem strokes, spinal cord injury, brachial plexus injury, CRPS, diabetic polyneuropathy, and fibromyalgia.

REFERENCES

1. Jones RC 3rd, Lawson E, Backonja M. Managing neuropathic pain. *Med Clin North Am.* 2016;100(1):151–167.
2. Scholten PM, Harden RN. Assessing and treating patients with neuropathic pain. *PM R.* 2015;7(11 Suppl):S257–S269.
3. Liebenson C. McKenzie self-treatments for sciatica. *J Bodyw Mov Ther.* 2005;9:40–42.
4. Casanova-Garcia C, Lerma Lara S, Perez Ruiz M, Ruano Dominguez D, Santana Sosa E. Nonpharmacological treatment for neuropathic pain in children with cancer. *Med Hypoth.* 2015;85(6):791–797.
5. Helmers LM, Donnelly KL, Verberne OM, Allen RJ. The effectiveness of desensitization therapy for individuals with complex regional pain syndrome: a systematic review. *Phys Ther Res Sympos.* 2015. Paper 13.
6. Moseley GL, Zalucki NM, Wiech K. Tactile discrimination, but not tactile stimulation alone, reduces chronic limb pain. *Pain.* 2008;137(3):600–608.
7. Weber DC, Hoppe KM. Physical agent modalities. In Braddom RL, Chan L, Harrast MA, et al., eds. *Physical Medicine and Rehabilitation.* 4th ed. Philadelphia: Saunders/Elsevier; 2011:449–481.
8. Akyuz G, Kenis O. Physical therapy modalities and rehabilitation techniques in the management of neuropathic pain. *Am J Phys Med Rehabil.* 2014;93(3):253–259.
9. Sturgeon JA. Psychological therapies for the management of chronic pain. *Psychol Res Behav Manage.* 2014;7:115–124.
10. Turk DC, Audette J, Levy RM, Mackey SC, Stanos S. Assessment and treatment of psychosocial comorbidities in patients with neuropathic pain. *Mayo Clin Proc.* 2010;85(3 Suppl):S42–S50.
11. Sawant A, Dadurka K, Overend T, Kremenchutzky M. Systematic review of efficacy of TENS for management of central pain in people with multiple sclerosis. *Mult Scler Relat Disord.* 2015;4(3):219–227.
12. Melzack R, Wall PD. Pain mechanisms: a new theory. *Science.* 1965;150(3699):971–979.
13. Brooks D. Electrophysical agents—contraindications and precautions: an evidence-based approach to

clinical decision making in physical therapy. *Physiother Can.* 2010;62(5):1–80.

14. Richerson S, Rosendale K. Does tai chi improve plantar sensory ability? A pilot study. *Diabetes Technol Ther.* 2007;9(3):276–286.

15. Field T. Knee osteoarthritis pain in the elderly can be reduced by massage therapy, yoga and tai chi: a review. *Complement Ther Clin Pract.* 2016;22:87–92.

16. Vallath N. Perspectives on yoga inputs in the management of chronic pain. *Indian J Palliat Care.* 2010;16(1):1–7.

17. Patil S, Sen S, Bral M, et al. The role of acupuncture in pain management. *Curr Pain Headache Rep.* 2016;20(4):22.

18. Sur B, Lee B, Yeom M, et al. Bee venom acupuncture alleviates trimellitic anhydride-induced atopic dermatitis-like skin lesions in mice. *BMC Complement Altern Med.* 2016;16(1):38.

19. Wu MS, Chen KH, Chen IF, et al. The efficacy of acupuncture in post-operative pain management: a systematic review and meta-analysis. *PloS One.* 2016;11(3):e0150367.

20. Yao C, Xu Y, Chen L, Jiang H, Ki CS, Byun JS, et al. Effects of warm acupuncture on breast cancer–related chronic lymphedema: a randomized controlled trial. *Curr Oncol.* 2016;23(1):27–34.

21. Fattal C, Kong ASD, Gilbert C, Ventura M, Albert T. What is the efficacy of physical therapeutics for treating neuropathic pain in spinal cord injury patients? *Ann Phys Rehabil Med.* 2009;52(2):149–166.

22. Kelly BM, Patel AT, Dodge CV. Upper limb orthotic devices. In Braddom RL, Chan L, Harrast MA, et al., eds. *Physical Medicine and Rehabilitation.* 4th ed. Philadelphia: Saunders/Elsevier; 2011:317–332.

23. Hudes K. Conservative management of a case of tarsal tunnel syndrome. *J Can Chiropr Assoc.* 2010;54(2):100–106.

24. Hennessey WJ. Lower limb orthotic devices. In Braddom RL, Chan L, Harrast MA, et al., eds. Physical Medicine and Rehabilitation. 4th ed. Philadelphia: Saunders/Elsevier; 2011:333–357.

25. Lefaucheur JP, Drouot X, Menard-Lefaucheur I, et al. Neurogenic pain relief by repetitive transcranial magnetic cortical stimulation depends on the origin and the site of pain. *J Neurol Neurosurg Psychiatry.* 2004;75(4):612–616.

26. Treister R, Lang M, Klein MM, Oaklander AL. Non-invasive transcranial magnetic stimulation (TMS) of the motor cortex for neuropathic pain—at the tipping point? *Rambam Maimonides Med J.* 2013;4(4):e0023.

27. Mhalla A, Baudic S, Ciampi de Andrade D, et al. Long-term maintenance of the analgesic effects of transcranial magnetic stimulation in fibromyalgia. *Pain.* 2011;152(7):1478–1485.

28. Hosomi K, Shimokawa T, Ikoma K, et al. Daily repetitive transcranial magnetic stimulation of primary motor cortex for neuropathic pain: a randomized, multicenter, double-blind, crossover, sham-controlled trial. *Pain.* 2013;154(7):1065–1072.

6

Pharmacological Treatment of Neuropathic Pain

RANDALL P. BREWER, RINOO V. SHAH, AND ELIZABETH CASSERLY

INTRODUCTION

Neuropathic pain was redefined in 2008 as "pain arising as a direct consequence of a lesion or disease affecting the somatosensory system" by the Neuropathic Pain Special Interest Group (NeuPSIG) of the International Association of Study of Pain (IASP).[1] Common etiologies of neuropathic pain include diabetic polyneuropathy (DPN), postherpetic neuralgia (PHN), lumbar nerve root irritation, post-stroke syndromes, human immunodeficiency virus (HIV) sensory neuropathy, and complex regional pain syndrome (CRPS) type II. Neuropathic pain can also be cancer related or caused by tumor invasion, surgery, or chemotherapy. Neuropathic pain can be classified as central neuropathic pain, such as post-stroke pain and spinal cord injury pain, or peripheral neuropathic pain, such as DPN or PHN.[2]

Neuropathic pain has been shown to reduce functionality and quality of life by causing physical and emotional harm to individuals. This loss in the individual's functionality places an emotional and financial burden on patients, their caregivers, and society.[3,4] Diabetic patients make up 8% of Americans. Between 26% and 47% of diabetic patients report the development of DPN during their lifetime.[5–7] A search of a US-based insurance company showed that patients with a neuropathic pain diagnosis had yearly charges that were 300% higher compared to matched controls.[8] The total healthcare costs related to neuropathic pain are estimated to be over 40 billion dollars annually.[9]

Regardless of the etiology, patients experiencing neuropathic pain commonly complain of burning, shooting or pricking pain, unpleasant sensations (dysesthesia), increased pain sensitivity to less painful stimuli (hyperalgesia), and pain induced by innocuous stimulation (allodynia).[10] Patients can experience some or all of these symptoms.

Neuropathic pain patients have been shown to have higher pain scores and lower health-related quality of life (HRQoL) compared to patients with other pain syndromes.[11] Treatment of neuropathic pain is challenging. The heterogeneity of neuropathic pain mechanisms makes it a complex disease process to treat, especially since anxiety and depression are commonly seen in these patients. Clinicians' familiarity with psychiatric medications plays a role in treatment as most patients with neuropathic pain have comorbid psychiatric diseases, requiring clinicians to take into account each medication's side-effect profile and drug–drug interactions, balancing patients' tolerability with clinical effectiveness.

Prior to initiation of a treatment modality, the patient should receive appropriate education to enable better communication between the practitioner and the patient, and better patient treatment compliance. Education should consist of explaining to the patient his or her disease process causing neuropathic pain and how to prevent further end-organ damage, if possible (e.g., glycemic control in a patient with DPN), the treatment plan, and what to expect from the medication, including side effects and administration directions. As with all pain treatment regimens, realistic goals and expectations should be set, as no modality will result in 100% alleviation of pain.

In this chapter we focus on the pharmacological treatment of neuropathic pain. The ideal treatment regimen should be individualized to achieve analgesia while balancing side effects, drug interactions, and relevant comorbidities.

TRICYCLIC ANTIDEPRESSANTS (TCAS)

Tricyclic antidepressants (TCAs) are the oldest and most widely researched antidepressants for the management of neuropathic pain and remain one of the first-line agents used.[12] TCAs inhibit the presynaptic reuptake of serotonin and noradrenaline. They also have antagonistic effects on postsynaptic muscarinic, alpha-adrenoceptor, and histamine H1 receptor, along with a blockade of membrane ion channels, reducing the entry of Na^+ and Ca^{2+} ions and thus reducing neuronal hyperexcitability.[13] Table 6.1 presents the mechanism of action of each neuropathic agent. TCAs modulate several neurotransmitters, allowing potentiation of the descending inhibitory pathways at different receptor sites. The drawback of TCAs, however, is that their side-effect profiles can limit the therapy, owing to their binding of multiple receptors. The main mechanism of action of TCAs is thought to increase the level of serotonin and noradrenaline by inhibiting their reuptake. TCAs have been used in the treatment of many neuropathic pain syndromes, such as painful diabetic neuropathy (PDN), PHN, and trigeminal neuralgia.[14–16] Table 6.2 provides the indications for TCAs as well as for the other neuropathic agents discussed in this chapter.

Common TCAs prescribed include amitriptyline, nortriptyline, imipramine, and desipramine. TCAs are rapidly absorbed after oral intake and metabolized through the CYP450 enzyme system. Nortriptyline is the active metabolite of amitriptyline, whereas desipramine is the active metabolite of imipramine. Amitriptyline and imipramine are tertiary amines, whereas nortriptyline and desipramine are secondary amines. Tertiary amines have fewer side effects compared to secondary amines, because secondary amines have a higher rate of binding a wider range of receptors.[17]

The adverse-effect profile of TCAs is multifaceted because of the numerous receptors involved in its pharmacodynamics. Anticholinergic effects result in drowsiness, confusion, blurry vision, dry mouth, tachycardia, and urinary retention in more than half of individuals.[18] Blockade of norepinephrine reuptake can result in impotence and trembling. Alpha-adrenergic blockade can result in orthostatic hypotension, tachycardia, and dizziness. The antihistamine H1 effects can result in sedation, somnolence, and weight gain. Table 6.3 lists the common side effects of TCAs and the other neuropathic agents discussed in this chapter. Cardiac toxicity can occur in patients with conduction abnormalities as TCAs have the potential to cause QTc interval prolongation at therapeutic doses.[19] The NeuPSIG guidelines recommend an electrocardiogram screen for patients with a history of cardiac disease and age over 40 years.

Dosage guidelines for TCAs recommend starting low-dose therapy of 10–25 mg at night time and titrating 10–25 mg every 3 to 7 days as tolerated by the patient.[20] Patients should be advised that the medication will take 6 to 8 weeks for full benefit and the medication should be taken every night whether the patient is hurting or not. The medication should not be considered a failure until the patient has been on the maximum dose for at least 2 weeks. Maximum dosage is routinely set at 150 mg daily. Titration schedules for TCAs and other neuropathic agents discussed in this chapter can be found in Table 6.4.

Evidence for TCAs in the treatment of neuropathic pain is of level 1 (good-quality patient-oriented evidence) in etiologies such as PHN and

TABLE 6.1. SUMMARY OF MECHANISMS OF ACTIONS OF PHARMACOLOGICAL AGENTS

Agents	Mechanism of Action
First-Line Medications (Strong Recommendations)	
Tricyclic antidepressants (TCAs)	Inhibition of reuptake of serotonin and/or norepinephrine Blockade of sodium channels Anticholinergic effects
Serotonin-noradrenaline reuptake inhibitors (SNRIs)	Inhibition of reuptake of serotonin and norepinephrine
Gabapentin/ Pregabalin	Decreased release of glutamate, norepinephrine, and substance P with ligands on α2δ-1 subunit of voltage-gated calcium channel
First-Line Medications (Weak Recommendations)	
Lidocaine patch 5%	Blockade of sodium channels
Capsaicin patch 8%	TRPV1 agonist
Second-Line Medication	
Tramadol	μ-Receptor agonist Inhibition of reuptake of serotonin and/or norepinephrine

TABLE 6.2. SUMMARY OF INDICATIONS FOR PHARMACOLOGICAL AGENTS FOR NEUROPATHIC PAIN

	TCAs	SNRIs	Gabapentin	Topical Lidocaine Patch 5%	Topical Capsaicin Patch 8%	Tramadol
Postherpetic neuralgia	+	–	+	+	+	+
Diabetic polyneuropathy	+	+				
Painful polyneuropathy	+	+	+	+		+
Phantom limb pain	–		Mixed			+
Neuropathic cancer pain	–		+			
Post-mastectomy pain	+	–				
Complex regional pain syndrome type 1			–			
Central post-stroke pain	+		+			
Spinal cord injury pain	–		+			

diabetic neuropathy.[21] Level 2 evidence (limited-quality patient-oriented evidence) for central neuropathic pain syndrome is seen with the use of TCAs.[19] Randomized control trials (RCTs) for HIV sensory neuropathy and chemotherapy-induced neuropathies have not shown positive results.[22]

SEROTONIN-NORADRENALINE REUPTAKE INHIBITORS (SNRIS)

Serotonin-noradrenaline reuptake inhibitors (SNRIs) were originally developed for psychiatric diagnoses, but patients on them also reported decreases in pain. Much like TCAs, they inhibit the presynaptic reuptake of serotonin and

TABLE 6.3. SUMMARY OF SIDE-EFFECT PROFILE OF PHARMACOLOGICAL AGENTS

	Side Effects	Precautions
Tricyclic antidepressants (TCAs)	Constipation, urinary retention, blurred vision, xerostomia, weight gain	Cardiovascular diseases (history of myocardial infarction (MI), conduction abnormalities, or stroke), diabetes mellitus, worsen psychosis, hepatic or renal impairment, seizure disorder
Serotonin-noradrenaline reuptake inhibitors (SNRIs)	Nausea, headache, dizziness, drowsiness, xerostomia, sexual dysfunction	Increased risk of suicidal thoughts/behavior, may worsen psychosis, hepatic impairment, serotonin syndrome reactions
Gabapentin	Sedation, dizziness, peripheral edema, weakness, weight gain	Increased risk of suicidal thoughts/behavior, renal impairment
Tramadol	Constipation, nausea, vomiting, dizziness, headache, flushing	Anaphylactoid reactions, serotonin syndrome reactions, history of substance abuse or heavy alcohol users, driving impairment, increased risk of suicidal thoughts/behavior
Topical lidocaine patch 5%	Erythema, rash	
Topical capsaicin patch 8%	Localized burning/stinging, erythema	

TABLE 6.4. DOSING GUIDELINES FOR PHARMACOLOGICAL AGENTS[21,22]

	Initial Dosage	Titration	Maximum Dosage
TCAs Nortriptyline (similar dosing for all TCAs)	10–25 mg nightly	Increase by10–25 mg daily weekly as tolerated	150 mg daily
SNRIs Duloxetine Venlafaxine	30 mg daily 37.5 mg daily	Increase to 60 mg daily after 1 week Increase by 75 mg weekly as tolerated	60 mg BID 300 mg daily
Calcium channel ligands Gabapentin Pregabalin	100–300 mg nightly or 100–300 TID 75 mg BID or 50 mg TID	Increase each dose by 100–300 mg as tolerated Increase daily dose to 300 mg after 1 week then increase by 150 weekly until maximum dosage is reached	3600 mg daily (1200 mg TID) 600 mg daily (200 mg TID or 300 mg BID)
Topical lidocaine patch 5%			3 patches daily, keep on for a maximum of 12 hours
Topical capsaicin patch 8%	Prior to placement of capsaicin patch, local anesthesia with lidocaine is recommended Application under vigilant monitoring for up to 60 minutes		Up to 60 minutes Single application can be expected to last for up to 12 weeks
Tramadol	50 mg daily or BID	Increase daily dose by 50–100 weekly as tolerated	400 mg daily (100 mg q8h daily); reduce maximum dose with age and metabolic impairments

BID, twice daily; q8h, every 8 hours; SNRIs, serotonin-noradrenaline reuptake inhibitors; TCAs, tricyclic antidepressants; TID, three times daily.

noradrenaline. They are considered "cleaner" drugs than TCAs because they do not bind the other receptors that TCAs do. Duloxetine and venlafaxine have the most evidence to support their use in treating neuropathic pain. Duloxetine has been studied in PHN, DPN, and peripheral polyneuropathy with good outcomes.[19,22] Duloxetine and venlafaxine have sequential binding of the serotonin and norepinephrine receptors. Duloxetine has a 10-to-1 affinity for serotonin receptor and must reach a therapeutic dose of 60 before neuropathic pain relief. Venlafaxine has a 30-to-1 affinity for the serotonin receptor and must reach a daily dose of 150 mg/day for neuropathic pain relief.[11,20]

A meta-analysis of 14 studies examining the use of SNRIs in neuropathic pain included 9 studies on duloxetine and 4 on venlafaxine. Seven of the studies on duloxetine were positive whereas only two of the studies on venlafaxine were. SNRIs are generally considered to be inferior to TCAs, with a number needed to treat of 6.4 compared to 3.6.[24]

SNRIs have fewer side effects than TCAs. Venlafaxine is known to raise blood pressure and cause gastrointestinal (GI) upset, dry mouth, and sexual dysfunction and should not be used in patients with uncontrolled blood pressure. Duloxetine can cause GI upset, headache, constipation, and dizziness. The most common side effects from duloxetine are nausea, vomiting, and insomnia. Patients often have less GI upset when the medication is taken with food.

Duloxetine therapeutic dosing is 60–120 mg, and venlafaxine therapeutic dosing is 150–300 mg. These are good options for patients with neuropathic pain and depression or anxiety. Much like TCAs, patients should be advised that the medication will take 6 to 8 weeks for full benefit, and the medication should be taken every night whether the patient is hurting or not. The medication should not be considered a failure until the patient has been on the maximum dose for at least 2 weeks.[24]

CALCIUM CHANNEL A2Δ-1 LIGANDS

Gabapentin was initially introduced as an anticonvulsant. However, Mellick et al. discovered in 1995 that calcium channel α2δ-1 ligands could be used as analgesics and since then they have become one of the major pharmacotherapies used for neuropathic pain.[23] They produce antiepileptic, analgesic, and sedentary effects.[24]

Gabapentin and pregabalin, despite the nomenclature, do not act as an agonist at the GABAA or GABAB receptor. They are structurally similar, and their mechanism of action is through modulating calcium influx through the calcium channel. Newer research has found that they bind and antagonize thrombospondin binding to α2δ-1 and inhibit synapse formation.[24] Gabapentin has a half-life of 5 to 7 hours, which requires every 8-hour dosing to be effective. Pregabalin has a longer half-life, which allows for dosing twice daily.

A typical regimen includes a low initial dose with careful titration until therapeutic effect is achieved or limited by side effects or maximum dosage is reached. A typical starting dose is 100–300 mg three times a day, titrating up weekly as tolerated with a maximum daily dosage of 3600 mg.[25] As with most pharmacotherapy agents for neuropathic pain, the limitation of gabapentin has been its side-effect profile. Sedation and dizziness are the most commonly reported side effects, followed by peripheral edema (8%) and weakness (6%).[26,27]

Pregabalin has similar side effects to gabapentin but can be titrated faster to an effective dose. Starting doses typically range from 50 to 75 mg twice daily. Gabapentin has a higher therapeutic dose than pregabalin. Patients should achieve 1800 mg/day of gabapentin for 6–8 weeks before considering the drug a failure. Pregabalin becomes therapeutic at 150 mg/day with a maximum dose of 600 mg/day. Both of these medications should be taken daily at the same time, even if the patient is not in pain. They are both eliminated through the kidneys 90% unchanged from the body and do not go through hepatic metabolism.[28]

A Cochrane review in 2014 of six studies with over 1800 participants showed at least 50% pain reduction in 34% of the gabapentin study group versus 21% in the placebo group for PHN.[26] Rauck et al. studied 165 patients with PDN and showed a pain reduction in the gabapentin group from 6.4 to 3.9 versus placebo, 6.5 to 5.1 ($p < 0.001$).[27] While gabapentin has not specifically received FDA approval for the treatment of PDN, it is considered a first-line treatment modality for PDN in most neuropathic pain guidelines.

A meta-analysis of 25 placebo-controlled randomized trials of pregabalin between 150 and 600 mg has 18 positive studies. There is a dose–response gradient with higher responses at 600 mg/day compared to 150 mg/day. Two trials studying HIV polyneuropathy were negative. The combined number needed to treat was 7.7 with a number needed to harm of 13.9. The most commonly studied neuropathic etiologies treated with gabapentin and pregabalin are PHN, PDN, mixed neuropathic pain, cancer-related neuropathic pain, and fibromyalgia.[43]

TRAMADOL

Tramadol is a synthetic codeine analog, making it a weak opioid with properties that inhibit the reuptake of norepinephrine and serotonin. Tramadol has mixed evidence for use in neuropathic pain, which is why it is recommended as a second-line medication. In a meta-analysis of tramadol studies, seven nonrandomized studies had positive outcomes using extended-release tramadol. The available evidence makes tramadol a second-line option owing to the lack of RCTs as well as its abuse potential.[25]

The best evidence is for long-acting tramadol, to be taken daily with a maximum dose of 400 mg/day. Tramadol is hepatically metabolized through cytochrome p450 3A4 and 2D9 into two inactive metabolites and excreted from the body. Tramadol should be used with caution with other serotonergic agents, as the combination can cause serotonin syndrome. Patients with renal and hepatic dysfunction will need dose adjustments, as the medication can cause seizures with high doses. Tramadol cannot be completely reversed with naloxone. This is important when a patient presents to the emergency department for tramadol overdose, as naloxone will only reverse the opioid overdose but not the serotonergic overdose.[47]

TOPICAL LIDOCAINE PATCH 5%

RCTs have shown that the 5% lidocaine patch is efficacious in reducing the intensity of localized neuropathic pain from PHN and DPN. An upregulation of sodium channels is thought to play a part in nociceptive pain pathways.[329,30] Topical lidocaine works by blocking these local sodium channels on nerve fibers (C-fibers and Aδ-fibers) that conduct nociception.[31] Treatment is typically well tolerated as it is devoid of systemic absorption and, hence, systemic side effects. Local side effects include erythema or rash. Guidelines recommend a maximum of three patches to be applied daily for up to 12 hours a day with a 12-hour off-period between patch applications. The patient should be advised that a trial period of at least 2 weeks is required before considering the medication a failure of therapy.[47]

TOPICAL CAPSAICIN PATCH 8%

Capsaicin (trans-8-methyl-N-vanillyl-6 nonenamide; 6-nonenamide, N-[(4hydroxy-3-methoxyphenyl) methyl]-8 methyl-, (6E) is the active pharmaceutical ingredient contained in the capsaicin 8% patch. The capsaicin content of chili peppers ranges from 0.1% to 1%. The patch is over 100 times greater in concentration than over-the-counter creams. The transient receptor potential cation channel subfamily V member 1 (TRPV1) is a ligand-gated, nonselective cation channel expressed on small-diameter sensory neurons, especially nociceptors that detect painful sensations. TRPV1 is predominantly expressed in unmyelinated C-fibers and small myelinated A-fibers.[32]

After placement of topical capsaicin, cutaneous nociceptors become less sensitive to a stimulus. Topical placement of capsaicin results in a reduction in spontaneous and evoked painful sensations. Desensitization or degeneration of nociceptive stimuli after placement of topical capsaicin is the hypothesis behind this treatment modality. The effects of topical capsaicin on nociceptor activity have been referred to as "desensitization" and are the rationale for the development of various topical capsaicin formulations for the management of chronic-pain syndromes.[33]

The capsaicin patch formulation is intended to rapidly deliver a high concentration devoid of systemic effects. Application to the site of maximum pain should be done under local anesthesia to help control the intense burning sensation that occurs with application of the patch.[34] Pain relief for up to 3 months has been reported with a single application of capsaicin 8% patch for 60 minutes.[35]

COMBINATION THERAPY

Treatment of neuropathic pain is centered on pharmacotherapy, as discussed in this chapter. Practical management strategies to optimize therapy should include combining two or more drugs to achieve analgesia through medication synergy. Combination therapy will also prevent monotherapy toxicities and improve patient tolerability by preventing dose escalations.

Clinical effectiveness has been seen with regimens combining antidepressants, opioids, and topical lidocaine with gabapentin.[36-38] The combination therapies of antidepressants and topical lidocaine have shown efficacy in RCTs in DPN and PHN patients.[39,40] Gilron et al. studied nortriptyline and gabapentin as a combination therapy for DPN and PHN and found that combination therapy of gabapentin and TCAs resulted in greater pain reduction (52.8% [SE 4.6]) than monotherapy with TCAs (38.8% [4.6], $p = 0.01$) or gabapentin (31.1% [4.6], $p = 0.0002$).[37] Combination therapy with venlafaxine also showed efficacy in treating PDN, with lower pain scores and improved quality of life, compared to gabapentin alone.[40] In a study published in the New England Journal of Medicine, Gilron et al. showed improved efficacy when gabapentin was combined with morphine, compared to either agent alone.[36]

Studies of calcium channel α2δ-1 ligands in combination with SNRIs or TCAs have shown that the use of both agents together allows for lower doses and results in decreased side effects of both agents. Tesfays et al. studied duloxetine and pregabalin in a randomized double-blind parallel group study and found that patients receiving duloxetine 60 mg and pregabalin 300 mg/day had lower pain scores than those of patients given either 120 mg/day of duloxetine or pregabalin 600 mg/day.[44] A second study of imipramine and pregabalin for painful polyneuropathy showed that patients on the combination therapy of imipramine and pregabalin had lower pain scores than with either agent used alone.[45] Calcium channel α2δ-1 ligands in combination with TCAs or SNRIs enhanced efficacy and tolerability as monotherapy and prevented patients from reaching maximum doses that might result in increased frequency of adverse events.

REFERENCES

1. Dworkin RH, Backonja M, Rowbotham M, et al. Advances in neuropathic pain. Diagnosis mechanisms, and treatment recommendations. *Arch Neurol.* 2003;60:1524–1534.

2. Gore M, Brandenburg NA, Hoffman DL, Tai KS, Stacey B. Burden of illness in painful diabetic peripheral neuropathy: the patients' perspectives. *J Pain.* 2006;7:892–900.

3. O'Connor AB. Neuropathic pain: a review of the quality of life impact, costs, and cost-effectiveness of therapy. *Pharmacoeconomics.* 2009;27:95–112.

4. Barrett AM, Lucero MA, Le T, Robinson RL, Dworkin RH, Chappell AS. Epidemiology, public health burden, and treat- ment of diabetic peripheral neuropathic pain: A review. *Pain Med,* 2007;8(suppl 2):S50–S62.

5. Boulton AJM, Malik RA, Arezzo JC, Sosenko JM. Diabetic somatic neuropathies. *Diabetes Care.* 2004;27:1458–1486.

6. Boulton AJM, Vinik AI, Arezzo JC, Bril V, Feldman EL, Freeman R, Malik RA, Maser RE, Sosenko JM, Ziegeler D. Diabetic neuropathies: A statement by the American Diabetes Association. *Diabetes Care.* 2005;28:956–962.

7. Berger A, Dukes EM, Oster G. Clinical characteristics and economic costs of patients with painful neuropathic disorders. *J Pain.* 2004;5:143–149.

8. Turk DC. Clinical effectiveness and cost-effectiveness of treatments for patients with chronic pain. *Clinical Journal of Pain.* Nov-Dec 2002;18(6):355–365.

9. Hansson P, Laceremza M, Marchettini P. Aspects of clinical and experimental neuropathic pain: The clinical perspective. In: Hansson P, Fields HL, Hill RG, Marchettini P (Eds.), *Neuropathic Pain: Pathophysiology and Treatment.* Vol 21. Seattle: IASP Press; 2001:1–18.

10. Torrance N, Smith BH, Watson MC, Bennett MI. Medication and treatment use in primary care patients with chronic pain of predominantly neuropathic origin. *Fam Pract.* 2007;24:481–485.

11. Jackson KC, St. Onge EL. Antidepressant pharmacotherapy: considerations for the pain clinician. *Pain Pract.* 2003;3:135–143.

12. Bielefeldt K, Ozaki N, Whiteis C, Gebhart GE. Amitriplyme inhibits voltage-sensitive sodium currents in rat gastric sensory neurons. *Dig Dis Sci.* 2002;47:959–966.

13. Wallace MS. Pharmacologic treatment of neuropathic pain. *Curr Pain Headache Rep.* 2001;5:138–150.

14. Abdi S, Lee DH, Chung JM. The anti-allodynic effects of amitriptyline, gabapentin, and lidocaine in a rat model of neuropathic pain. *Anesth Analg.* 1998;87:1360–1366.

15. Richeimer SH, Bajwa ZH, Kahraman SS, et al. Utilization patterns of tricyclic antidepressants in a multidisciplinary pain clinic: A survey. *Clin J Pain.* 1997;13:324–329.

16. Gillman PK. Tricyclic antidepressant pharmacology and therapeutic drug interactions updated. *Br J Pharmacol.* 2007;151(6):737–748.

17. Rintala DH, Holmes SA, Courtade D, et al. Comparison of the effectiveness of amitriptyline and gabapentin in chronic neuropathic pain in persons with spinal cord injury. *Arch Phys Med Rehabil.* 2007;88:1547–1560.

18. Harrigan RA, Brady WJ. ECG abnormalities in tricyclic antidepressant ingestion. *Am J Emerg Med.* 1999;17:387–393.

19. Dworkin RH, O'Connor AB, Backonja M, et al. Pharmacologic management of neuropathic pain: evidence-based recommendations. *Pain.* 2007;132(2007):237–251.

20. Bryson HM, Wilde MI. Amitriptyline: a review of its pharmacological properties and the therapeutic use in chronic pain states. *Drugs Aging.* 1996;8:459–476.

21. Attal N, Cruccua G, Haanpaa M, et al. EFNS guidelines on pharmacological treatment of neuropathic pain. *Eur J Neurol.* 2006;13:1153–1169.

22. Mellick GA, Mellicy LB, Mellick LB. Gabapentin in the management of reflex sympathetic dystrophy. *J Pain Symptom Manage.* 1995;10:265–266.

23. Eroglu C. Gabapentin receptor alpha2delta-1 is a neuronal thrombospondin receptor responsible for excitatory CNS synaptogenesis. Allen NJ, Susman MW, et al. *Cell.* 2009 Oct 16;139(2):380–392. doi:10.1016/j.cell.2009.09.025.

24. Attal N, Cruccu G, Baron R, et al. EFNS Guidelines on the Pharmacological Treatment of Neuropathic Pain: 2010 Revision. *Eur J Neurol.* 2010;17(9):1113–e88.

25. Goa KL, Sorkin EM. Gabapentin: A Review of Its Pharmacological Properties and Clinical Potential in Epilepsy. *Drugs.* 1993;46(3):409–427.

26. Moore RA, Wiffen PJ, Derry S, Toelle T, Rice ASC. Gabapentin for chronic neuropathic pain and fibromyalgia in adults. *Cochrane Database of Systematic Reviews.* 2014 Apr 27;(4): CD007938.

27. Rauck R, Makumi CW, Schwartz S, Graff O, Meno-Tetang G, Bell CF, et al. A randomized, controlled trial of gabapentin enacarbil in

subjects with neuropathic pain associated with diabetic peripheral neuropathy. *Pain Practice.* 2013;13(6):485–496.

28. Argoff CE, Galer BS, Jensen MP, Oleka N, Gammaitoni AR. Effectiveness of the lidocaine patch 5% on pain qualities in three chronic pain states: assessment with the neuropathic pain scale. *Curr Med Res Opin.* 2004;20 Suppl 2:S21–8.

29. Binder A, Bruxelle J, Rogers P, Hans G, Bo'sl I, Baron R. Topical 5% lidocaine (lignocaine) medicated plaster treatment for post-herpetic neuralgia: results of a double-blind, placebo-controlled, multinational efficacy and safety trial. *Clin Drug Investig.* 2009;29:393–408.

30. Demant DT, Lund K, Finnerup NB, Vollert J, Maier C, Segerdahl MS, Jensen TS, Sindrup SH. Pain relief with lidocaine 5% patch in localized peripheral neuropathic pain in relation to pain phenotype. *Pain.* 2015 Nov;156(11):2234–2244.

31. Gammaitoni AR, Alvarez NA, Bradley SG. Safety and tolerability of the lidocaine patch 5%, a targeted peripheral analgesic: a review of the litterature. *J Clin Pharmacol.* 2003;43:111–117.

32. Szolcsányi J. Forty years in capsaicin research for sensory pharmacology and physiology. *Neuropeptides.* 2004 Dec;38(6):377–384.

33. Holzer P. The pharmacological challenge to tame the transient receptor potential vanilloid-1 (TRPV1) nocisensor. *Br J Pharmacol.* 2008 Dec;155(8):1145–1162.

34. Anand P, Bley K. Topical capsaicin for pain management: therapeutic potential and mechanisms of action of the new high-concentration capsaicin 8% patch. *Br J Anaesth.* 2011 Oct;107(4):490–502.

35. Bardo-Brouard P, et al. High-concentration topical capsaicin in the management of refractory neuropathic pain in patients with neurofibromatosis type 1: a case series. *Curr Med Res Opin.* 2018;34(5):887–891.

36. Gilron I, Bailey JM, Tu D, Holden RR, Weaver DF, Houlden RL. Morphine, gabapentin, or their combination for neuropathic pain. *N Engl J Med.* 2005;352:1324–1334.

37. Gilron I, Bailey JM, Tu D, Holden RR, Jackson AC, Houlden RL. Nortriptyline and gabapentin, alone and in combination for neuropathic pain: a double-blind, randomised controlled crossover trial. *Lancet.* 2009;374:1252–1261.

38. Baron R, Mayoral V, Leijon G, Binder A, Steigerwald I, Serpell M. Efficacy and safety of combination therapy with 5% lidocaine medicated plaster and pregabalin in post-herpetic neuralgia and diabetic polyneuropathy. *Curr Med Res Opin.* 2009;25:1677–1687.

39. Simpson DA. Gabapentin and venlafaxine for the treatment of painful diabetic neuropathy. *J Clin Neuromusc Disease.* 2001;3:53–62.

40. Gilron I, Bailey JM, Tu D, Holden RR, Weaver DF, Houlden RL. Morphine, gabapentin, or their combination for neuropathic pain. *N Engl J Med.* 2005;352:1324–1334.

41. Freeman R, et al. Efficacy, safety, and tolerability of pregabalin treatment for painful diabetic peripheral neuropathy: findings from seven randomized, controlled trials across a range of doses. *Diabetes Care.* 2008;31(7):1448–1454.

42. Sansone and Sansone. Serotonin Norepinephrine Reuptake Inhibitors: A Pharmacological Comparison. *Innov Clin Neurosci.* 2014;11(3–4):37–42.

43. Lexicomp Online®, Drug Monographs®, Hudson, Ohio: Lexi-Comp, Inc.; March 6, 2018.

44. Tesfaye S, et al. Duloxetine and pregabalin: high-dose monotherapy or their combination? The "COMBO-DN study"—a multinational, randomized, double-blind, parallel-group study in patients with diabetic peripheral neuropathic pain. *Pain.* 2013;154(12):2616–2625.

45. Holbech JV, et al. Imipramine and pregabalin combination for painful polyneuropathy: a randomized controlled trial. *Pain.* 2015;156(5):958–966.

7

Interventional Treatment of Neuropathic Pain

JIANG WU AND JIANGUO CHENG

INTRODUCTION

Neuropathic pain can be severely disabling and is associated with impaired health-related quality of life, significant psychological and emotional distress, and high social and economic burden.[1–3] It has an estimated prevalence of 7%–9.8% of the US adult population. Up to 20% of patients with chronic pain may have some neuropathic component.[4,5] Only a minority of people who receive pharmacological and noninterventional conservative treatment experience meaningful analgesic benefit.[6]

Interventional treatments are defined as "invasive procedures involving delivery of drugs into targeted areas, or ablation/modulation of targeted structures for the treatment of persistent pain."[7] With better understanding of the pain mechanisms and technical advances and refinement, interventional pain approaches have emerged as efficacious and attractive treatment options for people living with refractory neuropathic pain. There is an emerging body of exciting and sufficient evidence to support specific interventional options for selected neuropathic pain states, particularly for refractory neuropathic pain, even though more well-designed randomized controlled trials (RCTs) or comparative studies are needed.[8,9] Here we summarize the scientific evidence on the efficacy of neural blockade and neural ablative procedures for managing neuropathic pain. A detailed discussion of the risk–benefit analysis and cost-effectiveness of these interventional techniques is beyond the scope of this chapter. Neuromodulatory approaches, such as spinal cord stimulation and peripheral nerve stimulation, are an important aspect of interventional management of neuropathic pain and will be discussed in this chapter.

NEURAL BLOCKADE TECHNIQUES

Nerve entrapment or compression in tissue planes and injury to nerves are considered triggering events for neuropathic pain.[10] Secretion of inflammatory mediators, increased excitability of nociceptors, and ectopic discharges from injured primary afferents[11,12] contribute to the development of neuropathic pain.[13,14] In addition to peripheral sensitization, changes in central pain processing and central sensitization play a critical role in the development and maintenance of neuropathic pain.[15] Peripheral nerves are amenable to nerve blockades, which may reduce peripheral as well as central sensitizations and provide pain reduction.

The Diagnostic Value of Neural Blockade

Diagnostic nerve blocks have a long history of clinical applications in determining if a particular nerve is involved in the patient's symptoms, by either signaling the pain from the innervated tissue or being the source of ectopic activity that leads to neuropathic pain. The information obtained from nerve blocks helps in confirming a clinical impression, selecting among different treatment options, or predicting the response to neuroablative therapies. However, interpretation of this information needs to take into account the caveats that the value of diagnostic blocks has not been carefully examined for most of the procedures, many details of diagnostic procedures for neuropathic pain are not clearly standardized, and the interpretation of even properly performed diagnostic blocks could be very challenging.

The value of diagnostic nerve blocks is best established in non-neuropathic axial spine pain, specifically with medial branch blocks for cervical and lumbar zygapophyseal (facet) joint pain. The evidence to support diagnostic blocks for neuropathic pain has been growing.

The selective nerve root block was developed as a technique to identify specific nerve roots responsible for intractable radicular symptoms, particularly for complicated clinical symptomatology, when the clinical picture and imaging studies indicate multilevel degenerative changes with possible compression of several nerve roots. The limited data, primarily from retrospective studies, have demonstrated relatively high positive predictive values, but low negative predictive values. The reported positive predictive values (defined as percent of patients with block indicating radiculopathy, in whom surgery confirmed radicular pathology at the level indicated by the block) range from 87% to 100%.[16-19] The reported negative predictive values (percent of patients with a negative response to the block and confirmed at the surgery to have normal nerve roots) in two studies are 20% and 38% of the small number of patients operated on.[16,17]

The ultrasound-guided, selective peripheral nerve block might provide valuable diagnostic information when more standard testing, such as electromyography (EMG), ultrasonography, computer tomography (CT), and/or magnetic resonance imaging (MRI), has led to ambiguity in diagnosing peripheral neuropathies. For example, in a patient with classic neuropathic pain after below-knee amputation, successful diagnostic, ultrasound-guided, selective common peroneal nerve block helped confirm the diagnosis and subsequent surgical resection of a painful neuroma to relieve severe neuropathic pain.[20] A multicenter retrospective study examined the diagnostic role of occipital nerve blocks in predicting the outcome of pulsed radiofrequency (PRF) for occipital neuralgia and reported that about half the subjects experienced a positive outcome (≥50% pain relief coupled with procedure satisfaction lasting at least 3 months).[21]

Despite the fact that the diagnostic value of the classic stellate ganglion block and lumbar sympathetic block to differentiate sympathetically independent pain from sympathetically maintained pain is limited, with weak evidence to support them,[22] sympathetic blocks have a unique and long tradition in the dual roles of both diagnostic and therapeutic tools in the management of complex regional pain syndrome (CRPS).

The Therapeutic Value of Neural Blockade

Although the exact mechanism of improved pain in response to local anesthetic injection with steroids is unknown, the reversal of diverse neuroplastic changes has been observed clinically. It is presumed that application of steroids to injured nerve fibers may suppress both peripheral and central sensitizations, alleviating edema and resulting in a reduction of both spontaneous and evoked pain.[23] Here we discuss the therapeutic value of neural blocks in a few examples of common neuropathic pain conditions.

Peripheral Compression or Trauma-Related Neuropathic Pain

Chronic peripheral neuropathic pain secondary to trauma or compression and Morton's neuroma has been treated with perineural steroids.[24-26] A recent systemic review revealed a modest but clinically meaningful pain reduction following injection of steroids from baseline (25%).[27] A few RCTs showed that combining steroids with local anesthetic may increase efficacy,[28] and local anesthetic injections without steroid may confer long-term analgesic benefits.[29] Double-blind and placebo-controlled studies indicate that the analgesia resulting from steroid injection is possibly dose dependent. A larger reduction in pain scores is associated with higher doses of steroids,[30-32] and lower doses of steroids are associated with earlier return of pain scores.[28,33,34] It is noteworthy that studies with a high risk of bias[28,32,34] were associated with a significant analgesic effect in favor of perineural steroids, that the placebo analgesic effect was strong, and that some of the analgesic benefits may be due to systemic uptake of the perineurally injected steroids.[35]

Three high-quality RCTs on carpal tunnel syndrome with local anesthetic and steroid injections demonstrated clinical improvement at 1 month or less following use of local corticosteroids.[36,37] There was significantly more improvement in the steroid injection group, compared with the oral corticosteroid group, within 8 weeks.[38] The favorable outcomes support the notion that carpel tunnel injection is an option for the improvement of functional status, before considering more definite surgical decompression. Additionally, a meta-analysis of 10 studies with 633 patients concluded that the ultrasound-guided in-plane approach was most effective among the four injection techniques for carpal tunnel syndrome.[39]

Emerging evidence strongly suggests the efficacy of botulinum toxin type A (BTA) for several neuropathic pain conditions. A randomized, prospective double-blind, parallel group study in 29 patients with neuropathic pain conditions assessed the effectiveness of intradermal injection of BTA and reported significant improvement in average pain scores, brush allodynia, and cold pain threshold despite transiently aggravating immediate postprocedural pain.[40]

Herpes Zoster and Postherpetic Neuralgia

Epidural or paravertebral nerve blocks provide symptomatic relief of acute pain associated with herpes zoster. An RCT demonstrated decreased pain and allodynia via epidural blocks with local anesthetics combined with steroids soon after the onset of herpes zoster.[41] Another RCT reported a modest benefit at 1 month with a single epidural injection of methylprednisolone and bupivacaine within 7 days of the onset of herpes zoster.[42] A third RCT found significantly lower incidence of acute herpes zoster–related pain at 1 month and also lower incidence of postherpetic neuralgia (PHN) at 3, 6, and 12 months post-therapy in the paravertebral group (repetitive paravertebral injections with local anesthetics/steroids and acyclovir/analgesics) compared with the standard therapy group (acyclovir/analgesics).[43] These results are consistent with the results of several previous observational and cohort studies evaluating epidural local anesthetics alone or combined with steroids in herpes zoster.[44]

The efficacy of intrathecal methylprednisolone acetate (IT MPA) in the treatment of PHN appeared to be inconsistent in three published RCTs,[45-47] and the use of intrathecal methylprednisolone or sympathetic nerve blocks in PHN is not recommended.[48] In contrast, the efficacy of BTA in the treatment of PHN is supported by two RCTs. One reported better pain relief, improved sleep hours, and reduced opioid consumption in the BTA group over the 3-month follow-up.[49] These favorable outcomes were reproduced in a subsequent RCT.[50] These results were consistent with the results of two retrospective observational studies with small numbers of patients.[51,52]

Lumbosacral and Cervical Radiculopathy

Epidural steroid injection (ESI) is a viable treatment option for acute radiculopathy for short-term benefit. A short-term pain-reducing benefit (>2 weeks but <12 months) from transforaminal ESI in patients with acute or subacute radicular pain was supported by three systemic reviews and meta-analysis of RCTs.[53-55] The benefit of ESI differs among different administration techniques—the transforaminal approach has the greatest likelihood (70% of patients) of having beneficial effects lasting up to 3 months. The conclusions about the value of epidural steroids are also heavily influenced by the specialty of the authors, with more positive outcomes reported by pain physicians than by non-pain physicians.[56] Important factors that influence clinical outcomes include appropriate patient selection with specific radicular pain, proper use of imaging guidance, sufficient volume of injectate, and suitable selection and application of refined technical modalities.

Appropriate use of ESI represents a relatively safe and inexpensive option to facilitate recovery and reduce the need for surgical intervention. A double-blind RCT reported that 29% of patients in the ESI group underwent surgery, compared with a 67% operative rate in the control group without ESI at follow-up periods ranging between 13 and 28 months; the avoidance of surgery persisted in most patients available at a subsequent 5-year follow-up.[57] A small preventive effect of epidural steroids from the need for surgery in the short term (<1 year) was also reported in a meta-analysis and systemic review of randomized trials.[58]

Complex Regional Pain Syndrome (CRPS)

Sympathetic block is a reasonable treatment option for patients with CRPS refractory to pharmacological and nonpharmacological conservative treatments, especially when conducted early in the disease course to provide a "window of opportunity" for more aggressive rehabilitation therapy before consideration of a more invasive option such as spinal cord stimulation (SCS).[59] In patients who respond favorably to sympathetic block, the pain relief generally outlasts the effects of the local anesthetic and may be long-lasting in some cases.[60,61] A modest benefit, 3 days after a local anesthetic sympathetic block, was reported in a randomized crossover study.[60] A long-term RCT reported significant reduction in average pain items, pain dimensions (McGill Pain Questionnaire), evoked-pain symptom subscores, and depression scores in the thoracic sympathetic block group for upper limb type

I CRPS at 12-month follow-up compared to the control group.[62] About 76% of patients receiving three stellate ganglion blocks at weekly intervals for upper extremity CRPS reported complete or partial pain relief over a 6-month observation period in a case series study.[63]

Given the role of the proliferation of adrenergic receptors and catecholamine release as a possible molecular basis underlying sympathetically mediated pain, BTA injection has been used to enhance the analgesia of local anesthetic from sympathetic ganglion block. A profoundly prolonged analgesia from BTA (71 days of the median time to analgesia failure after lumbar sympathetic block with BTA comparing with fewer than 10 days after standard lumbar sympathetic block) was reported in patients with CRPS from a double-blind, crossover RCT.[64] The effective and durable lumbar sympathetic blockade with a mixture of local anesthetic and botulinum toxin type B (BTB) was reproduced in two patients with CRPS.[65]

Trigeminal Neuralgia and Trigeminal Neuropathy

Trigeminal ganglion block with local anesthetics is a treatment option for medically refractory trigeminal neuralgia, based on conclusions from multiple uncontrolled case series.[66-71] Also, there is a surge of evidence supporting the efficacy of BTA in treating trigeminal neuralgia. Favorable effects without serious side effects of subcutaneous BTA injections were described in 20 reports, including three double-blind studies[72-74] and one single-blind study.[75] Significant reduction in pain frequency and intensity and a high number of pain responders were reported in the group receiving subcutaneous injection of BTA in dosages up to 75 U in the affected trigeminal area, compared with the saline control group, in an RCT.[72] The comparable efficacy of low-dose (25 U) and high-dose (75 U) BTA was observed, with fewer side effects in the low-dose group.[73] A delayed but clinically significant improvement in visual analog scale (VAS) scores at 3 months after injection was reported in the 50 U BTA group, compared to placebo control.[74] A reduction of 6.5 points in VAS after subcutaneous injections of 40–60 U BTA was demonstrated, compared with 3 points in the placebo group, in a single-blind RCT study.[75]

Painful Diabetic and Other Peripheral Neuropathies

BTA injection could also provide prolonged symptomatic pain relief for painful diabetic neuropathy (PDN). A double-blind crossover study reported pain reduction and sleep quality improvement at 12 weeks after intradermal Botox injection (4 U per site) into the hyperesthetic and allodynic foot regions.[76] A marked decrease in both tactile perception and mechanical pain was reported at weeks 1, 4, 8, and 12 after treatment compared with baseline in another study with a similar size and design.[77] A third RCT demonstrated sustained analgesic effects over 24 weeks from the first administration in the group receiving repeated subcutaneous administration of BTA of up to 300 U, compared to the placebo group.[78] A meta-analysis revealed improvement of 1.96 VAS points following PDN treatment with BTA.[79]

NEURAL DESTRUCTIVE TECHNIQUES, PULSE RADIOFREQUENCY

Neural destructive techniques may be pursued for longer-term pain relief if a diagnostic nerve block confirms that the pain is in the sensory distribution of a single nerve, which is both distal and purely sensory in function, or forms a neuroma as a result of nerve injury.[80,81] These neural ablative modalities include chemical denervation, cryoablation, and thermal radiofrequency ablation of the peripheral nerve. Neuroablation may be considered for severe malignant neuropathic pain that is refractory to conservative pain management. Given the potential risk of increased post-ablation neuropathic pain with the possible exception of cryoablation,[82] caution should be exercised when selecting the chemical, thermal, or cryo approaches.[83] PRF has emerged more recently as a potentially safer mode of radiofrequency treatment for refractory nonmalignant neuropathic pain conditions. It is considered more neuromodulative than neurodestructive, by exposing the neural tissue to a high-frequency electric field instead of to neuroablative temperature (>45°C).[84,85]

Postherpetic Neuralgia

Accumulating evidence supports the efficacy of PRF of the intercostal nerve(s) or dorsal root ganglion (DRG) in treating PHN. A double-blind RCT assessed the efficacy of PRF treatment of intercostal nerves at the level of zoster lesion for

PHN affecting thoracic dermatomes. Compared to the sham group, post-procedure pain scores and tramadol use were significantly lower, and several health-related quality-of-life measures were significantly improved through 6 months after treatment in the PRF group.[86] The efficacy of PRF treatment of the affected cervical, thoracic, or lumbar DRG for patients with refractory PHN was examined in an open-label, prospective study. A persistent 55% of the reduction in pain score was demonstrated at 4 weeks after PRF and maintained at the subsequent 12-week follow-up.[87] Interestingly, PRF of the DRG was more effective than a continuous epidural block in treating the acute phase of herpes zoster and preventing the development of PHN.[88] There was a more significant decrease in the numerical rating scale (NRS) score and analgesic consumption in the PRF group than in the continuous epidural group. Thus, PRF of the DRG may be a useful option for reducing the progression of neuropathic changes caused by the persistent transmission of a pain signal after the acute phase of herpes zoster.[88]

Cervical and Lumbosacral Radiculopathy
The efficacy of DRG PRF has been examined in patients with lumbosacral and cervical radicular pain.[89–91] In contrast to the lack of evidence for conventional radiofrequency lesioning in the treatment of chronic lumbar radiculopathy,[92] there is promising evidence for the beneficial effects of PRF of the DRG or segmental nerve roots in the treatment of both chronic lumbar radiculopathy and cervical radicular pain. A long-term pain reduction up to 12 months after PRF in the treatment of lumbosacral radicular pain was reported in a small–sample size RCT, compared to a control group that received nerve root blocks with local anesthetics.[93] Favorable safety profile and beneficial effects of PRF therapy in the treatment of lumbosacral radiculopathy were also supported in a clinical audit, as well as in a systematic review.[94,95] Compared to sham therapy, short-term efficacy of PRF of the cervical DRG and segmental nerve roots 2–3 months after treatment was reported.[96] The outcomes were not significantly different between the two groups with electrode tip temperature of 40°C and 67°C.[97] The efficacy of PRF treatment in cervical radicular pain was reproduced in two clinical trials[98,99] and supported by a prospective observational study.[100] Long-term efficacy of up to 12 months was reported in a prospective observational study.[101]

A comparative effectiveness study suggests that PRF of the DRG appears to be as effective as transforaminal epidural steroid injection in terms of attenuating cervical and lumbar radicular pain caused by disc herniation, and its use would avoid the adverse effects of using steroids.[102] Furthermore, combining cervical nerve root block with PRF appears to be a safe and more efficacious technique for cervical radicular pain.[103] The combination therapy yielded better outcomes than either cervical nerve root block or PRF alone. Clearly, the use of PRF to the DRG in cervical radicular pain is compelling.[104] It is appealing because long-lasting effects are reported without complications. It has progressively gained a place in the management of chronic radicular pain.[105]

Sympathetically Maintained Pain
Ablative sympathectomy techniques have been advocated for many years in an effort to produce a permanent interruption in the transmission of sympathetically maintained pain. Promising short-term outcomes were reported in either uncontrolled case series or poorly controlled comparative studies.[106] A large case series described percutaneous radiofrequency ablation of the upper thoracic sympathetic supply by destroying the entire fusiform ganglion.[107] The lesion effectiveness was defined by significant diminishment of the sympathetic activity, but no clinical analgesic or functional outcomes were reported. Thus, there is no high-level evidence to support these techniques' widespread use in nonmalignant, nonterminal pain, and post-ablation pain remains a real concern.[82,108] Clearly, more research is needed before definitive recommendations can be made.

Radiofrequency Thermocoagulation for Trigeminal Neuralgia
Minimally invasive interventional pain therapies and surgery are available when conservative therapy fails. Younger patients may benefit from microvascular decompression, which is described in Chapter 8. Elderly patients with poor surgical risk may be more suitable for percutaneous trigeminal nerve rhizolysis.[109] Under monitored anesthesia care, a stimulating electrode is introduced through a needle placed in the foramen ovale with the aid of fluoroscopy. The patient is awakened from anesthesia for mapping of the sensory and motor responses. A thermocouple lead is used to lesion the nerve.

The advantage of dermatomal mapping in radiofrequency ablation is that it is more selective than balloon compression. Pain relief following radiofrequency approaches 90%, with nearly 60% of patients still pain-free at 60 months. The estimated recurrence rate of 25% is likely lower than for glycerol rhizotomy. Complications with radiofrequency ablation include masticatory weakness, dysesthesia, and corneal numbness (if V1 is targeted). There is also a risk of vascular injury.

REFERENCES

1. Attal N, Lanteri-Minet M, Laurent B, Fermanian J, Bouhassira D. The specific disease burden of neuropathic pain: results of a French nationwide survey. *Pain*. 2011;152(12):2836–2843.
2. Schaefer C, Mann R, Sadosky A, et al. Burden of illness associated with peripheral and central neuropathic pain among adults seeking treatment in the United States: a patient-centered evaluation. *Pain Med*. 2014;15(12):2105–2119.
3. Schaefer C, Sadosky A, Mann R, et al. Pain severity and the economic burden of neuropathic pain in the United States: BEAT neuropathic pain observational study. *Clinicoecon Outcomes Res*. 2014;6:483–496.
4. Bouhassira D, Lanteri-Minet M, Attal N, Laurent B, Touboul C. Prevalence of chronic pain with neuropathic characteristics in the general population. *Pain*. 2008;136:380–387.
5. Yawn BP, Wollan PC, Weingarten TN, Watson JC, Hooten WM, Melton LJ 3rd. The prevalence of neuropathic pain: clinical evaluation compared with screening tools in a community population. *Pain Med*. 2009;10(3):586–593.
6. Harden RN. Chronic neuropathic pain. Mechanisms, diagnosis, and treatment. *Neurologist*. 2005;11(2):111–122.
7. Accident Compensation Corporation. ACC guideline. Interventional guidelines for pain management. 2016.Accessed Sept. 1, 2016.
8. Liu T, Yu CP. Placebo analgesia, acupuncture and sham surgery. *Evid Based Complement Alternat Med*. 2011;2011:943147.
9. McGuirk S, Fahy C, Costi D, Cyna AM. Use of invasive placebos in research on local anaesthetic interventions. *Anaesthesia*. 2011;66(2):84–91.
10. Kehlet H, Jensen TS, Woolf CJ. Persistent postsurgical pain: risk factors and prevention. *Lancet*. 2006;367(9522):1618–1625.
11. Zimmermann M. Pathobiology of neuropathic pain. *Eur J Pharmacol*. 2001;429(1–3):23–37.
12. Moalem G, Tracey DJ. Immune and inflammatory mechanisms in neuropathic pain. *Brain Res Rev*. 2006;51(2):240–264.
13. Sommer C, Kress M. Recent findings on how proinflammatory cytokines cause pain: peripheral mechanisms in inflammatory and neuropathic hyperalgesia. *Neurosci Lett*. 2004;361(1–3):184–187.
14. Zhang JM, An J. Cytokines, inflammation, and pain. *Int Anesthesiol Clin*. 2007;45(2):27–37.
15. Maeda Y, Kettner N, Holden J, et al. Functional deficits in carpal tunnel syndrome reflect reorganization of primary somatosensory cortex. *Brain*. 2014;137(Pt 6):1741–1752.
16. Haueisen DC, Smith BS, Myers SR, Pryce ML. The diagnostic accuracy of spinal nerve injection studies. Their role in the evaluation of recurrent sciatica. *Clin Orthop Relat Res*. 1985;198:179–183.
17. Dooley JF, McBroom RJ, Taguchi T, Macnab I. Nerve root infiltration in the diagnosis of radicular pain. *Spine (Phila Pa 1976)*. 1988;13(1):79–83.
18. Schutz H, Lougheed WM, Wortzman G, Awerbuck BG. Intervertebral nerve-root in the investigation of chronic lumbar disc disease. *Can J Surg*. 1973;16(3):217–221.
19. Krempen JF, Smith BS, DeFreest LJ. Selective nerve root infiltration for the evaluation of sciatica. *Orthop Clin North Am*. 1975;6(1):311–315.
20. Saxena S, So S, Williams BA, Mangione MP. The role of diagnostic ultrasound-guided selective common peroneal nerve block in a patient with negative imaging but with classic neuropathic pain after below knee amputation. *A Case Rep*. 2014;3(2):20–22.
21. Huang JH, Galvagno SM,Jr, Hameed M, et al. Occipital nerve pulsed radiofrequency treatment: a multi-center study evaluating predictors of outcome. *Pain Med*. 2012;13(4):489–497.
22. Boas RA. Sympathetic nerve blocks: in search of a role. *Reg Anesth Pain Med*. 1998;23(3):292–305.
23. Johansson A, Bennett GJ. Effect of local methylprednisolone on pain in a nerve injury model. A pilot study. *Reg Anesth*. 1997;22(1):59–65.
24. Wang JC, Chiou HJ, Lu JH, Hsu YC, Chan RC, Yang TF. Ultrasound-guided perineural steroid injection to treat intractable pain due to sciatic nerve injury. *Can J Anaesth*. 2013;60(9):902–906.
25. Johansson A, Sjolund B. Nerve blocks with local anesthetics and corticosteroids in chronic pain: a clinical follow-up study. *J Pain Symptom Manage*. 1996;11(3):181–187.
26. Markovic M, Crichton K, Read JW, Lam P, Slater HK. Effectiveness of ultrasound-guided corticosteroid injection in the treatment of Morton's neuroma. *Foot Ankle Int*. 2008;29(5):483–487.
27. Bhatia A, Flamer D, Shah PS. Perineural steroids for trauma and compression-related peripheral

neuropathic pain: a systematic review and meta-analysis. *Can J Anaesth*. 2015;62(6):650–662.

28. Karadas O, Tok F, Akarsu S, Tekin L, Balaban B. Triamcinolone acetonide vs procaine hydrochloride injection in the management of carpal tunnel syndrome: randomized placebo-controlled study. *J Rehabil Med*. 2012;44(7):601–604.

29. Andreae MH, Andreae DA. Local anaesthetics and regional anaesthesia for preventing chronic pain after surgery. *Cochrane Database Syst Rev*. 2012;10:CD007105.

30. Ambrosini A, Vandenheede M, Rossi P, et al. Suboccipital injection with a mixture of rapid- and long-acting steroids in cluster headache: a double-blind placebo-controlled study. *Pain*. 2005;118(1–2):92–96.

31. Eker HE, Cok OY, Aribogan A, Arslan G. Management of neuropathic pain with methylprednisolone at the site of nerve injury. *Pain Med*. 2012;13(3):443–451.

32. Singh PM, Dehran M, Mohan VK, Trikha A, Kaur M. Analgesic efficacy and safety of medical therapy alone vs combined medical therapy and extraoral glossopharyngeal nerve block in glossopharyngeal neuralgia. *Pain Med*. 2013;14(1):93–102.

33. Thomson CE, Beggs I, Martin DJ, et al. Methylprednisolone injections for the treatment of Morton neuroma: a patient-blinded randomized trial. *J Bone Joint Surg Am*. 2013;95(9):790–8, S1.

34. Karadas O, Tok F, Ulas UH, Odabasi Z. The effectiveness of triamcinolone acetonide vs. procaine hydrochloride injection in the management of carpal tunnel syndrome: a double-blind randomized clinical trial. *Am J Phys Med Rehabil*. 2011;90(4):287–292.

35. Farrar JT, Young JP,Jr, LaMoreaux L, Werth JL, Poole RM. Clinical importance of changes in chronic pain intensity measured on an 11-point numerical pain rating scale. *Pain*. 2001;94(2):149–158.

36. Armstrong T, Devor W, Borschel L, Contreras R. Intracarpal steroid injection is safe and effective for short-term management of carpal tunnel syndrome. *Muscle Nerve*. 2004;29(1):82–88.

37. Dammers JW, Veering MM, Vermeulen M. Injection with methylprednisolone proximal to the carpal tunnel: randomised double blind trial. *BMJ*. 1999;319(7214):884–886.

38. Wong SM, Hui AC, Tang A, et al. Local vs systemic corticosteroids in the treatment of carpal tunnel syndrome. *Neurology*. 2001;56(11):1565–1567.

39. Chen PC, Chuang CH, Tu YK, Bai CH, Chen CF, Liaw M. A bayesian network meta-analysis: comparing the clinical effectiveness of local corticosteroid injections using different

treatment strategies for carpal tunnel syndrome. *BMC Musculoskelet Disord*. 2015;16:394.

40. Ranoux D, Attal N, Morain F, Bouhassira D. Botulinum toxin type A induces direct analgesic effects in chronic neuropathic pain. *Ann Neurol*. 2008;64(3):274–283.

41. Pasqualucci A, Pasqualucci V, Galla F, et al. Prevention of post-herpetic neuralgia: acyclovir and prednisolone versus epidural local anesthetic and methylprednisolone. *Acta Anaesthesiol Scand*. 2000;44(8):910–918.

42. van Wijck AJ, Opstelten W, Moons KG, et al. The PINE study of epidural steroids and local anaesthetics to prevent postherpetic neuralgia: a randomised controlled trial. *Lancet*. 2006;367(9506):219–224.

43. Ji G, Niu J, Shi Y, Hou L, Lu Y, Xiong L. The effectiveness of repetitive paravertebral injections with local anesthetics and steroids for the prevention of postherpetic neuralgia in patients with acute herpes zoster. *Anesth Analg*. 2009;109(5):1651–1655.

44. Kumar V, Krone K, Mathieu A. Neuraxial and sympathetic blocks in herpes zoster and postherpetic neuralgia: an appraisal of current evidence. *Reg Anesth Pain Med*. 2004;29(5):454–461.

45. Kikuchi A, Kotani N, Sato T, Takamura K, Sakai I, Matsuki A. Comparative therapeutic evaluation of intrathecal versus epidural methylprednisolone for long-term analgesia in patients with intractable postherpetic neuralgia. *Reg Anesth Pain Med*. 1999;24(4):287–293.

46. Kotani N, Kushikata T, Hashimoto H, et al. Intrathecal methylprednisolone for intractable postherpetic neuralgia. *N Engl J Med*. 2000;343(21):1514–1519.

47. Rijsdijk M, van Wijck AJ, Meulenhoff PC, Kavelaars A, van der Tweel I, Kalkman CJ. No beneficial effect of intrathecal methylprednisolone acetate in postherpetic neuralgia patients. *Eur J Pain*. 2013;17(5):714–723.

48. van Rijn MA, Munts AG, Marinus J, et al. Intrathecal baclofen for dystonia of complex regional pain syndrome. *Pain*. 2009;143(1–2):41–47.

49. Xiao L, Mackey S, Hui H, Xong D, Zhang Q, Zhang D. Subcutaneous injection of botulinum toxin A is beneficial in postherpetic neuralgia. *Pain Med*. 2010;11(12):1827–1833.

50. Apalla Z, Sotiriou E, Lallas A, Lazaridou E, Ioannides D. Botulinum toxin A in postherpetic neuralgia: a parallel, randomized, double-blind, single-dose, placebo-controlled trial. *Clin J Pain*. 2013;29(10):857–864.

51. Liu HT, Tsai SK, Kao MC, Hu JS. Botulinum toxin A relieved neuropathic pain in a case of postherpetic neuralgia. *Pain Med*. 2006;7(1):89–91.

52. Sotiriou E, Apalla Z, Panagiotidou D, Ioannidis D. Severe post-herpetic neuralgia successfully treated with botulinum toxin A: three case reports. *Acta Derm Venereol.* 2009;89(2):214–215.

53. Levin JH. Prospective, double-blind, randomized placebo-controlled trials in interventional spine: what the highest quality literature tells us. *Spine J.* 2009;9(8):690–703.

54. Pinto RZ, Maher CG, Ferreira ML, et al. Epidural corticosteroid injections in the management of sciatica: a systematic review and meta-analysis. *Ann Intern Med.* 2012;157(12):865–877.

55. Quraishi NA. Transforaminal injection of corticosteroids for lumbar radiculopathy: systematic review and meta-analysis. *Eur Spine J.* 2012;21(2):214–219.

56. Cohen SP, Bicket MC, Jamison D, Wilkinson I, Rathmell JP. Epidural steroids: a comprehensive, evidence-based review. *Reg Anesth Pain Med.* 2013;38(3):175–200.

57. Riew KD, Park JB, Cho YS, et al. Nerve root blocks in the treatment of lumbar radicular pain. A minimum five-year follow-up. *J Bone Joint Surg Am.* 2006;88(8):1722–1725.

58. Bicket MC, Horowitz JM, Benzon HT, Cohen SP. Epidural injections in prevention of surgery for spinal pain: systematic review and meta-analysis of randomized controlled trials. *Spine J.* 2015;15(2):348–362.

59. Harden RN, Oaklander AL, Burton AW, et al. Complex regional pain syndrome: practical diagnostic and treatment guidelines, 4th edition. *Pain Med.* 2013;14(2):180–229.

60. Price DD, Long S, Wilsey B, Rafii A. Analysis of peak magnitude and duration of analgesia produced by local anesthetics injected into sympathetic ganglia of complex regional pain syndrome patients. *Clin J Pain.* 1998;14(3):216–226.

61. Burton AW, Conroy BP, Sims S, Solanki D, Williams CG. Complex regional pain syndrome type II as a complication of subclavian catheter insertion. *Anesthesiology.* 1998;89(3):804.

62. Rocha Rde O, Teixeira MJ, Yeng LT, et al. Thoracic sympathetic block for the treatment of complex regional pain syndrome type I: a double-blind randomized controlled study. *Pain.* 2014;155(11):2274–2281.

63. Ackerman WE, Zhang JM. Efficacy of stellate ganglion blockade for the management of type 1 complex regional pain syndrome. *South Med J.* 2006;99(10):1084–1088.

64. Carroll I, Clark JD, Mackey S. Sympathetic block with botulinum toxin to treat complex regional pain syndrome. *Ann Neurol.* 2009;65(3):348–351.

65. Choi E, Cho CW, Kim HY, Lee PB, Nahm FS. Lumbar sympathetic block with botulinum toxin type B for complex regional pain syndrome: a case study. *Pain Physician.* 2015;18(5):E911–E916.

66. Cetas JS, Saedi T, Burchiel KJ. Destructive procedures for the treatment of nonmalignant pain: a structured literature review. *J Neurosurg.* 2008;109(3):389–404.

67. Cruccu G, Gronseth G, Alksne J, et al. AAN-EFNS guidelines on trigeminal neuralgia management. *Eur J Neurol.* 2008;15(10):1013–1028.

68. Gronseth G, Cruccu G, Alksne J, et al. Practice parameter: the diagnostic evaluation and treatment of trigeminal neuralgia (an evidence-based review): report of the Quality Standards Subcommittee of the American Academy of Neurology and the European Federation of Neurological Societies. *Neurology.* 2008;71(15):1183–1190.

69. Lopez BC, Hamlyn PJ, Zakrzewska JM. Systematic review of ablative neurosurgical techniques for the treatment of trigeminal neuralgia. *Neurosurgery.* 2004;54:973–983.

70. Lopez BC, Hamlyn PJ, Zakrzewska JM. Stereotactic radiosurgery for primary trigeminal neuralgia: state of the evidence and recommendations for future reports. *J Neurol Neurosurg Psychiatry.* 2004;75(7):1019–1024.

71. Zakrzewska JM, Akram H. Neurosurgical interventions for the treatment of classical trigeminal neuralgia. *Cochrane Database Syst Rev.* 2011;(9):CD007312.

72. Wu CJ, Lian YJ, Zheng YK, et al. Botulinum toxin type A for the treatment of trigeminal neuralgia: results from a randomized, double-blind, placebo-controlled trial. *Cephalalgia.* 2012;32(6):443–450.

73. Zhang H, Lian Y, Ma Y, et al. Two doses of botulinum toxin type A for the treatment of trigeminal neuralgia: observation of therapeutic effect from a randomized, double-blind, placebo-controlled trial. *J Headache Pain.* 2014;15:65.

74. Zuniga C, Piedimonte F, Diaz S, Micheli F. Acute treatment of trigeminal neuralgia with onabotulinum toxin A. *Clin Neuropharmacol.* 2013;36(5):146–150.

75. Shehata HS, El-Tamawy MS, Shalaby NM, Ramzy G. Botulinum toxin-type A: could it be an effective treatment option in intractable trigeminal neuralgia? *J Headache Pain.* 2013;14:92.

76. Yuan RY, Sheu JJ, Yu JM, et al. Botulinum toxin for diabetic neuropathic pain: a randomized double-blind crossover trial. *Neurology.* 2009;72(17):1473–1478.

77. Chen WT, Yuan RY, Chiang SC, et al. Onabotulinumtoxin A improves tactile and mechanical pain perception in painful diabetic polyneuropathy. *Clin J Pain.* 2013;29(4):305–310.

78. Attal N, de Andrade DC, Adam F, et al. Safety and efficacy of repeated injections of botulinum toxin A in peripheral neuropathic pain (BOTNEP): a randomised, double-blind, placebo-controlled trial. *Lancet Neurol.* 2016;15(6):555–565.

79. Lakhan SE, Velasco DN, Tepper D. Botulinum toxin-A for painful diabetic neuropathy: a meta-analysis. *Pain Med.* 2015;16(9):1773–1780.

80. Balcin H, Erba P, Wettstein R, Schaefer DJ, Pierer G, Kalbermatten DF. A comparative study of two methods of surgical treatment for painful neuroma. *J Bone Joint Surg Br.* 2009;91(6):803–808.

81. Stokvis A, van der Avoort DJ, van Neck JW, Hovius SE, Coert JH. Surgical management of neuroma pain: a prospective follow-up study. *Pain.* 2010;151(3):862–869.

82. Kapetanos AT, Furlan AD, Mailis-Gagnon A. Characteristics and associated features of persistent post-sympathectomy pain. *Clin J Pain.* 2003;19(3):192–199.

83. Zhou L, Kambin P, Casey KF, et al. Mechanism research of cryoanalgesia. *Neurol Res.* 1995;17(4):307–311.

84. Chua NH, Vissers KC, Sluijter ME. Pulsed radiofrequency treatment in interventional pain management: mechanisms and potential indications—a review. *Acta Neurochir (Wien).* 2011;153(4):763–771.

85. Van Boxem K, Huntoon M, Van Zundert J, Patijn J, van Kleef M, Joosten EA. Pulsed radiofrequency: a review of the basic science as applied to the pathophysiology of radicular pain: a call for clinical translation. *Reg Anesth Pain Med.* 2014;39(2):149–159.

86. Ke M, Yinghui F, Yi J, et al. Efficacy of pulsed radiofrequency in the treatment of thoracic postherpetic neuralgia from the angulus costae: a randomized, double-blinded, controlled trial. *Pain Physician.* 2013;16(1):15–25.

87. Kim YH, Lee CJ, Lee SC, et al. Effect of pulsed radiofrequency for postherpetic neuralgia. *Acta Anaesthesiol Scand.* 2008;52(8):1140–1143.

88. Kim ED, Lee YI, Park HJ. Comparison of efficacy of continuous epidural block and pulsed radiofrequency to the dorsal root ganglion for management of pain persisting beyond the acute phase of herpes zoster. *PLoS One.* 2017;12(8):e0183559.

89. Byrd D, Mackey S. Pulsed radiofrequency for chronic pain. *Curr Pain Headache Rep.* 2008;12(1):37–41.

90. van Boxem K, van Eerd M, Brinkhuizen T, Patijn J, van Kleef M, van Zundert J. Radiofrequency and pulsed radiofrequency treatment of chronic pain syndromes: the available evidence. *Pain Pract.* 2008;8(5):385–393.

91. Malik K, Benzon HT. Radiofrequency applications to dorsal root ganglia: a literature review. *Anesthesiology.* 2008;109(3):527–542.

92. Chou R. 2009 clinical guidelines from the American Pain Society and the American Academy of Pain Medicine on the use of chronic opioid therapy in chronic noncancer pain: what are the key messages for clinical practice? *Pol Arch Med Wewn.* 2009;119(7–8):469–477.

93. Fujii H, Kosogabe Y, Kajiki H. Long-term effects of pulsed radiofrequency on the dorsal root ganglion and segmental nerve roots for lumbosacral radicular pain: a prospective controlled randomized trial with nerve root block. *Masui.* 2012;61(8):790–793.

94. Van Boxem K, van Bilsen J, de Meij N, et al. Pulsed radiofrequency treatment adjacent to the lumbar dorsal root ganglion for the management of lumbosacral radicular syndrome: a clinical audit. *Pain Med.* 2011;12(9):1322–1330.

95. Nagda JV, Davis CW, Bajwa ZH, Simopoulos TT. Retrospective review of the efficacy and safety of repeated pulsed and continuous radiofrequency lesioning of the dorsal root ganglion/segmental nerve for lumbar radicular pain. *Pain Physician.* 2011;14(4):371–376.

96. van Kleef M, Liem L, Lousberg R, Barendse G, Kessels F, Sluijter M. Radiofrequency lesion adjacent to the dorsal root ganglion for cervicobrachial pain: a prospective double-blind randomized study. *Neurosurgery.* 1996;38(6):1127–1131; discussion 1131–1132.

97. Slappendel R, Crul BJ, Braak GJ, et al. The efficacy of radiofrequency lesioning of the cervical spinal dorsal root ganglion in a double blinded randomized study: no difference between 40 degrees C and 67 degrees C treatments. *Pain.* 1997;73(2):159–163.

98. Van Zundert J, Lame IE, de Louw A, et al. Percutaneous pulsed radiofrequency treatment of the cervical dorsal root ganglion in the treatment of chronic cervical pain syndromes: a clinical audit. *Neuromodulation.* 2003;6(1):6–14.

99. Van Zundert J, Patijn J, Kessels A, Lame I, van Suijlekom H, van Kleef M. Pulsed radiofrequency adjacent to the cervical dorsal root ganglion in chronic cervical radicular pain: a double-blind sham controlled randomized clinical trial. *Pain.* 2007;127(1–2):173–182.

100. Choi GS, Ahn SH, Cho YW, Lee DK. Short-term effects of pulsed radiofrequency on chronic refractory cervical radicular pain. *Ann Rehabil Med.* 2011;35(6):826–832.

101. Yoon YM, Han SR, Lee SJ, Choi CY, Sohn MJ, Lee CH. The efficacy of pulsed radiofrequency

treatment of cervical radicular pain patients. *Korean J Spine*. 2014;11(3):109–112.

102. Lee DG, Ahn SH, Lee J. Comparative effectivenesses of pulsed radiofrequency and transforaminal steroid injection for radicular pain due to disc herniation: a prospective randomized trial. *J Korean Med Sci*. 2016;31(8):1324–1330.

103. Wang F, Zhou Q, Xiao L, et al. A randomized comparative study of pulsed radiofrequency treatment with or without selective nerve root block for chronic cervical radicular pain. *Pain Pract*. 2017;17(5):589–595.

104. Facchini G, Spinnato P, Guglielmi G, Albisinni U, Bazzocchi A. A comprehensive review of pulsed radiofrequency in the treatment of pain associated with different spinal conditions. *Br J Radiol*. 2017;90(1073):20150406.

105. Vanneste T, Van Lantschoot A, Van Boxem K, Van Zundert J. Pulsed radiofrequency in chronic pain. *Curr Opin Anaesthesiol*. 2017;30(5):577–582.

106. Straube S, Derry S, Moore RA, Cole P. Cervicothoracic or lumbar sympathectomy for neuropathic pain and complex regional pain syndrome. *Cochrane Database Syst Rev*. 2013;9:CD002918.

107. Wilkinson HA. Percutaneous radiofrequency upper thoracic sympathectomy. *Neurosurgery*. 1996;38(4):715–725.

108. Mockus MB, Rutherford RB, Rosales C, Pearce WH. Sympathectomy for causalgia. patient selection and long-term results. *Arch Surg*. 1987;122(6):668–672.

109. Emril DR, Ho KY. Treatment of trigeminal neuralgia: role of radiofrequency ablation. *J Pain Res*. 2010;3:249–254.

8

Surgical Treatment of Neuropathic Pain

JIANGUO CHENG AND WENBAO WANG

INTRODUCTION

Surgical treatment of intractable neuropathic pain includes neuroablative and neuromodulatory approaches. Early treatments focus on neuroablation of the pain pathways, such as with percutaneous cordotomy, spinothalamic tractotomy, anterolateral cordotomy, dorsal root entry zone lesioning, commissural myelotomy, cingulotomy, and thalamotomy. These techniques have largely fallen out of favor and are rarely used in patients with cancer pain. Neuromodulation techniques, such as spinal cord stimulation, dorsal root ganglion stimulation, and peripheral nerve stimulation, have evolved significantly in recent years to become important treatment options for neuropathic pain conditions refractory to conservative therapies.[1] Another form of neuromodulation is intrathecal drug delivery through programmable pumps.[2] These neuromodulatory techniques can be safe, efficacious, and cost-effective in appropriately selected patients, especially in those with failed back surgical syndrome, complex regional pain syndrome (CRPS), and other well-defined neuropathic pain conditions. Deep brain stimulation and motor cortex stimulation are options for central neuropathic pain states. Surgical approaches, such as microvascular decompression and Gamma Knife radiosurgery (GKRS), are also excellent options for the treatment of refractory trigeminal neuralgia and glossopharyngeal neuralgia. There are a number of other surgical approaches that are beyond the scope of this chapter but are used in treating neuropathic pain, such as neuroma excision and release of nerve entrapment/compression or spinal stenosis through carpel tunnel surgery, minimally invasive lumbar decompression, foraminotomy, discectomy, laminectomy, or other spine surgeries.

SPINAL CORD STIMULATION (SCS)

The "gate control theory," by Melzack and Wall in 1965, hypothesized that electrical stimulation of the dorsal columns depolarized large A-β fibers that activate inhibitory interneurons and "close the gate" to prevent the transmission of pain-inducing nociceptive signals from A-delta and C-fiber afferent fibers.[3] In light of this theory, Norman Shealy first intrathecally implanted a dorsal column simulator in a terminally ill cancer patient in Cleveland and demonstrated temporary but compete abolition of pain in 1967.[4] With FDA approval in 1968, Medtronic first offered these devices for the treatment of pain. However, the early procedures suffered from many serious complications, including spinal fluid leakage and compression of the spinal cord. Significant advancement has been made in the last 50 years,[5] particularly in the last 10 years.[6] SCS is now widely used as a relatively safe and effective long-term treatment option for chronic neuropathic pain.

The most common indications of SCS in the United States are lumbar post-laminectomy syndrome, CRPS, radiculopathy, and polyneuropathy.[7] Other challenging diagnoses successfully treated with SCS include postherpetic neuralgia (PHN), post-thoracotomy syndrome, phantom limb pain, stroke central pain syndrome, spinal cord injury, and multiple sclerosis (MS). SCS is also used to alleviate pain from peripheral arterial occlusive disease and chronic refractory angina pectoris.[7,8]

There is strong evidence (level I–II) from randomized controlled trials and systematic reviews supporting SCS for lumbar failed back surgery syndrome (FBSS) when conservative management has failed.[9,10] A recent systematic review and meta-analysis of conventional SCS indicated that the majority of patients experienced significant pain relief.[11] A recent randomized controlled trial reported that patients with a history of spinal surgery and unremitting leg and back pain benefited significantly from SCS, particular high-frequency (HF) stimulation.[12,13] The beneficial effects were maintained for a mean follow-up period of 24 months.[9,13] Both conventional SCS and HF stimulation are effective treatment options for patients with neuropathic pain that is notoriously difficult to treat. The data supporting SCS in its multiple forms are compelling, thus this therapy should be considered earlier in the treatment continuum, rather than regarded as simply an end-stage salvage therapy.

Conventional SCS typically delivers electrical pulses at a frequency below 1200 Hz and more commonly around 50 Hz.[14] It produces paresthesia (generally at frequencies below 300 Hz) to "map" the painful area. Although conventional SCS typically can reliably cover leg pain, it often fails to cover axial back pain.[9] HF-10 SCS (high-frequency, 10,000 Hz) was introduced to clinical practice recently to overcome this limitation.[12] Patients do not experience paresthesia in HF-10 SCS, as the stimulus intensity is below the paresthesia threshold.[14] "Paresthesia mapping" is not necessary during trial or implant surgery, making a "wake-up" test unnecessary. In the SENZA trial, HF-10 SCS was compared with conventional paresthesia-based SCS in patients with back and leg pain due to post-laminectomy syndrome, radiculopathy, or degenerative disc disease. In the HF-10 group, more than 80% of patients reported greater than 50% back pain reduction over a 12-month follow-up period. In contrast, in the conventional SCS group, about 50% of patients reported greater than 50% back pain reduction. Similarly, rates of greater than 50% leg pain reduction were approximately 80% in the HF10 group and 50%–55% in the conventional SCS group. The superior analgesic efficacy of HF-10 therapy was sustained at 24 months.[13]

Dorsal root ganglion (DRG) stimulation is a new modality of neuromodulation. Electrodes are placed in close proximity to DRG where the cell bodies of the peripheral nerve system reside.[15,16] Much less electrical current is required, as energy scattering is reduced by thinner layers of cerebrospinal fluid (CSF) surrounding the DRGs. Strictly speaking, it is a form of peripheral nerve stimulation. However, it is considered a form of SCS for regulatory reasons. In a multicenter, randomized comparative effectiveness trial,[15] DRG stimulation was compared to conventional SCS in 152 patients with CRPS in the leg. DRG stimulation provided greater than 50% pain relief in 81.2% patients versus 55.7% for conventional SCS. There were no differences in device-related complications between the two groups. DRG stimulation was associated with less postural variation in paresthesia and greater improvement in quality of life. DRG stimulation for FBSS was reported in a retrospective study: stimulation of the L2 or L3 DRG produced at least 50% pain reduction in 7 of 12 patients with chronic low back pain.[17] These data suggest that DRG stimulation is a superior option for managing CRPS and may be effective in other chronic neuropathic pain conditions as well.

In addition to the development of DRG stimulation, other new advances are being made in SCS technology, such as burst stimulation SCS, high-density SCS, wireless SCS, and closed-loop control of SCS, to improve efficacy and reduce complications.[6]

The most common complication in SCS is lead migration or misplacement (12.2%; range 5%–21%), with no significant difference between systems that are implanted surgically (14%) or percutaneously (12%).[18] Other device-related complications include implantable pulse generator failure (0.4%), migration (0.2%), and wire breakage (1.5%). In one series, loss of therapeutic efficacy was observed in 4% of cases (range 0%–14%). Pain at the sites of device implantation occurred in 9% of cases, and this was more frequent among devices placed surgically (12%) than those placed percutaneously (7%). Wound complications of infection and dehiscence were observed in 5% of patients (range 0%–14%). Such problems were noted more frequently among devices placed surgically (5%) than those placed percutaneously (2%).[18]

The technical details and intricacies are beyond the scope of this chapter. Here we briefly describe the process of SCS therapy, which usually takes a three-step approach. Patient selection is a key factor in determining the clinical outcomes of SCS. A pre-trial psychological evaluation is typically required to exclude patients who have significant psychological or psychiatric comorbidities and are therefore less ideal candidates for this type of treatment.[19] Once a patient is deemed a good candidate, a trial is performed to evaluate the individual response to this therapy.

The trial is typically performed through a percutaneous approach under moderate sedation or monitored anesthesia care (MAC). The patient is placed in a prone position, which is optimized for lead entry to the targeted epidural space. Fluoroscopy is used to guide the entry-level and lead placement. Via a paramedian approach, a Tuohy needle is introduced into the epidural space with a loss-of-resistance technique. A lead is passed through the needle and threaded to a target level appropriate for intended coverage. Multiple leads may be necessary for adequate coverage and satisfactory outcomes. The leads are connected to the external stimulator and intraoperative test stimulation is performed, with the exception of HF stimulation. With satisfactory coverage, the leads are connected to an external pulse generator, and stimulation parameters are programmed for a trail period of typically 7 to 10 days. Outcome measures typically include percent pain reduction, functional improvement (sleep, daily activity), and analgesic assumption. If the patient responds well to therapy with satisfactory outcomes by the end of the trial, an implant surgery will be performed, typically 6–8 weeks after removal of the trial lead(s).

Permanent leads can be placed percutaneously (percutaneous leads) or with laminectomy (pedal leads). Spine operative site and implantable pulse generator (IPG) site are marked. It is recommended that intravenous (IV) antibiotic be given 30 minutes before the incision is made. The patient is placed in a prone position. Under MAC supplemented with local anesthetic infiltration, an incision is made over the lead entry level and the leads are placed at the exact position as the trial. An intraoperative test is performed to confirm optimal coverage. The leads are anchored to the fascia. An IPG pocket is created at the previously designed place. Leads are tunneled to the IPG sites and connected to the IPG. Incisions are closed with sutures.

In rare circumstances, the trial leads may be used as permanent leads (the tunneled trial). For this purpose, the leads are buried subcutaneously by making an incision, and an extension is used to connect to the external pulse generator for testing. The leads are anchored to the fascia using permanent anchoring techniques. The extension lead is passed through a tunnel to the opposite site of the ultimate internal pulse generator pocket location. By doing so, the trial leads are not exposed to air during the trial and can be used as permanent leads once the trial proves to be a success.

PERIPHERAL NERVE STIMULATION (PNS)

Peripheral neuromodulation involves applying electrical current to stimulate a specific nerve, such as the occipital nerve, the ilioinguinal nerve, or the vagus nerve.[20] PNS can be achieved percutaneously or through implanted devices. Since the first report of a full permanent implant, by Sweet and Wall in 1968,[21] PNS has evolved and expanded over the course of the past few decades. It has become one of the most attractive therapies in neuromodulation and an effective treatment modality in management of chronic neuropathic pain.

For a long period, peripheral neurostimulation implantations were carried out via open surgery, until Weiner and Reed introduced a lead percutaneously in the proximity of the greater occipital nerve, in 1999.[22] This report suggests that occipital nerve stimulation (ONS) reduced not only pain from occipital neuralgia but also headaches from chronic migraine. It led to increased interest in this therapeutic modality. A randomized controlled trial demonstrated that ONS dramatically reduced pain from chronic migraine in about 40% of patients.[23] This is in sharp contrast to medical management, which did not achieve significant pain reduction or migraine frequency in any of the patients. A prospective study of 37 patients demonstrated significant long-term beneficial effects of ONS on migraine.[24] A systematic review and meta-analysis of five randomized controlled trials and seven case series confirmed the beneficial effects of ONS in reducing migraine pain and frequency.[25] In addition, ONS has been successfully used for treating cluster headaches in controlled and noncontrolled studies.[20,26,27] Infection and lead migration are common. Lead migration has a rate as high as 24%, and often requires lead revision.

Other than the occipital nerve, PNS for neuropathic pain has been studied for a number of specific targets, including branches of the trigeminal nerve; the median, ulnar, sciatic, ilioinguinal, and genitofemoral nerves; and the brachial and lumbar plexuses, with varying success.[20,28] Ultrasound imaging guidance for lead placement may help improve accuracy and reduce complications, such as visceral and blood vessel injuries. The indications include facial pain, neuropathic pain after trauma or surgery in areas of specific nerve innervation, CRPS type II, and amputation pain (both residual limb and phantom limb pain).[28]

Peripheral nerve field stimulation (PNFS) is achieved by placing electrodes near the area of pain without direct contact with the peripheral nerve. The electrodes are tunneled and connected to an IPG in a distant area. PNFS has been shown to reduce chronic low back pain, decrease analgesic requirement, and improve quality of life in a prospective, multicenter study involving 118 patients,[29] as well as in a recent review.[30] It was also beneficial in treating chronic chest pain in a prospective study of 20 patients,[31] chronic headaches in a study of 60 patients,[32] and neuropathic pain in extremities.[33] This method has the benefit of reducing potential nerve damage, compared to direct stimulation of a peripheral nerve that requires closer proximity to the nerve of interest when conducting surgery. Adverse effects can include electrode migration.

MOTOR CORTEX STIMULATION

Tsubokawa and colleagues published the first study of motor cortex stimulation in 1991.[34] The exact mechanism of action is largely unknown. Functional imaging studies have provided insights into the mechanisms by which motor cortex stimulation works to inhibit pain signal transmission in patients with central neuropathic pain.[35]

The most common indications are central pain, especially pain related to a thalamic lesion and trigeminal neuropathic pain.[36] In contrast, SCS is generally used for pain in the extremities or trunk. The central pain usually follows ischemic or hemorrhagic stroke or, less commonly, from MS or trauma. Other indications reported in the literature include phantom limb pain, brachial plexus avulsion, spinal cord injury, PHN, and peripheral nerve lesions including nerve root or nerve trunk pain.

A minimal craniotomy is performed over the motor cortex contralateral to the side of pain, using neuronavigation. A plate electrode is inserted into the epidural space overlying the region of the motor cortex that corresponds to the location of neuropathic pain and can usually be identified preoperatively with functional MRI. Motor-evoked responses can be used intraoperatively to confirm the location. The electrode is generally tested externally for several days before returning to the operating room for internalization and connection to an IPG.

A review of 14 studies involving a total of 210 cases of motor cortex stimulation implanted for different conditions suggests that overall, 57.6% of the patients had "good" postoperative pain relief (defined as pain relief ≥40% or 50%, depending on the studies), while about 30% of the patients had at least 70% improvement.[37] In the 152 patients in the studies who had a follow-up of longer than 1 year, 45.4% had a "good postoperative outcome." Outcomes are best in patients with trigeminal neuropathic pain. Reported complications include hardware-related complications, stroke, abscess, seizures, and intracranial bleeding.

DEEP BRAIN STIMULATION (DBS)

Deep brain stimulation (DBS) was extensively used in the 1970s and 1980s for a variety of indications. However, the use of DBS for pain greatly diminished after its approval for this indication was rescinded by the FDA. Currently, DBS is considered an investigational off-label surgical option for patients with chronic pain refractory to both pharmacological and surgical therapies. Indications include post-stroke pain, phantom limb pain/stump pain, and history of spinal injury or brachial plexus injury.[38–41]

A stimulating electrode is implanted through a burr hole using stereotactic navigation. The most commonly targeted regions are the periventricular gray/periaqueductal gray area and the ventral posterior lateral and medial thalamus. Once the electrode is in place, it is secured and connected to an IPG that delivers electrical impulses to the brain at a set frequency, pulse width, and intensity.

The response of patients with refractory pain following DBS has been variable. In a study of 85 patients over 12 years, DBS was used for various etiologies: 9 amputees, 7 brachial plexus injuries, 31 after stroke, 13 with spinal pathology, 15 with head and face pain, and 10 with miscellaneous pain.[40] Contralateral DBS targeted the periventricular gray area ($n = 33$), the ventral posterior nuclei of the thalamus ($n = 15$), or both targets ($n = 37$). Mean follow-up was 19.6 months. Almost 70% (69.4%) of patients retained implants 6 months after surgery. Thirty-nine of 59 (66%) of those implanted gained benefit and efficacy varied by etiology, improving outcomes in 89% after amputation and 70% after stroke. In this cohort, greater than 30% improvement sustained in visual analog scale (VAS) score, McGill Pain Questionnaire, Short-Form 36-question (SF-36) quality-of-life survey, and EuroQol-5D Questionnaire was observed in 15 patients with more than 42 months of follow-up, with several outcome measures improving from those assessed at 1 year. In a recent report,[39] contralateral, ventroposterolateral sensory thalamic DBS was performed in 16 patients with chronic neuropathic pain over 29 months: 10 with brachial plexus injury and 6 with phantom limb pain, all due to trauma. A postoperative trial of externalized DBS failed in 1 patient with brachial plexus injury, while 15 patients proceeded to implantation. No surgical complications or stimulation side effects were noted. After 36 months, mean pain relief was sustained, and the median (and interquartile range) of the improvement of VAS score was 52.8% (45.4%), University of Washington Neuropathic Pain Score was 30.7% (49.2%), Brief Pain Inventory (BPI) was 55.0% (32.0%), and SF-36 was 16.3% (30.3%). Potential complications of DBS include stroke, intracranial hemorrhage, neurological deficits, hardware failure/infection, lead dislocation/fracture, and unintentional motor or sensory disturbances.

INTRATHECAL DRUG DELIVERY

Opioids or ziconitide can be directly delivered to the intrathecal space surrounding the spinal cord.[2,42] Such a delivery route helps minimize the dose required to achieve analgesic effects. In 1973, the opioid receptor was first identified in the dorsal horn of the spinal cord. This finding constitutes the foundation for intrathecal opioid therapy. Dupen developed the first "permanent" catheter for intraspinal drug delivery in the 1980s, and Medtronic released the first FDA-approved externally programmable intrathecal drug delivery pump in 1991. Ziconitide was first tested in humans for neuropathic pain in 1997[43,44] and is added to the armamentarium of managing neuropathic pain and cancer-related pain.[2]

The indications for use of the intrathecal drug delivery system (IDDS) are neuropathic pain and cancer-related pain,[45] which typically has a significant neuropathic component.[2,46] IDDS may be considered when patients require high-dose opioid therapy but are unable to tolerate the medication because of side effects. In the United States, the most common indication for intrathecal therapy is chronic intractable noncancer pain, such as FBSS, spinal stenosis, intractable low back pain, and CRPS.[42] Contraindication for use of IDDS may include systemic infection, coagulopathy, allergy to medication being used, inappropriate drug habituation (untreated), failure to obtain pain relief in a screening trial, and poor personal hygiene.

Psychological evaluation and appropriate patient selection are critical to patient outcomes. Selection criteria for intrathecal pump placement include stable medical condition amenable to surgery; clear organic pain generator; no psychological or sociological contraindications; no familial contraindication, such as severe codependent behavior; documented responsible behavior and stable social situation; good pain relief with oral or parenteral opioids therapy; baseline neurological exam and psychological evaluation; failure of more conservative therapy; constant or almost-constant pain requiring round-the-clock opioid therapy; no tumor encroachment of the thecal sac in cancer patients; life expectancy greater than 3 months; no practical issues that might interfere with device placement, maintenance, or assessment (e.g., morbid obesity, severe cognitive impairment); and positive response to an intrathecal trial.

Common intrathecal trial approaches include single-shot injection, multiple bolus injections, and continuous infusion. Opioids that are used for intrathecal therapy include morphine (FDA approved) and several other off-label drugs such as hydromorphine, fentanyl, and sufentanil.[42] These drugs are commonly used as a single agent or in combination with a local anesthetic, bupivacaine. Nonopioid drugs include ziconitide, clonidine, and bupivacaine. In general, a greater than 50% pain reduction is expected for a successful trial without major side effects.

An intrathecal pump is placed in patients after a successful trial. Briefly, the pump reservoir site is marked on the patient's abdomen. IV antibiotic should be given 30 minutes before the incision is made. The patient is placed in the lateral decubitus position with pump site in the nondependent position. The intrathecal catheter is placed through a spinal needle and catheter guide wire. A purse-string suture is tied around the fascia surrounding the catheter. An anchor is attached to the fascia via nonabsorbable sutures. A subcutaneous pocket in the abdominal wall is prepared that is large enough to accommodate the pump. A subcutaneous tunnel is formed from the spinal incision site to the pocket. The catheter is passed through the tunnel and connected to the pump. The pump is positioned inside the pocket with nonabsorbable suture. The incisions are closed with sutures.

For cancer pain, the success rate of intrathecal delivery is around 85%. One study showed that patients with cancer receiving intrathecal morphine survived longer, had fewer side effects, and reported less pain.[42] The efficacy of IDDS for treatment of chronic noncancer pain seems less clear and robust. Complications include intrathecal infection, bleeding, pump reservoir site hematoma, leakage of CSF, catheter failure, and catheter tip granulomas.

PERCUTANEOUS CERVICAL CORDOTOMY (PCC)

Percutaneous cervical cordotomy (PCC) is performed to lesion the spinothalamic tract in the spinal cord and disrupt pain processing before it is integrated in the brain. It may be indicated in patients with cancer-related pain that is unilaterally localized below the C5 dermatome, such as unilateral chess wall pain, and extremity pathologies (unilateral/bilateral) in cancer patients with a life expectancy of less than 1 year.[47,48] It has a special place in the treatment of a large group of patients suffering from pain associated with primary lung cancer, including mesothelioma and Pancoast syndrome. PCC should also be considered for treating metastatic carcinoma pain. Contraindications include expected survival of less than 3 months, coagulation disorder, severely reduced ventilator function (FEV_1 <12 mg kg^{-1}), the patient not being able to cooperate, severe pulmonary dysfunction, and bilateral upper extremity pathologies.

PCC can be performed under fluoroscopy,[49] CT,[50] or microendoscopy[51] guidance. CT-guided PCC offers the advantage of superior topographical orientation in the spinothalamic tract. The patient is awake so is able to provide feedback during the procedure. A radiofrequency needle is directed under CT guidance following intrathecal contrast administration into the C1–C2 interspace contralateral to the side of the pain. Following flow of CSF, a stimulating electrode is then advanced into the lateral spinothalamic tract. After electrophysiological verification, two to three lesions are made using radiofrequency ablation (80°C for 60 seconds)[52] until the patient reports diminished sensation in the area of pain.[48] The procedure can be repeated on the other side a minimum of 1 week later.

Impressive outcomes have been reported.[53] It is estimated that 80% of patients report a satisfactory reduction in pain at 6 months. Mild weakness of the leg contralateral to the side of the pain, due to damage of the corticospinal tract, and, rarely, in the arm is seen in up to 8%–10% of patients in the first few days. Prolonged weakness has been reported in only 1–2%. Weakness usually improves within 48 hours, but occasionally can take up to a month to settle. Other complications include painful dysesthesia, weakness of bowel and bladder control, hemiparesis, mirror-image pain, headache, and adhesive arachnoiditis. Respiratory dysfunction is the main cause of procedure-related mortality (1%–6%). But in recent studies that used more accurate ablation techniques, no respiratory dysfunction occurred.

DORSAL ROOT ENTRY ZONE (DREZ) LESIONING

Dorsal root entry zone lesioning (DREZotomy) is a modality used to treat intractable pain caused by insults to neural structures.[54-56] DREZ lesioning is excellent for brachial plexus avulsion pain, patients with segmental pain at the level of their spinal cord injury, radiation plexopathy, and inoperable upper thoracic tumors that compress the brachial plexus (Pancoast tumor). DREZ lesioning is good for pain involving one upper extremity. The following findings wound indicate poor outcomes with DREZ lesioning: constant burning pain in the limb; pain that extends outside the region of the limb, such as shoulder, trunk, or pelvis; and burning pain in the lower extremities that is well below the level of a spinal cord injury.

Under general anesthesia, the patient is placed in the prone position. A laminectomy or hemilaminectomy at the site of the pain is performed initially. The dura is opened in the midline and a radiofrequency electrode is inserted at the DREZ. Multiple lesions 1–2 mm apart are made targeting dorsal rootles, substantia gelatinosa, and Lissauer's tract.

A recent study reported on 40 patients who underwent microsurgical DREZotomy for relief of intractable pain; there were 27 brachial plexus injuries (BPIs), 6 spinal cord injuries, 3 neoplasms, and 4 other causes.[54] A significant reduction in pain was observed for both average and maximal pain. Favorable outcome (≥50% pain reduction) was observed in 67.5% of patients, with the best outcome for BPI-related pain. Injury of the spinal nerve root (root avulsion or injury) was significantly associated with good pain relief. Electrical pain and lower number of painful dermatomes were significantly associated with good maximal pain relief. The study's authors concluded that this procedure is an effective for treatment of intractable pain in well-selected patients, particularly in cases with brachial plexus avulsion pain. Another study of 83 patients reported the outcomes of nucleus caudalis (NC) or spinal DREZ.[55] Indications for NC DREZ lesioning included trigeminal neuropathic pain (6), trigeminal deafferentation pain (3), glossopharyngeal or occipital neuralgia (3), PHN (3), and trauma (1). Indications of spinal DREZ lesioning included brachial plexus avulsion (20), PHN (19), spinal cord injury (11), phantom limb pain (8), pelvic pain (5), and CRPS (4).[55] Pain relief was most significant among patients with trigeminal pain, traumatic brachial plexus avulsion injuries, spinal cord injury, and traumatic phantom limb pain. Mean pain reduction averaged 58.3% at a mean follow-up of 8.3 years. Complications included three cases of paresis, three cases of neuropathy/radiculopathy, two cases of ataxia, three general medical conditions (colitis, two; atelectasis, one), and two cases of persistent incisional site pain. Pain relief lasted an average of 4.3 years. Thus, spinal and NC DREZ lesioning can provide effective relief in well-selected patients with intractable pain arising from trigeminal neuralgia, spinal cord injury, brachial plexus avulsions, PHN, and phantom limb pain.

COMMISSURAL MYELOTOMY

As a method to abolish midline visceral pain, commissural myelotomy transects the ascending visceral pain fibers and spinothalamic tract fibers that cross midline from the dorsal horn to the contralateral spinothalamic pathway. This procedure interrupts painful bilateral signals from the viscera and is used in patients with midline or bilateral abdominal or pelvic pain from cervical, pancreatic, or gastric cancers as well as sacral or bilateral leg pain.

Both CT-guided percutaneous and open myelotomy techniques have been described. In open surgery, a midline incision is made and a laminectomy performed, usually from T10 to L1. The thecal sac is opened, the midline septum is exposed, and a radiofrequency or mechanical lesion is made through the dorsal median sulcus.

Outcomes data are limited to case reports.[57] Eight articles on 175 cases of complete commissural myelotomy reported complete relief of pain was achieved in an average of 92% of the cases. In the cases where follow-up was longer and up to 11 years, 59% of 63 patients with malignant tumors and 48% of 21 patients with pain from nonmalignant causes had a "good" outcome. Leg weakness (unilateral or bilateral) occurred in 27% of patients. Diminished proprioception

in the lower extremities is common but difficult to measure. About 9% of patients developed dysesthesias resulting in either gait disturbances or, worse, burning sensation in the legs.

CINGULOTOMY

Cingulotomy is reserved for patients with metastatic cancer and medically refractory pain at multiple sites who are not candidates for other surgical interventions.[58] The anterior cingulate gyrus is a limbic structure located superior to the corpus callosum. It participates in the processing of behavior and emotion, including the affective aspect of chronic pain. Radiofrequency bilateral lesioning of the anterior cingulate is performed stereotactically with MRI guidance through paramedian burr holes.

Cingulotomy has been reported to be safe and effective in resolving chronic refractory pain.[58] It did not affect patient cognition or the sensory conductive pathway. However, patients who had recurrent intractable pain after a cingulotomy did not respond well to the reoperation. In a review of 11 articles with a total of 224 patients, greater than 60% of patients across all studies were reported to have significant pain relief postoperatively as well as at 1 year after surgery.[59] Common transient adverse effects included urinary incontinence and confusion/disorientation, which subsided within days postoperatively. Serious or permanent adverse effects included seizure in less than 5%, hemiparesis in less than 1%, and personality change in less than 1% of operations reported across all studies, all of which occurred primarily in operations where MRI guidance was not used.

MICROVASCULAR DECOMPRESSION (MVD) FOR TRIGEMINAL NEURALGIA AND GLOSSOPHARYNGEAL NEURALGIA

Trigeminal neuralgia and glossopharyngeal neuralgia are characterized by severe, episodic pain in the trigeminal nerve or glossopharyngeal nerve distribution and are most commonly managed by medical therapy. Glossopharyngeal neuralgia is sometimes confused with trigeminal neuralgia, characterized by excruciating pain in the throat and ear. For patients with refractory pain or those who have developed tolerance to medications, interventional or surgical treatment is available. These procedures include microvascular decompression, trigeminal or glossopharyngeal nerve blocks, and/or percutaneous radiofrequency rhizotomy. Percutaneous glycerol rhizotomy, percutaneous balloon compression, and stereotactic radiosurgery have also been used to treat refractory trigeminal neuralgia.[60]

Neurovascular compression is sometimes seen, and the pain is typically relieved with MVD of cranial nerve V for trigeminal neuralgia or cranial nerve IX for glossopharyngeal neuralgia. MVD remains the gold-standard operative therapy.[60] While it is the most invasive treatment option, it has also been shown to provide long-lasting relief. It is generally considered the preferred option in younger patients with few comorbidities and evidence of neurovascular compression. Patients are operated on under general anesthesia. A rectosigmoid craniotomy is used to gain entry into the posterior fossa. After opening the dura, the offending vessel is dissected off the trigeminal nerve or glossopharyngeal nerve, and a piece of Telfa or other nonabsorbent material is put in its place.

Patients often report significant improvement of their pain shortly after surgery, but more delayed improvements may also be seen. MVD is associated with long-term pain relief and a low rate of pain recurrence, compared to other modalities, along with a relatively low risk of complications. In studies of trigeminal neuralgia with follow-up of up to 10 years, 65%–70% of patients were still pain-free. Repeat MVD surgery is less likely to be effective and has an increased risk of facial weakness. Sensory loss is reported to be 5%–10% and CSF leak occurs in 7% of patients. Hearing loss and facial weakness may be seen. The mortality rate has been reported to be 0.37%.

STEREOTACTIC RADIOSURGERY

Stereotactic radiosurgery using a Gamma Knife (GK) or cyberknife system is a noninvasive technique used to treat refractory trigeminal neuralgia[61–63] and glossopharyngeal neuralgia.[64,65] The trigeminal nerve is lesioned at the root entry zone and the glossopharyngeal nerve is lesioned at the glossopharyngeal meatus using focused radiation with doses between 70 and 90 Gy. Pain relief is delayed several weeks, unlike with other procedures that may acutely relieve the pain. Most studies report that 50%–80% of patients achieve good pain control at long-term follow-up.[66] Increased radiation doses are associated with an increase in paresthesias or dysesthesias. Repeat treatment with GK is an option for recurrent or refractory cases. Compared to MVD, GK treatment is associated with a lower rate of long-term pain-free outcomes.[61–63,66] Overall, the low complication rate, coupled with short recovery, makes this an excellent option for higher-risk surgical patients or for those who prefer to avoid more invasive surgical options.

REFERENCES

1. Nizard J, Raoul S, Nguyen JP, Lefaucheur JP. Invasive stimulation therapies for the treatment of refractory pain. *Discov Med*. 2012;14:237–246.
2. Pope JE, Deer TR, Bruel BM, Falowski S. Clinical uses of intrathecal therapy and its placement in the pain care algorithm. *Pain Pract*. 2016;16(8):1092–1106.
3. Melzack R, Wall PD. Pain mechanisms: a new theory. *Science*. 1965;150:971–979.
4. Shealy CN, Mortimer JT, Reswick JB. Electrical inhibition of pain by stimulation of the dorsal columns: preliminary clinical report. *Anesth Analg*. 1967;46:489–491.
5. Mekhail NA, Cheng J, Narouze S, Kapural L, Mekhail MN, Deer T. Clinical applications of neurostimulation: forty years later. *Pain Pract*. 2010;10:103–112.
6. Xu J, Liu A, Cheng J. New advancements in spinal cord stimulation for chronic pain management. *Curr Opin Anaesthesiol*. 2017;30(6):710–717.
7. Mekhail NA, Mathews M, Nageeb F, Guirguis M, Mekhail MN, Cheng J. Retrospective review of 707 cases of spinal cord stimulation: indications and complications. *Pain Pract*. 2011;11:148–153.
8. Deer TR, Mekhail N, Provenzano D, et al. The appropriate use of neurostimulation of the spinal cord and peripheral nervous system for the treatment of chronic pain and ischemic diseases: the Neuromodulation Appropriateness Consensus Committee. *Neuromodulation*. 2014;17:515–550; discussion 550.
9. Kumar K, Taylor RS, Jacques L, et al. The effects of spinal cord stimulation in neuropathic pain are sustained: a 24-month follow-up of the prospective randomized controlled multicenter trial of the effectiveness of spinal cord stimulation. *Neurosurgery*. 2008;63:762–770; discussion 770.
10. Kumar K, Taylor RS, Jacques L, et al. Spinal cord stimulation versus conventional medical management for neuropathic pain: a multicentre randomised controlled trial in patients with failed back surgery syndrome. *Pain*. 2007;132:179–188.
11. Grider JS, Manchikanti L, Carayannopoulos A, et al. Effectiveness of spinal cord stimulation in chronic spinal pain: a systematic review. *Pain Physician*. 2016;19:E33–E54.

12. Kapural L, Yu C, Doust MW, et al. Novel 10-kHz high-frequency therapy (HF10 therapy) is superior to traditional low-frequency spinal cord stimulation for the treatment of chronic back and leg pain: the SENZA-RCT randomized controlled trial. *Anesthesiology.* 2015;123:851–860.

13. Kapural L, Yu C, Doust MW, et al. Comparison of 10-kHz high-frequency and traditional low-frequency spinal cord stimulation for the treatment of chronic back and leg pain: 24-month results from a multicenter, randomized, controlled pivotal trial. *Neurosurgery.* 2016;79:667–677.

14. Miller JP, Eldabe S, Buchser E, Johanek LM, Guan Y, Linderoth B. Parameters of spinal cord stimulation and their role in electrical charge delivery: a review. *Neuromodulation.* 2016;19:373–384.

15. Deer TR, Levy RM, Kramer J, et al. Dorsal root ganglion stimulation yielded higher treatment success rate for complex regional pain syndrome and causalgia at 3 and 12 months: a randomized comparative trial. *Pain.* 2017;158:669–681.

16. Harrison C, Epton S, Bojanic S, Green AL, FitzGerald JJ. The efficacy and safety of dorsal root ganglion stimulation as a treatment for neuropathic pain: a literature review. *Neuromodulation.* 2018;21(3):225–233.

17. Huygen F, Liem L, Cusack W, Kramer J. Stimulation of the L2-L3 dorsal root ganglia induces effective pain relief in the low back. *Pain Pract.* 2018;18(2):205–213.

18. Shamji MF, Westwick HJ, Heary RF. Complications related to the use of spinal cord stimulation for managing persistent postoperative neuropathic pain after lumbar spinal surgery. *Neurosurg Focus.* 2015;39:E15.

19. Campbell CM, Jamison RN, Edwards RR. Psychological screening/phenotyping as predictors for spinal cord stimulation. *Curr Pain Headache Rep.* 2013;17:307.

20. Goroszeniuk T, Pang D. Peripheral neuromodulation: a review. *Curr Pain Headache Rep.* 2014;18:412.

21. Wall PD, Sweet WH. Temporary abolition of pain in man. *Science.* 1967;155:108–109.

22. Weiner RL, Reed KL. Peripheral neurostimulation for control of intractable occipital neuralgia. *Neuromodulation.* 1999;2:217–221.

23. Saper JR, Dodick DW, Silberstein SD, McCarville S, Sun M, Goadsby PJ. Occipital nerve stimulation for the treatment of intractable chronic migraine headache: ONSTIM feasibility study. *Cephalalgia.* 2011;31:271–285.

24. Rodrigo D, Acin P, Bermejo P. Occipital nerve stimulation for refractory chronic migraine: results of a long-term prospective study. *Pain Physician.* 2017;20:e151–e159.

25. Chen YF, Bramley G, Unwin G, et al. Occipital nerve stimulation for chronic migraine—a systematic review and meta-analysis. *PLoS One.* 2015;10:e0116786.

26. Burns B, Watkins L, Goadsby PJ. Treatment of medically intractable cluster headache by occipital nerve stimulation: long-term follow-up of eight patients. *Lancet.* 2007;369:1099–1106.

27. Brewer AC, Trentman TL, Ivancic MG, et al. Long-term outcome in occipital nerve stimulation patients with medically intractable primary headache disorders. *Neuromodulation.* 2013;16:557–562; discussion 563–554.

28. Chakravarthy K, Nava A, Christo PJ, Williams K. Review of recent advances in peripheral nerve stimulation (PNS). *Curr Pain Headache Rep.* 2016;20:60.

29. Kloimstein H, Likar R, Kern M, et al. Peripheral nerve field stimulation (PNFS) in chronic low back pain: a prospective multicenter study. *Neuromodulation.* 2014;17:180–187.

30. Verrills P, Russo M. Peripheral nerve stimulation for back pain. *Prog Neurol Surg.* 2015;29:127–138.

31. Mitchell B, Verrills P, Vivian D, DuToit N, Barnard A, Sinclair C. Peripheral nerve field stimulation therapy for patients with thoracic pain: a prospective study. *Neuromodulation.* 2016;19:752–759.

32. Verrills P, Rose R, Mitchell B, Vivian D, Barnard A. Peripheral nerve field stimulation for chronic headache: 60 cases and long-term follow-up. *Neuromodulation.* 2014;17:54–59.

33. Pope JE, Carlson JD, Rosenberg WS, Slavin KV, Deer TR. Peripheral nerve stimulation for pain in extremities: an update. *Prog Neurol Surg.* 2015;29:139–157.

34. Tsubokawa T, Katayama Y, Yamamoto T, Hirayama T, Koyama S. Chronic motor cortex stimulation for the treatment of central pain. *Acta Neurochir Suppl.* 1991;52:137–139.

35. Garcia-Larrea L, Peyron R. Motor cortex stimulation for neuropathic pain: from phenomenology to mechanisms. *NeuroImage.* 2007;37(Suppl 1):S71–S79.

36. Nguyen JP, Nizard J, Keravel Y, Lefaucheur JP. Invasive brain stimulation for the treatment of neuropathic pain. *Nat Rev Neurol.* 2011;7:699–709.

37. Fontaine D, Hamani C, Lozano A. Efficacy and safety of motor cortex stimulation for chronic neuropathic pain: critical review of the literature. *J Neurosurg.* 2009;110:251–256.

38. Pereira EA, Boccard SG, Linhares P, et al. Thalamic deep brain stimulation for neuropathic pain after amputation or brachial plexus avulsion. *Neurosurg Focus.* 2013;35:E7.

39. Abreu V, Vaz R, Rebelo V, et al. Thalamic deep brain stimulation for neuropathic pain: efficacy at three years' follow-up. *Neuromodulation.* 2017;20:504–513.

40. Boccard SG, Pereira EA, Moir L, Aziz TZ, Green AL. Long-term outcomes of deep brain stimulation for neuropathic pain. *Neurosurgery*. 2013;72:221–230; discussion 231.

41. Gray AM, Pounds-Cornish E, Eccles FJ, Aziz TZ, Green AL, Scott RB. Deep brain stimulation as a treatment for neuropathic pain: a longitudinal study addressing neuropsychological outcomes. *J Pain*. 2014;15:283–292.

42. Pope JE, Deer TR, Amirdelfan K, McRoberts WP, Azeem N. The pharmacology of spinal opioids and ziconotide for the treatment of non-cancer pain. *Curr Neuropharmacol*. 2017;15:206–216.

43. McGuire D, Bowersox S, Fellmann JD, Luther RR. Sympatholysis after neuron-specific, N-type, voltage-sensitive calcium channel blockade: first demonstration of N-channel function in humans. *J Cardiovasc Pharmacol*. 1997;30:400–403.

44. Brose WG, Gutlove DP, Luther RR, Bowersox SS, McGuire D. Use of intrathecal SNX-111, a novel, N-type, voltage-sensitive, calcium channel blocker, in the management of intractable brachial plexus avulsion pain. *Clin J Pain*. 1997;13:256–259.

45. Bruel BM, Burton AW. Intrathecal therapy for cancer-related pain. *Pain Med*. 2016;17:2404–2421.

46. Fallon MT. Neuropathic pain in cancer. *Br J Anaesth*. 2013;111:105–111.

47. Bellini M, Barbieri M. Percutaneous cervical cordotomy in cancer pain. *Anaesthesiol Intensive Ther*. 2016;48:197–200.

48. Bain E, Hugel H, Sharma M. Percutaneous cervical cordotomy for the management of pain from cancer: a prospective review of 45 cases. *J Palliat Med*. 2013;16:901–907.

49. Sanders M, Zuurmond W. Safety of unilateral and bilateral percutaneous cervical cordotomy in 80 terminally ill cancer patients. *J Clin Oncol*. 1995;13:1509–1512.

50. Kanpolat Y, Ugur HC, Ayten M, Elhan AH. Computed tomography-guided percutaneous cordotomy for intractable pain in malignancy. *Neurosurgery*. 2009;64:ons187–193; discussion ons193–184.

51. Fonoff ET, Lopez WO, de Oliveira YS, Teixeira MJ. Microendoscopy-guided percutaneous cordotomy for intractable pain: case series of 24 patients. *J Neurosurg*. 2016;124:389–396.

52. Shepherd TM, Hoch MJ, Cohen BA, et al. Palliative CT-guided cordotomy for medically intractable pain in patients with cancer. *Am J Neuroradiol*. 2017;38:387–390.

53. Raslan AM, Cetas JS, McCartney S, Burchiel KJ. Destructive procedures for control of cancer pain: the case for cordotomy. *J Neurosurg*. 2011;114:155–170.

54. Piyawattanametha N, Sitthinamsuwan B, Euasobhon P, Zinboonyahgoon N, Rushatamukayanunt P, Nunta-Aree S. Efficacy and factors determining the outcome of dorsal root entry zone lesioning procedure (DREZotomy) in the treatment of intractable pain syndrome. *Acta Neurochir (Wien)*. 2017;159(12):2431–2442.

55. Chivukula S, Tempel ZJ, Chen CJ, Shin SS, Gande AV, Moossy JJ. Spinal and nucleus caudalis dorsal root entry zone lesioning for chronic pain: efficacy and outcomes. *World Neurosurg*. 2015;84:494–504.

56. Konrad P. Dorsal root entry zone lesion, midline myelotomy and anterolateral cordotomy. *Neurosurg Clinics North Am*. 2014;25:699–722.

57. Viswanathan A, Burton AW, Rekito A, McCutcheon IE. Commissural myelotomy in the treatment of intractable visceral pain: technique and outcomes. *Stereotact Funct Neurosurg*. 2010;88:374–382.

58. Wang GC, Harnod T, Chiu TL, Chen KP. Effect of an anterior cingulotomy on pain, cognition, and sensory pathways. *World Neurosurg*. 2017;102:593–597.

59. Sharim J, Pouratian N. Anterior cingulotomy for the treatment of chronic intractable pain: a systematic review. *Pain Physician*. 2016;19:537–550.

60. Bick SKB, Eskandar EN. Surgical treatment of trigeminal neuralgia. *Neurosurg Clin North Am*. 2017;28:429–438.

61. Wang DD, Raygor KP, Cage TA, et al. Prospective comparison of long-term pain relief rates after first-time microvascular decompression and stereotactic radiosurgery for trigeminal neuralgia. *J Neurosurg*. 2017:1–10.

62. Regis J, Tuleasca C, Resseguier N, et al. Long-term safety and efficacy of Gamma Knife surgery in classical trigeminal neuralgia: a 497-patient historical cohort study. *J Neurosurg*. 2016;124:1079–1087.

63. Berger I, Nayak N, Schuster J, Lee J, Stein S, Malhotra NR. Microvascular decompression versus stereotactic radiosurgery for trigeminal neuralgia: a decision analysis. *Cureus*. 2017;9:e1000.

64. Pommier B, Touzet G, Lucas C, Vermandel M, Blond S, Reyns N. Glossopharyngeal neuralgia treated by Gamma Knife radiosurgery: safety and efficacy through long-term follow-up. *J Neurosurg*. 2018;128(5):1372–1379.

65. Kano H, Urgosik D, Liscak R, et al. Stereotactic radiosurgery for idiopathic glossopharyngeal neuralgia: an international multicenter study. *J Neurosurg*. 2016;125:147–153.

66. Borius PY, Tuleasca C, Muraciole X, et al. Gamma Knife radiosurgery for glossopharyngeal neuralgia: a study of 21 patients with long-term follow-up. *Cephalalgia*. 2018;38(3):543–550.

9

Postsurgical Neuralgia

JOHN P. KENNY IV AND DALIA ELMOFTY

CASE

A 65-year-old man presents to the pain clinic 3 months after a laparoscopic Heller myotomy for the treatment of achalasia. The patient reports that his postoperative pain, located primarily at the port sites, was poorly controlled. He was discharged home on postoperative day 3 with an oral analgesic regimen of hydrocodone-acetaminophen 5–325 mg every 6 hours as needed. Over the next 2 weeks, the pain subsided in two of the three port sites; however, he has noticed that the pain at his left upper abdomen is worsening. In the following 10 weeks, the pain changes in character from a constant ache to a sharp and burning sensation radiating to the midline and around his back. A computerized tomography (CT) scan of his abdomen and pelvis reveals no abnormality. He is diagnosed with chronic abdominal wall pain and started on a neuropathic oral analgesic regimen of gabapentin 300 mg three times a day and amitriptyline 10 mg at bedtime.

DISCUSSION

Chronic postsurgical pain is a common, yet poorly defined phenomenon occurring after surgical procedures. It affects a patient's quality of life, productivity, personal relationships, and finances. One type of chronic postsurgical pain is postsurgical neuralgia (PSN), which is a result of peripheral nerve dysfunction. Studies have described its prevalence from 10% to 50% depending on the location of the operative site. One recent systematic literature review estimated that one in five patients undergoing surgery will develop chronic incisional pain.[1] Identification of high-risk patients and subsequent prevention is critical. Patient characteristics associated with a propensity to develop chronic pain include demographic and psychological factors. Young, obese females with anxiety, depression, or both and catastrophizing behavior are at higher risk than others.[2]

DEFINITION

The International Association for the Study of Pain (IASP) defines neuralgia as pain in the distribution of a nerve or nerves that may be paroxysmal in nature.[3] Chronic pain is pain without biological value that has persisted beyond the normal tissue healing time.[3] Chronic postsurgical pain (CPSP) has been described by the following criteria[4]: (1) pain that develops after a surgical procedure, (2) pain lasting at least 2 months, (3) infection as a cause has been excluded, and (4) pain continuing from a preexisting condition has been excluded.

Multiple postsurgical pain syndromes have been described according to the type of surgical procedure performed: mastectomy, thoracotomy, sternotomy, herniorraphy, and cholecystectomy. A strong correlation exists between patient characteristics and PSN.[2]

PREVALENCE

Historically the prevalence of CPSP has been considered to be 20%; however, there is wide variability in the rates (see Table 9.1) and in the assessment tools to obtain the percentages. A recent systematic review of 281 studies that used the neuropathic pain probability grading system to determine the prevalence of postsurgical neuropathic pain found rates of between 6% and 68%, depending on the surgical procedure.[1] Rates were 66% after thoracic surgery, 68% after breast surgery, 31% after hernia repairs, 7.5%–14% after thyroid procedures, and 6% after total hip or knee arthroplasty.[1,5] Other studies have estimated different rates: amputation 30%–50%,[6] breast surgery 20%–30%,[7] thoracotomy 30%–40%,[8] inguinal hernia repair 10%,[9] coronary artery bypass grafting (CABG) surgery 30%–50%,[10] and

TABLE 9.1. INCIDENCE OF CHRONIC POSTSURGICAL PAIN

Surgery Type	Incidence (%)
Breast surgery[1,7]	20–68
Thoracic surgery[1,8]	30–66
Limb amputation[6]	30–50
Coronary artery bypass surgery[10]	30–50
Inguinal hernia surgery[1,9]	10–31
Thyroid surgery[5]	7.5–14
Caesarean section surgery[11]	10
Knee or hip arthroplasty surgery[1]	6

TABLE 9.2. RISK FACTORS FOR CHRONIC POSTSURGICAL PAIN

Surgery-Specific Factors[22]
- Thoracotomy
- Mastectomy
- Axillary lymph node dissection
- Sternotomy
- Herniorraphy
- Amputation

Patient Factors[2,25,26]
- Old or young age
- Obesity
- Female gender
- Employment
- Private insurance

Psychological and Medical Factors[2]
- Anxiety
- Depression
- Stress
- Catastrophizing behavior
- Preoperative pain at site
- Smoker

caesarean section 10%.[11] The variability in prevalence rates can be attributed to a lack of standard criteria to classify PSN, patient characteristics, and surgical technique. Prevalence changes at different time points after surgery. As expected, the rates are reduced over time. A prospective study of patients undergoing thoracotomy found the prevalence of surgical site pain at 3 months was 80%, at 6 months was 75%, and at 1 year was 61%.[12] Another retrospective study determined that the rates of thoracotomy pain were 70% at 1 month and 41% at 1 year.[8] The intensity of pain also lessens over time. Two retrospective studies evaluating chronic post-mastectomy pain determined the prevalence to be 68% at 6 months, and 27% at approximately 3 years.[13,14] The time course of pain, including onset, duration, and change in intensity, is often unpredictable. Although pain intensity decreases in most patients at 6 months, 9% of patients in one study reported increases in pain.[14] In a prospective study of 318 post-sternotomy patients, the incidence of chronic pain was still 28% 1 year after surgery.[15] Chronic post-herniorraphy pain has been described in numerous studies, with a reported incidence of between 9% and 34%.[16,17] When specifically evaluating for pain associated with nerve injury, the prevalence has been reported at between 1% and 5% at 1 year.[18,19]

RISK FACTORS

Because the treatment of PSN can be difficult, prevention should be the first step in management. Since not all patients will develop PSN, identifying those at risk is essential (see Table 9.2). Certain surgical procedures, such as thoracotomy, mastectomy, sternotomy, and herniorraphy, are associated with high rates of pain. Newer data suggest patient-specific risk factors for PSN. These risk factors are young age, obesity, female sex, and psychological characteristics such as anxiety, depression, stress, and catastrophizing.[2]

Regarding chronic post-mastectomy pain, a retrospective cohort study identified young age and high body mass index (BMI) as risk factors for developing PSN.[14] Pain at the site before surgery is also a risk factor.[20] In a prospective questionnaire-based study of patients undergoing mastectomy, history of chronic pain, multiple surgeries, preoperative pain at the incision site, high BMI, history of smoking, and older age were risk factors for PSN.[21]

Factors specific to the treatment and perioperative course of mastectomy surgery have been associated with chronic pain. Patients who undergo axillary lymph node dissection are at higher risk of developing chronic pain.[22] Postoperatively, uncontrolled acute pain and adjuvant radiation therapy are also associated with the development of chronic pain.[23,24]

Risk factors for chronic pain after inguinal hernia repair are similar to those for chronic post-mastectomy pain: young age, obesity, preoperative pain at the surgical site, chronic pain syndromes, employment status, and private insurance.[25,26] Direct nerve injury also positively correlated with PSN. The use of mesh was thought to be a risk factor; however, recent data suggest otherwise.[27] A large study demonstrated no difference in PSN after laparoscopic and open mesh repair.[28] Similarly, young age and a high BMI were identified as risk factors for chronic pain after sternotomy.

ETIOLOGY AND PATHOPHYSIOLOGY

Neuralgia is caused by injury to a nerve, which results in dysfunction and dysesthesia. The modes of injury during surgery include transection, constriction, traction, crush, and inflammation. Currently, the association between the mechanism and extent of nerve injury that produces symptoms is poorly understood. Four main mechanisms have been implicated in the sensation of pain in the context of neuralgia: ion channel dysfunction, ectopic mechanical signals, pain fiber cross-stimulation by nonpain fibers, and central nervous system dysfunction.

PSN pain starts with a surgical insult that discharges high-threshold nociceptors and increases nerve impulses in the short term. The increase in pain impulses combined with an inflammatory response results in peripheral sensitization. In the spinal cord, inhibitory pathways are decreased and primary afferent nerves sprout into the dorsal root ganglion.[29]

Post-mastectomy pain can arise from multiple factors, including intercostobrachial neuralgia, motor nerve injury, phantom breast, and neuroma formation.[7,30] The most common cause of post-mastectomy pain is intercostobrachial neuralgia when the nerve is injured during axillary node dissection. The prevalence is 13% to 68%.[7] The medial and lateral pectoral, long thoracic and thoracodorsal nerves also may be injured with forceful traction during surgery. Although damage to motor nerves is unlikely to result in chronic pain, it is believed that damage to the nervi nervorum surrounding motor nerves can cause neuropathic pain.[31]

The relatively small intercostal space leaves the intercostal nerves highly susceptible to injury during both open and closed thoracic procedures.[32] During video-assisted thoracotomies, trocars have been implicated in causing nerve damage. Damage to intercostal nerves and the brachial plexus has also been implicated in post-sternotomy pain. Burning anterior chest wall pain, also known as internal mammary artery syndrome, is thought to be a result of damage to the intercostal nerves during dissection of the internal mammary artery.[33] Nerve entrapment during closure may be another cause of pain.

In post-herniorraphy pain the ilioinguinal, iliohypogastric, genitofemoral, lateral femoral cutaneous, or femoral nerves can be damaged during traction, dissection, or repair.[34] Surgeons avoid the "triangle of pain," a space defined by the gonadal vessels medially, the reflected peritoneum laterally, and the iliopubic tract superiorly. Entry into the triangle of pain may damage the femoral, femoral branch of the genitofemoral, or the lateral femoral cutaneous nerve.

The nerves most often implicated in the development of PSN are the intercostobrachial, intercostal, iliohypogastric, ilioinguinal, and genitofemoral. The rigidity of the chest wall, in comparison to the pliability of the abdominal wall, may be the reason for the higher prevalence of PSN after thoracic surgeries.[35]

CLINICAL CHARACTERISTICS

The negative symptom of PSN is an area of anesthesia or analgesia; positive symptoms include paresthesias and stereotypical neuropathic pain.[36] This pain is continuous and paroxysmal and is described as burning, shooting, or aching. Other positive neuropathic symptoms are hyperalgesia, allodynia, anesthesia dolorosa, and hyperpathia.

The type and intensity of symptoms vary from patient to patient, even with similar nerve injuries. Some pain syndromes, however, have a classic presentation. Chronic burning pain in the anterior chest wall is associated with left internal mammary artery dissection in CABG surgery. Lingual nerve injury during surgical extraction of the mandibular third molar often causes paresthesias rather than pain.[37] Anesthesia dolorosa along the distribution of the affected nerve is characteristic of intercostal nerve injury during thoracotomy. Patients with post-sternotomy pain complain of pain in the chest, head, neck, shoulder, or between the scapulae.

Individual sensory nerves may be injured during breast cancer surgeries. Injury to the intercostobrachial nerve during breast surgery produces aching, burning, or stabbing pain in the upper medial arm.[38] Notalgia paresthetica results from injury to the long thoracic nerve. Symptoms of the injury are burning pain between the medial border of the scapula and the spine on the ipsilateral side.[39]

DIAGNOSTIC MODALITIES

The diagnosis of neuralgia can be difficult and relies on a thorough history and physical examination. Obtaining a detailed description of the characteristics of the pain is helpful in making a diagnosis. Pain assessment scales, such as the McGill Pain Questionnaire, can be useful in characterizing the pain. Nerve conduction studies may identify a single nerve responsible for the symptoms.[40] A detailed evaluation of the pain, including intensity and aggravating and alleviating factors, will help determine the adequacy of any treatment.

PREVENTION

Once PSN develops, it can be difficult to treat; therefore, the identification of patients at risk for PSN is an important element in management. Prevention of PSN can minimize its burden on the healthcare system and improve the quality of life of patients.

In animals opioids, local anesthetics, NMDA receptor antagonists, and anti-inflammatory drugs are effective in preventing pain-like behavior.[35] No single pharmacological technique or intervention has been shown to prevent PSN alone. A multimodal approach to prevention may be the most beneficial. Promising results have been found with ketamine, pregabalin, or gabapentin, although data are insufficient to determine doses and treatment duration with these medications at this time. In one study, however, 2 weeks of perioperative pregabalin for patients undergoing total knee arthroplasty decreased neuropathic pain from 5% to zero at 6 months.[41] In a meta-analysis that studied pregabalin and gabapentin for the prevention of chronic postsurgical pain, six of the eight gabapentin trials demonstrated a moderate-to-large reduction in chronic pain, and the pregabalin studies were even more promising.[42] In a randomized, double-blinded clinical trial, perioperative administration of venlafaxine reduced the incidence of postsurgical mastectomy pain at 6 months.[43]

There have been multiple studies investigating the efficacy of epidural anesthesia on the prevention of chronic postsurgical pain. When thoracic epidurals were used for the prevention of chronic PSN in patients undergoing thoracotomy, at 6 months 12% of patients had moderate pain or less. The investigators compared this result to the 22% to 67% prevalence of post-thoracotomy pain found in the general population and determined that epidurals can be protective.[44] Another prospective randomized, double-blinded study comparing the effect of timing the initiation of epidural analgesia on chronic pain found that pain scores at 6 months were lower if the epidural was started 20 minutes before the incision than after completion of thoracotomy.[45]

Studies of paravertebral and intercostal nerve blocks for the prevention of PSN are conflicting. In one randomized trial, preincisional paravertebral blocks in patients reduced the rates of chronic post-mastectomy pain compared to patients without the nerve block.[46] In another study, however, intercostal nerve blocks did not reduce chronic post-thoracotomy pain.[47]

TREATMENT

Only a few randomized control trials have investigated the treatment of chronic PSN. Data from the treatment of other neuropathic pain syndromes is typically used to guide treatment of PSN. Treatment strategies can be divided into four categories: pharmacological, nerve stimulation, nerve blocks, and surgical. All chronic pain interventions should be accompanied by physical or occupational therapy, and patients should be referred to a pain psychiatrist or psychologist for cognitive-behavioral therapy and coping skills.[48]

Pharmacological

According to the neuropathic pain literature, no single medication is effective alone; however, a combination has been shown to be beneficial. Typical neuropathic pain medications include anticonvulsants, antidepressants, and opioids.

Antidepressants are of benefit in the treatment of chronic pain. Tricyclic antidepressants, such as amitriptyline and nortriptyline, have side effects. The tertiary amine amitriptyline can cause drowsiness and may be useful for patients with sleep disturbances because of pain. Nortriptyline, a secondary amine, may combat fatigue. In a randomized, double-blinded, placebo-controlled trial, amitriptyline had good pain-relieving effects in breast cancer patients with chronic neuropathic pain. Of the 15 patients, 8 had greater than 50% improvement in pain on a visual analog scale.[49] As for the 7 patients with less than 50% improvement in pain, amitriptyline dosing was limited by the side effects experienced by the patients. In a subsequent study, venlafaxine was chosen as an alternative because it was better tolerated by patients.[50] That randomized, double-blind, crossover study found no difference in average daily pain scores between patients given venlafaxine or placebo, but maximum daily pain intensity was reduced with venlafaxine.[50] The norepinephrine and dopamine reuptake inhibitor bupropion also was effective in the treatment of neuropathic pain.[51]

In two randomized control trials dedicated to studying the treatment of post-mastectomy pain, capsaicin cream was the intervention. In the first, with 99 patients, pain was reduced by 53% with 0.075% capsaicin cream and by 17% with placebo.[52] In the second, in 62% of patients pain was reduced by greater than 50% with treatment and by 30% with placebo.[53]

Gabapentin is one of the most commonly prescribed medications to treat neuropathic pain. In one randomized control study of responsiveness to gabapentin in 60 patients with post-traumatic neuralgia, there was a slight benefit from gabapentin over placebo.[54] Others have found a similar modest improvement in pain scores and sleep with once-daily dosing of gabapentin in patients with postherpetic neuralgia.[55]

Multiple small, randomized control trials have been conducted on the treatment of post-traumatic neuralgia using various intravenous medications. Although there was no single superior drug identified, these studies showed superiority at treating individual symptoms. Ketamine infusions were helpful in reducing spontaneous pain and tactile allodynia.[56–59] Alfentanil infusions were efficacious in reducing the area of tactile allodynia and the threshold of cold allodynia.[56,60] Lidocaine and magnesium infusions were not beneficial in pain reduction.[55,57,61]

Nerve Stimulation

Neuromodulation with spinal cord and peripheral nerve stimulators has been used for decades in the treatment of chronic neuropathic pain. Its utility for PSN has been extrapolated from the neuropathic pain literature. Peripheral nerve stimulators placed at occipital and trigeminal nerves were beneficial in patients for whom conservative treatments were not successful.[62,63]

Percutaneous electrical nerve stimulation (PENS) has been investigated for the treatment of neuropathic pain.[64] With PENS fine needles are placed percutaneously into trigger points, and electrical stimulation is applied to the area for a period of time. Of 66 patients included in a multicenter, prospective, observational study, 24 were suffering from chronic postsurgical pain. PENS relieved pain, and relief was long-lasting. PENS appears to be a safe and feasible alternative therapy.

Nerve Blocks

Neuralgia is caused by the dysfunction of an individual nerve. Identifying the culprit nerve and blocking its activity is an attractive therapy. Peripheral nerve blocks have been used for years in the treatment of neuralgia. These blocks can be achieved with local anesthetics, steroids, phenol, ethanol, thermal ablation, or surgical lysis. One study determined that parasternal nerve blocks to treat post-sternotomy pain were effective in 89% of 54 patients.[65] Initially, bupivacaine blocks were employed, then phenol blocks for nonresponders, followed by alcohol blocks for the remaining nonresponders. Another study found that some patients with post-mastectomy pain respond to stellate ganglion blocks.[66] The proposed mechanism for pain relief with this block is sympathetic mediation, and the stellate ganglion targets the sympathetic fibers from the upper extremities and axilla.

Surgical Intervention

Surgical procedures to treat PSN include nerve transection, neurolysis, venous wrapping, and nerve-to-nerve anastomosis.[67] Some surgical interventions are more beneficial in treating neuralgia depending on the mechanism of initial nerve injury. For instance, adhesive neuralgia responds well to vein wrapping procedures. Patients had substantial improvement in symptoms from pain associated with scar entrapment in the lower extremities.[68] These procedures are not curative, and therefore careful selection of patients is needed when considering surgical treatment of PSN.

Although spinal cord stimulation and intrathecal drug delivery have been studied for the treatment of neuropathic pain, there have are no large studies specifically targeting PSN. Smaller studies and case reports describe the efficacy of spinal cord stimulation in post-thoracotomy and post-mastectomy pain syndromes.[69,70]

GUIDING QUESTIONS
- What patient characteristics are risk factors for postsurgical neuralgia?
- What surgical characteristics are associated with it?

- What classes of medications have shown promise in preventing postsurgical neuralgia?
- What medications are effective in treating it?
- What nonpharmacological methods are used to treat postsurgical neuralgia?

KEY POINTS

- Chronic postsurgical pain causes significant strain on the patient and the healthcare system.
- Surgery-specific risk factors for postsurgical neuralgia are breast surgery, thoracic surgery, amputation, sternotomy, and inguinal herniorraphy.
- Patient-specific risk factors are young or old age, female gender, obesity, history of depression or anxiety, catastrophizing behavior, or preoperative pain at the surgical site.
- Because it is difficult to treat, prevention of postsurgical neuralgia is important.
- In animals, opioids, local anesthetics, NMDA receptor antagonists, and anti-inflammatory drugs were effective in the prevention of pain-like behavior.
- Pharmacological treatment is multimodal.
- Typical neuropathic pain medications include anticonvulsants, antidepressants, and opioids.

REFERENCES

1. Haroutiunian S, Nikolajsen L, Finnerup NB, Jensen TS. The neuropathic component in persistent postsurgical pain: a systematic literature review. *Pain.* 2013;154:95–102.
2. Rashiq S, Dick BD. Post-surgical pain syndromes: a review for the non-pain specialist. *Can J Anaesth.* 2014;61(2):123–130.
3. IASP Task Force on Taxonomy. Part III: pain terms, a current list with definitions and notes on usage. In: Merskey H, Bogduk N, eds. *Classification of Chronic Pain.* 2nd ed. Seattle, WA: IASP Press; 1994:209–214.
4. Macrae WA, Davies HT. Chronic postsurgical pain. In: Crombie IK, Croft PR, et al., eds. *Epidemiology of Pain.* Seattle: IASP Press; 1999.
5. Payakachat N, Ounpraseuth S, Suen JY. Late complications and long-term quality of life for survivors (>5 years) with history of head and neck cancer. *Head Neck.* 2013;35(6):819–825.
6. Nikolajsen L, Jensen TS. Phantom limb pain. *Br J Anaesth.* 2001; 87:107–116.
7. Jung BF, Ahrendt GM, Oaklander AL, Dworkin RH. Neuropathic pain following breast cancer surgery: proposed classification and research update. *Pain.* 2003;104:1–13.
8. Gotoda Y, Kambara N, Sakai T, et al. The morbidity, time course and predictive factors for persistent post-thoracotomy pain. *Eur J Pain.* 2001;5:89–96.
9. Aasvang E, Kehlet H. Chronic postoperative pain: the case of inguinal herniorrhaphy. *Br J Anaesth.* 2005;95:69–76.
10. Bruce J, Drury N, Poobalan AS, et al. The prevalence of chronic chest and leg pain following cardiac surgery: a historical cohort study. *Pain.* 2003;104:265–273.
11. Nikolajsen L, Sorensen HC, Jensen TS, Kehlet H. Chronic pain following caesarean section. *Acta Anaesthesiol Scand.* 2004;48:111–116.
12. Perttunen K, Tasmuth T, Kalso E. Chronic pain after thoracic surgery: a follow-up study. *Acta Anaesthesiol Scand.* 1999;43:563–567.
13. Carpenter JS, Andrykowski MA, Sloan P, et al. Postmastectomy/postlumpectomy pain in breast cancer survivors. *J Clin Epidemiol.* 1998;51:1285–1292.
14. Smith WC, Bourne D, Squair J, Phillips DO, Chambers WA. A retrospective cohort study of post mastectomy pain syndrome. *Pain.* 1999;83:91–95.
15. Van Leersum NJ, van Leersum RL, Verwey HF, Klautz RJM. Pain symptoms accompanying chronic poststernotomy pain: a pilot study. *Pain Med.* 2010;11:1628–1634.
16. Grant AM, Scott NW, O'Dwyer PJ. Five-year follow-up of a randomized trial to assess pain and numbness after laparoscopic or open repair of groin hernia. *Br J Surg.* 2004;91:1570–1574.
17. Aasvang EK, Bay-Nielsen M, Kehlet H. Pain and functional impairment 6 years after inguinal herniorrhaphy. *Hernia.* 2006;10:316–321.
18. Topal B, Hourlay P. Totally preperitoneal endoscopic inguinal hernia repair. *Br J Surg.* 1997;84:61–63.
19. Horton MD, Florence MG. Simplified preperitoneal Marlex hernia repair. *Am J Surg.* 1993;165:595–599.
20. Andersen KG, Kehlet H. Persistent pain after breast cancer treatment: a critical review of risk factors and strategies for prevention. *J Pain.* 2011;12(7):725–746.
21. Sipila R, Estlander AM, Tasmuth T, Kataja M, Kalso E. Development of a screening instrument for risk factors of persistent pain after breast cancer surgery. *Br J Cancer.* 2012;107:1459–1466.
22. Peintinger F, Reitsamer R, Stranzl H, Ralph G. Comparison of quality of life and arm complaints

after axillary lymph node dissection vs sentinel lymph node biopsy in breast cancer patients. *Br J Cancer*. 2003;89:648–652.

23. Howlader N, Noone AM, Krapcho M, et al., eds. *SEER Cancer Statistic Review, 1975–2009*. Bethesda, MD: National Cancer Institute; 2012.

24. Ishiyama H, Niino K, Hosoya T, Hayakawa K. Results of a questionnaire survey for symptom of late complications caused by radiotherapy in breast conserving therapy. *Breast Cancer*. 2006;13:197–201.

25. Fränneby U, Sandblom G, Nordin P, Nyrén O, Gunnarsson U. Risk factors for long-term pain after hernia surgery. *Ann Surg*. 2006;244(2):212–219.

26. Courtney CA, Duffy K, Serpell MG. Outcome of patients with severe chronic pain following repair of groin hernia. *Br J Surg*. 2002;89:1310–1314.

27. Koninger J, Redecke J, Butters M. Chronic pain after hernia repair: a randomized trial comparing Shouldice, Lichtenstein and TAPP. *Langenbecks Arch Surg*. 2004;389:361–365.

28. Neumayer L, Giobbie-Hurder A, Jonasson O, et al. Open mesh versus laparoscopic mesh repair of inguinal hernia. *N Engl J Med*. 2004;350:1819–1827.

29. Bridges D, Thompson SW, Rice AS. Mechanisms of neuropathic pain. *Br J Anaesth*. 2001;87(1):12–26.

30. Barelka P, Carroll IR. Chronic pain after surgery for breast cancer. In: Dirbas F, Scott-Conner C, eds. *Breast Surgical Techniques and Interdisciplinary Management*. New York: Springer; 2011:1029–1037.

31. Bove GM, Light AR. The nervi nervorum: missing link for neuropathic pain? *Pain Forum*. 1997;6:181–190.

32. Wallace AM, Wallace MS. Post mastectomy and post thoracotomy pain. *Anesthesiol Clin North Am*. 1997;15(2):353–370.

33. Mailis A, Chan J, Basinski A, et al. Chest wall pain after aortocoronary bypass surgery using internal mammary artery graft: a new pain syndrome? *Heart Lung*. 1989;18:553–558.

34. Ferzli GS, Edwards ED, Khoury GE. Chronic pain after inguinal herniorrhaphy. *J Am Coll Surg*. 2007;205(2):333–341.

35. Eisenberg E. Post-surgical neuralgia. *Pain*. 2004;111(1–2):3–7.

36. Yarnitsky D, Eisenberg E. Neuropathic pain: between positive and negative ends. *Pain Forum*. 1998;7:241–242.

37. Bataineh AB. Sensory nerve impairment following mandibular third molar surgery. *J Oral Maxillofac Surg*. 2001;59:1012–1017.

38. Vecht CJ. Arm pain in the patient with breast cancer. *J Pain Symptom Manage*. 1990;5:109–117.

39. Tacconi P, Manca D, Tamburini G, Cannas A, Giagheddu M. Notalgia paresthetica following neuralgic amyotrophy: a case report. *Neurol Sci*. 2004;25:27–29.

40. Daniel HC, Narewska J, Serpell M, Hoggart B, Johnson R, Rice ASC. Comparison of psychological and physical function in neuropathic pain and nociceptive pain: implications for cognitive behavioral pain management programs. *Eur J Pain*. 2008;12:731–741.

41. Buvanendran A, Kroin JS, Della Valle CJ, Kari M, Moric M, Tuman KJ. Perioperative oral pregabalin reduces chronic pain after total knee arthroplasty: a prospective, randomized, controlled trial. *Anesth Analg*. 2010;110:199–207.

42. Clarke H, Bonin RP, Orser BA, Englesakis M, Wijeysundera DN, Katz J. The prevention of chronic postsurgical pain using gabapentin and pregabalin: a combined systematic review and met analysis. *Anesth Analg*. 2012;115(2):428–442.

43. Amr Y, Yousef A. Evaluation of the efficacy of the perioperative administration of venlafaxin or gabapentin on acute or chronic post-mastectomy pain. *Clin J Pain*. 2012;26(5):381–385.

44. Tiippana E, Nilsson E, Kalso E. Post-thoracotomy pain after thoracic epidural analgesia: a prospective follow-up study. *Acta Anaesthesiol Scand*. 2003;47:433–438.

45. Obata H, Saito S, Fujita N, Fuse Y, Ishizaki K, Goto F. Epidural block with mepivacaine before surgery reduces long-term post-thoracotomy pain. *Can J Anaesth*. 1999;46(12):1127–1132.

46. Ibarra MM, S-Carralero GC, Vincente GU, et al. Chronic postoperative pain after general anesthesia with or without a single-dose pre-incisional paravertebral nerve block in radical breast cancer surgery. *Rev Esp Anestesiol Reanim*. 2011;58:290–294.

47. Wildgaard K, Ravn J, Kehlet H. Chronic post-thoracotomy pain: a critical review of pathogenic mechanisms and strategies for prevention. *Eur J Cardiothorac Surg*. 2009;36:170–180.

48. Songer D. Psychotherapeutic approaches in treatment of pain. *Psychiatry*. 2005;2(5):19–24.

49. Kalso E, Tasmuth T, Neuvonen PJ. Amitriptyline effectively relieves neuropathic pain following treatment of breast cancer. *Pain*. 1996;64:293–302.

50. Tasmuth T, Härtel B, Kalso E. Venlafaxine in neuropathic pain following treatment of breast cancer. *Eur J Pain*. 2002;6(1):17–24.

51. Semenchuk MR, Sherman S, Davis B. Double-blind, randomized trial of bupropion SR for the treatment of neuropathic pain. *Neurology*. 2001;57:1583–1588.

52. Ellison N, Loprinzi CL, Kugler J, et al. Phase III placebo-controlled trial of capsaicin

cream in the management of surgical neuropathic pain in cancer patients. *J Clin Oncol.* 1997;15:2974–2980.

53. Watson CP, Evans RJ. The postmastectomy pain syndrome and topical capsaicin: a randomized trial. Pain 1992;51:375–379.

54. Serpell MG. Neuropathic pain study group. Gabapentin in neuropathic pain syndromes: a randomized, double-blind, placebo-controlled trial. *Pain.* 2002;99:557–566.

55. Wallace MS, Irving G, Cowles VE. Gabapentin extended-release tablets for the treatment of patients with postherpetic neuralgia: a randomized, double-blind, placebo-controlled, multicentre study. *Clin Drug Investig.* 2010;30(11):765–776.

56. Jorum E, Warncke T, Stubhaug A. Cold allodynia and hyperalgesia in neuropathic pain: the effect of N-methyl-D-aspartate (NMDA) receptor antagonist ketamine—a double-blind, cross-over comparison with alfentanil and placebo. *Pain.* 2003;101:229–235.

57. Kvarnstrom A, Karlsten R, Quiding H, Emanuelsson BM, Gordh T. The effectiveness of intravenous ketamine and lidocaine on peripheral neuropathic pain. *Acta Anaesthesiol Scand.* 2003;47:868–877.

58. Felsby S, Nielsen J, Arendt-Nielsen L, Jensen TS. NMDA receptor blockade in chronic neuropathic pain: a comparison of ketamine and magnesium chloride. *Pain.* 1996;64:283–291.

59. Max MB, Byas-Smith MG, Gracely RH, Bennett GJ. Intravenous infusion of the NMDA antagonist, ketamine, in chronic posttraumatic pain with allodynia: a double-blind comparison to alfentanil and placebo. *Clin Neuropharmacol.* 1995;18:360–368.

60. Leung A, Wallace MS, Ridgeway B, Yaksh T. Concentration-effect relationship of intravenous alfentanil and ketamine on peripheral neurosensory thresholds, allodynia and hyperalgesia of neuropathic pain. *Pain.* 2001;91:177–187.

61. Wallace MS, Dyck JB, Rossi SS, Yaksh TL. Computer-controlled lidocaine infusion for the evaluation of neuropathic pain after peripheral nerve injury. *Pain.* 1996;66:69–77.

62. Johnson MD, Burchiel KJ. Peripheral stimulation for treatment of trigeminal postherpetic neuralgia and trigeminal posttraumatic neuropathic pain: a pilot study. *Neurosurgery.* 2004;55(1):135–142.

63. Jasper JF, Hayek SM. Implanted occipital nerve stimulators. *Pain Physician.* 2008;11(2):187–200.

64. Rossi M, DeCarolis G, Liberatoscioli G, Iemma D, Nosella P, Nardi LF. A novel mini-invasive approach to the treatment of neuropathic pain: the PENS Study. *Pain Physician.* 2016;19(1):E121–E128.

65. Defalque RJ, Bromley JJ. Poststernotomy neuralgia: a new pain syndrome. *Anesth Analg.* 1989;69:81–82.

66. Abbas DN, Abd el Ghafar EM, Ibrahim WA, Omran AF. Fluoroscopic stellate ganglion block for post-mastectomy pain: a comparison of the classic anterior approach and the oblique approach. *Clin J Pain.* 2011;27:207–213.

67. Schon LC, Anderson CD, Easley ME, et al. Surgical treatment of chronic lower extremity neuropathic pain. *Clin Orthop.* 2001;389:156–164.

68. Easley ME, Schon LC. Peripheral nerve vein wrapping for intractable lower extremity pain. *Foot Ankle Int.* 2000;21(6):492–500.

69. de Leon-Casasol OA. Spinal cord and peripheral nerve stimulation techniques for neuropathic pain. *J Pain Symptom Manage.* 2009;38(25):S28–S38.

70. Graybill J, Conermann MD, Kabazie ME, Chandy S. Spinal cord stimulation for treatment of pain in a patient with post-thoracotomy pain syndrome. *Pain Physician.* 2011;14:441–445.

10

Post-Traumatic Neuralgia

MAGDALENA ANITESCU, JOSHUA FRENKEL, AND BRADLEY A. SILVA

CASE

A 25-year-old man has had left arm pain for 8 weeks. The pain began after a motorcycle accident in which he dislocated his left shoulder. He was taken to a local emergency department where his shoulder dislocation was reduced. A workup at the time, including imaging, revealed a likely torn ligament within his left rotator cuff. There were no other significant injuries and he was discharged home with instructions to take ibuprofen as needed. The pain after the injury felt like throbbing over his shoulder, and it responded well to ibuprofen. Approximately 3 weeks after the accident, the throbbing began to subside. However, he began to feel a different type of pain, a constant burning with intermittent, shooting, electric-shock sensations. The new pain around his left shoulder radiates down his arm. The intensity is 7/10. He feels no weakness or numbness in the extremity. His only medication, ibuprofen, no longer provides pain relief. On physical examination the skin is warm, dry, and nontender to palpation. Strength is 5/5 bilaterally, but sensation is decreased on the lateral surface of the left arm. Magnetic resonance imaging of the left upper extremity reveals enhanced T2 signal and enhancement of the upper trunk of the brachial plexus. He is diagnosed with post-traumatic neuralgia, specifically, a neurapraxia of the upper trunk of the left brachial plexus. A prescription for gabapentin 400 mg three times a day is given along with appointments for both physical and occupational therapy.

INTRODUCTION

Post-traumatic neuralgia develops after an acute physical injury to the peripheral nervous system. While all trauma can cause acute nociceptive pain, it is damage to nerves and their supporting structures that leads to chronic neuropathic pain. The etiology of post-traumatic neuralgia can be broadly divided into iatrogenic and noniatrogenic causes.

Peripheral nerve injuries, regardless of etiology, generally fall into one of four types.[1] Stretch injuries, when traction forces exceed the nerve's elastic capacity, can cause complete interruption of the nerve (e.g., brachial plexus avulsion) or damage without loss of continuity (e.g., brachial plexus stretch from traumatic birth due to shoulder dystocia). Laceration injuries can cause both complete and partial nerve transection. Finally, compression and mechanical deformation are two injury types that often occur in combination (e.g., tourniquet use or nerve entrapment). These injury types are distinct from stretch and laceration injuries in that they do not involve nerve interruption, but instead cause nerve ischemia within the compression site and degenerative changes along the edges of the compressed area.

A nerve consists of multiple axons bound by distinct layers of connective tissue sheaths. Each axon, along with Schwann cells and myelin, if present, is first encased in a basal membrane sheath surrounded by a layer of connective tissue called the *endoneurium*. Bundles of axons, known as *fascicles*, are then encased in a sheath called the *perineurium*. Finally, multiple fascicles, surrounded by connective tissue are encased in an outermost sheath, the *epineurium*.

Stretching a peripheral nerve can cause rupture of nerve tissue, beginning with the axon, then the basal membrane, endoneurium, perineurium, and epineurium.[2] Laceration also can cause varying degrees of nerve damage, beginning from the epineurium and moving inward. The likelihood of neurological recovery depends on the degree of nerve damage. The Seddon classification of nerve damage appears in Table 10.1.[3] In the mildest of the three injury types, *neurapraxia*, myelin dysfunction is transient and

TABLE 10.1. SEDDON CLASSIFICATION OF NERVE DAMAGE

Seddon Classification	Pathology	Able to be First Identified	NCS Findings	Earliest EMG Findings	Serial Study Findings
Neurapraxia	Localized myelin dysfunction	Acutely	Conduction block, focal slowing	Reduced recruitment of MUPs	Usually full recovery
Axonotmesis	Axonal damage with intact neural tube	3 weeks after injury	Low-amplitude or absent responses	Fibrillations, reduced recruitment of large, complex MUPs; if severe—no activation in first weeks/ months after injury	Reinnervation
Neurotmesis	Axonal and neural tube damage	3 weeks after injury	Absent responses	Fibrillations, no activation of MUPs	No reinnervation

EMG, electromyography; MUP, motor unit potential; NCS, nerve conduction studies.
Obtained from Watson JC, Huntoon MA. Neurologic evaluation and management of perioperative nerve injury. *Reg Anesth Pain Med.* 2015;40:491–501.

the nerve axon is not interrupted. Neurological impairment is transient. In *axonotmesis*, continuity of the axon is lost without damage to the connective tissue sheath. The sheath framework maintains a path for the regenerating axons to reach their target end-organ. Regeneration, reinnervation, and functional recovery can take from weeks to months. In the third type of nerve damage, *neurotmesis*, both the axon and the connective tissue sheath are interrupted. Loss of the sheath framework along with formation of scar tissue prevents the axons from regenerating along the correct path to reinnervate their target organ. Without surgical intervention, neurological dysfunction will be permanent.

After peripheral nerve injury, the portion of the axon distal to the lesion degenerates (Wallerian degeneration); the portion that remains intact with the neural cell body will regenerate as a growth cone with axon sprouts that are guided by Schwann cells toward the target organ. The severity of the injury dictates the changes that impact regeneration. For instance, if the connective tissue sheath is severed (i.e., neurotmesis), inflammatory processes cause the formation of disorganized fibrosis at the site. The axon growth cone cannot regenerate toward the target organ. The reported rate of axon regeneration varies from 0.5 to 9 mm per day.[1] This variability is due to numerous factors: (1) the rate of growth decreases as the distance from the cell body to growth cone increases; (2) the rate of

regeneration depends on the type and severity of injury, duration of denervation, and condition of surrounding tissues; and (3) differences in animal models, types of nerve injury, and methods of measuring regeneration have yielded different results. Finally, axon regeneration does not necessarily return neurological function. Organs undergo degenerative morphological changes with prolonged denervation. For instance, while the synaptic folds of motor endplates survive for at least 1 year after denervation, muscle fibers lose a mean value of 70% of their cross-sectional area within 2 months of injury.[1] End-organ changes that prevent reinnervation abort axon regeneration.

IATROGENIC PERIPHERAL NERVE INJURY

The etiology behind iatrogenic nerve injury is broad, ranging from mechanical causes (such as compression, traction, injection, and transection) to ischemic and neurotoxic causes. With regard to anesthetic causes, the incidence of long-term nerve injury after peripheral nerve block is approximately 2–4 per 10,000 blocks, a rate that has not decreased over 10 years despite the fact that the primary nerve localization tool transitioned from peripheral nerve stimulation to ultrasound.[4] Postoperative neurological symptoms after peripheral nerve blockade typically dissipate over time. Iatrogenic peripheral nerve injury is responsible for significant morbidity, healthcare costs, and litigation. In the American Society of Anesthesiologists (ASA) closed-claims database, nerve damage is the second most common category of claims, accounting for 16% of all cases.[5] The top three most frequent sites of injury are the ulnar nerve, the brachial plexus, and the lumbosacral nerve roots.

With regard to surgical causes, orthopedic procedures likely carry the greatest risk of nerve injury because the surgical field is close to narrow joint spaces through which peripheral nerves traverse. Thus, surgery of the shoulder, elbow, hip, knee, and ankle can lead to nerve injuries. For arthroscopic procedures, nerve injury ranges from 0.1%–10% for shoulders and 0.4%–13.3% for hips.[4]

Risk Factors

The risk factors associated with iatrogenic peripheral nerve injury can be perioperative or patient oriented.[6] Perioperative risk factors are anesthetic, surgical, or positional. Anesthetic risk factors are associated with placement of peripheral nerve blocks and vascular catheterization.[7] In both situations, direct needle trauma to a nerve can lead to injury. Likewise, hematoma formation during needle placement can cause neural ischemia. Peripheral nerve blocks complicated by neurotoxicity from local anesthetics pose the highest risk for injury after intrafascicular injection.

Surgical risk factors follow from surgical technique or implantation of foreign bodies. Retraction can cause varying degrees of stretch injury. Surgical dissection and port insertion can lead to direct nerve trauma or transection. Two examples are brachial plexus compression from wide sternal retraction during median sternotomy[7] and ilioinguinal nerve transection during open inguinal hernia repair.[8] In orthopedics, extremity traction and tourniquet placement can lead to stretch and compression injuries, respectively.

Implantation of foreign bodies also poses risk in a wide variety of surgical specialties. Polypropylene mesh used during hernia repair can compress the ilioinguinal nerve, resulting in inflammatory degeneration of the myelin sheath.[9] The associated fibrosis leads to nerve injury. During orthopedic procedures, placement of pins and plates can penetrate nerves or compress them.

Inappropriate patient positioning can subject nerves to compression and stretch injuries.

In animal studies, a nerve stretched by a mean of 15% or more from baseline length causes complete cessation of intraneural microcirculation.[10] External compression of as little as 20 mmHg can inhibit intraneural microcirculation, 30 mmHg can limit axonal transport, and 50 mmHg can alter myelin sheath structure.[11] The two most commonly reported peripheral nerve injuries in the ASA closed-claims database—ulnar neuropathy and brachial plexopathy—are associated with positioning injuries. The most common cause of ulnar neuropathy is compression at the elbow from either prolonged elbow flexion or external pressure. Brachial plexus stretch injury results from arm abduction greater than 90 degrees, lateral rotation of the arm, or depression of the shoulder girdle.[12]

The patient characteristics that increase the risk of perioperative nerve injury are male gender, older age, smoking history, and high body mass index (BMI). Preexisting neurological disease also may affect the development of post-traumatic neuralgia. Termed the "double-crush" phenomenon, preexisting neurological injury limits the neurological reserve of affected nerves, thus increasing the risk of developing new deficits from a subsequent nerve injury (Figure 10.1).[13] The underlying neurological disease may be subclinical, and research suggests that a wide range of etiologies may predispose to the double-crush phenomenon, including metabolic, ischemic, mechanical, toxic, and autoimmune processes. For instance, diabetic patients both have a higher incidence of carpal tunnel syndrome and are at greater risk of developing postanesthetic peripheral nerve injury.[14] In animal models, electrophysiological studies of nerve damage have shown that the level of nerve function is less than would be expected by simple additive damage of each injury.[15]

Diagnosis

Early recognition of perioperative nerve injury is critical to guide diagnosis and management strategies. In some cases, supportive care and symptom management are all that is possible. In other situations, however, emergent imaging and intervention may alter the long-term neurological prognosis. Unfortunately, many barriers exist that can delay early recognition of injury.[6] Acutely, in the post-anesthesia care unit, sedation, analgesics, and regional anesthesia may mask neurological symptoms. Conversely, a patient may incorrectly attribute symptoms of

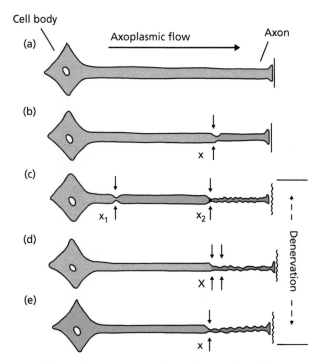

FIGURE 10.1. Neural lesions resulting in denervation. Axoplasmic flow is indicated by the degree of shading. Complete loss of axoplasmic flow results in denervation (**C, D, E**). A. Normal neuron. **B.** Mild neuronal injury at a single site (x) is insufficient to cause denervation distal to the insult. **C.** Mild neuronal injury at two separate sites (x1 and x2) may cause distal denervation (i.e., "double crush"). **D.** Severe neuronal injury at a single site (X) may also cause distal denervation. **E.** Axon with a diffuse preexisting underlying disease process (toxic, metabolic, ischemic) may have impaired axonal flow throughout the neuron, which may or may not be symptomatic, but predisposes the axon to distal denervation after a single minor neural insult at x (i.e., "double crush").

Obtained from Neal JM, Barrington MJ, Brull R, et al. The second ASRA practice advisory on neurologic complications associated with regional anesthesia and pain medicine: executive summary 2015. *Reg Anesth Pain Med.* 2015;40:401–430. Note: this article obtained permission from the Mayo Foundation for Medical Education and Research.

nerve injury to residual nerve blockade or may assume that neurological symptoms are expected after surgery. Apart from the perioperative setting, diagnosis becomes even more challenging, as patients often have trouble constructing an accurate timeline of the onset of symptoms as they recover from the effects of anesthesia over the first few postoperative days. Diagnosis can be further complicated by a lack of standardized follow-up by anesthesiologists postoperatively. In the ambulatory setting, for example, patients are often discharged before complete recovery from anesthesia or with peripheral nerve catheters in place that may mask traumatic neurological injury.

Once a nerve injury is suspected, a focused history and physical examination can help define the nature and location of the injury. For instance, urgent imaging is indicated for suspected hematoma-induced nerve compression. Likewise, surgical re-exploration may be needed for suspected retained foreign objects or nerve compression secondary to sutures or clips. If immediately reversible causes are not suspected, electrophysiological studies, such as electromyography (EMG) and nerve conduction studies (NCS), can be beneficial to localize and categorize the severity of injury. Acutely, NCS can identify neurapraxia by conduction block or focal slowing, or reveal preexisting neurological disease. These studies, however, are more useful 14–21 days after injury. Axonotmetic and neurotmetic lesions can be distinguished with serial studies used to detect the presence of axon regeneration and reinnervation into target tissue. With axonotmesis, responses are either low amplitude or absent with NCS. The EMG shows reduced recruitment of motor unit potentials.

With neurotmesis, responses are absent with NCS. EMG shows no activation of motor unit potentials.

NONIATROGENIC PERIPHERAL NERVE INJURY

Post-traumatic neuralgia can develop after physical injuries from falls, motor vehicle accidents (MVA), penetrating trauma, and blunt-force trauma.[16] The pathophysiology of chronic neuropathic pain can be similar for both iatrogenic and noniatrogenic nerve injuries, but some stark differences are apparent. The often abrupt and violent nature of noniatrogenic trauma can lead to more significant injury to the nerve. The incidence of noniatrogenic traumatic nerve injury is approximately 3%–5% in trauma centers.[17,18] Approximately 60% of these patients have head injuries. MVAs are a major cause of morbidity and are responsible for disabling over 3.2 million people.[19] Iatrogenic trauma accounts for 10%–15% of peripheral nerve injuries and noniatrogenic trauma for 85%–90% of peripheral nerve injuries.[20]

Noniatrogenic trauma is most common in young adult males. Of the sites of injury, 63.5% are found in the peripheral nerves. The top three nerves in order of frequency are the radial, ulnar, and median. Next is the brachial plexus at 36% (trunks > cords > roots), and last, the lumbrosacral plexus at 0.5%. Not surprisingly, these injuries cause acute nociceptive pain and also lead to chronic neuropathic pain. One study found the rate of chronic neuropathic pain as high as 50%, with approximately 79% of the patients rating the pain as moderate to severe in intensity.[16]

Traumatic Brachial Plexopathy

A focused analysis of a specific type of noniatrogenic injury is an example that can be extrapolated to different regions of the peripheral nervous system. Brachial plexus injuries present unique pathophysiological and diagnostic challenges, based on their location at the interface between the peripheral and central nervous systems. Noniatrogenic traumatic brachial plexus injuries are the most common type of plexopathy.[21] In comparing injuries from gunshot wounds and MVAs, the trunks are the most frequent site of damage within the plexus (52%), followed by the cords (36%) and roots (12%).[22] Supraclavicular injuries are widespread, severe, and have a worse prognosis than infraclavicular

injuries.[23] The brachial plexus is particularly vulnerable to stretch-type injuries in falls and MVAs, and the manner in which the traction occurs can determine whether the upper plexus or the lower plexus is affected.[24] Upper plexus injury prevails with violent lateral neck flexion with the arm adducted; the first rib acts as a fulcrum, directing the force in line with the upper roots. Lower plexus injury is recognized after violent arm abduction overhead; the coracoid process acts as a fulcrum in line with the lower roots.

Brachial plexus injuries are classified into three types based on their location relative to the dorsal root ganglion: stretch lesion, postganglionic lesion (rupture), and preganglionic lesion (avulsion) (Figure 10.2).[25,26] Stretch lesions weaken the nerve anywhere along its course. Postganglionic lesions form when traction creates discontinuity of the nerve. Preganglionic lesions, called *avulsion*, are created when the root is torn out of the spinal cord.

Diagnostic evaluation of noniatrogenic injuries can be challenging immediately after trauma. Neurological assessment of a brachial plexus injury may be limited during the resuscitation period or if the patient is obtunded. In patients able to follow commands, specific motor and sensory deficits help localize the lesion. Upper plexus impairment may limit arm abduction and pronation of the forearm (waiter's tip position). Sensory deficits may be found on the extensor surface of the forearm. Lower plexus impairment reduces motor function of the intrinsic hand muscles and flexors. Sensory deficits appear along the ulnar surface of the forearm. Finally, the presence of Horner's syndrome indicates a lesion at C8–T1. Neuropathic pain is present in 30%–90% of patients with a traumatic brachial plexus lesion.

In the acute period, imaging studies are critical to detect structural damage. Ultrasound can reveal nerve transection. Chest radiography elicits clavicle, humerus, or vertebral fractures that may impinge on the plexus. CT or MRI studies may be needed in patients who are unable to communicate symptoms.[27] CT myelography is 85% accurate in detecting root avulsion, which may be evident as a meningocele at the affected level, or when intrathecal contrast migrates into the epidural space through the open dura around an avulsed root.[28] MRI can provide evidence of non-avulsed nerve damage by the presence of hematoma, soft tissue edema, or increased T2 signal and enhancement.[29] Electrophysiological

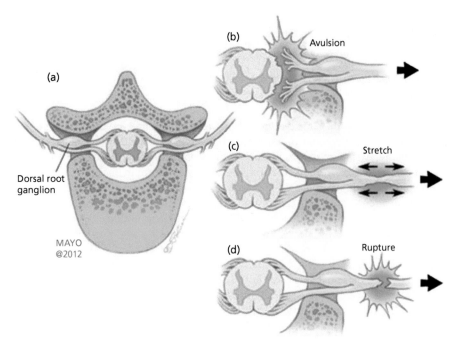

FIGURE 10.2. Cross-section views of the major types of brachial plexus stretch injuries. Normal spinal column anatomy is shown in **A** with the spinal cord in the center and the nerves in yellow.

Obtained from Mayo Foundation for Medical Education and Research.

studies help in the localization and long-term management of noniatrogenic injury. Correct diagnosis of the type of brachial plexus injury is important because the surgical treatment of pre- versus post-ganglion injuries differs.

MANAGEMENT OF POST-TRAUMATIC NEURALGIA

Management of post-traumatic neuralgia usually requires consultation with other specialists, including a neurologist, neurosurgeon, and pain medicine physician. Indications for a consultation with a neurologist are found in Table 10.2.[6] Neurological consultation can be helpful in differentiating peripheral nerve injury from other neurological dysfunction (e.g., stroke). Neurosurgical consultation may be indicated acutely in cases requiring emergent decompression (e.g., hematoma) or if serial electrophysiological studies fail to demonstrate sufficient axonal regeneration for spontaneous recovery.

Because pain is a prominent symptom of post-traumatic neuralgia, a pain medicine consultation for a full evaluation may reveal unrecognized neurological, musculoskeletal, or psychological injury. In some situations, the severity of injury may be known, but the patient's expectations of full recovery may be unrealistic. Pain physicians assist in developing treatment goals and expectations. Indications for prompt pain medicine consultation are listed in Table 10.2.

Treatment of post-traumatic neuralgia with a multidisciplinary approach has two central goals: restoring nerve function and minimizing chronic neuropathic pain. Physical therapy reduces the development of contractures, muscle atrophy, and secondary pain. In cases of stretch injury, therapy alone can improve symptoms and function.

Surgical therapy is usually indicated if there has been no improvement in nerve function (i.e., reinnervation). Most centers wait 3–6 months to monitor for signs of spontaneous recovery. In the case of lacerating lesions, exploration within the first 72 hours and end-to-end anastomoses may be optimal. Absent spontaneous recovery, the risk of delayed intervention is permanent muscle atrophy and contractures.

Preganglionic lesions (i.e. avulsion) require a nerve transfer; postganglionic lesions can be repaired with a nerve graft. In a nerve transfer, a nerve of less significant functional importance (e.g., intercostal nerve) is anastomosed to the distal stump of an avulsed root. In grafting, a nerve graft bridges the proximal and

TABLE 10.2. INDICATIONS FOR NEUROLOGICAL CONSULTATION FOR POST-TRAUMATIC NEURALGIA

Indications for Early Neurological Consultation for Peripheral Nerve Injury	Indications for Early Pain Clinic Consultation for Peripheral Nerve Injury
If neurological deficits are as follows: • Severe • Functionally limiting • Progressive • Multifocal or difficult to localize • Unexplained neurological impairment outside the block region or region of common compression • Associated with severe pain (disproportionate to typical postoperative course) • Associated with an intervening return to neurologic baseline after surgery before development of peripheral nerve injury	If pain is one of the following: • Severe • Functionally limiting • Progressive • Multifocal or difficult to localize (may indicate comorbidity such as anxiety or complex regional pain syndrome) • Unexplained neurological impairment outside the block region or region or common compression • Associated with severe pain (disproportionate to typical postoperative course) • Associated with allodynia, edema, hyperhidrosis, uninvolved extremity • Failure to respond to initial therapies • Increasing or problematic opioid escalations

Obtained from Watson JC, Huntoon MA. Neurologic evaluation and management of perioperative nerve injury. *Reg Anesth Pain Med.* 2015;40:491–501.

distal stumps. Nerve grafting in postganglionic lesions can improve function in 40%–75% of patients.[30]

Neuropathic pain is managed with pharmacotherapy and procedural therapies. Various organizations have created treatment algorithms for chronic neuropathic pain. They typically follow a tiered approach, beginning with single first-line agents, before multiple first-line agents, then second- and third-line agents as needed (Table 10.3).[6] Pharmacological agents include secondary amine tricyclic antidepressants (e.g., nortriptyline, desipramine), calcium channel α-2-δ ligand anticonvulsants (e.g., pregabalin, gabapentin), opioids, ketamine, and topical lidocaine.

Procedural interventions may be indicated when pharmacotherapy fails. Blocks, ablation, or neurostimulation are designed to interfere with or interrupt pain pathways (see Chapter 8). The injection of anesthetic medication in a block—for example, a stellate ganglion block for post-traumatic complex regional pain syndrome—blocks transmission of sympathetic nerve fibers. Ablation destroys abnormally hyperactive neurons. Lesioning of the dorsal root entry zone (DREZotomy) is a procedure used for refractory neuropathic pain after brachial plexus avulsion.[31] DREZotomy destroys portions of the dorsal rootlets and neurons in the substantia gelatinosa by means of microsurgical, radiofrequency, or laser ablation.[32]

TABLE 10.3. MANAGEMENT OF NEUROPATHIC PAIN

Step 1: Assess pain, establish cause and probable neuropathic mechanism, and identify comorbidities

Step 2: Initiate therapy with first-line agent:
• Secondary amine tricyclic antidepressant (nortriptyline, desipramine)
• Calcium channel α2-δ ligand (gabapentin, pregabalin)
• Topical lidocaine for localized peripheral neuropathic conditions, alone or combined with other primary agents
• Nonpharmacological therapies, when indicated
• Opioid analgesics may be used, generally in combination

Step 3:
• Reassess and continue if efficacious
• Consider addition of other first-line agents or combinations for partial/incomplete responders

Step 4: Consider referral to specialty pain clinic or neurological subspecialist if ongoing poor response

Obtained from Watson JC, Huntoon MA. Neurologic evaluation and management of perioperative nerve injury. *Reg Anesth Pain Med.* 2015;40:491–501. Note: this table was modified from Dworkin RH, O'Connor AB, Audette J, et al. Recommendations for the pharmacologic management of neuropathic pain: an overview and literature update. *Mayo Clin Proc.* 2010;85(Suppl):S3–S14.

During neurostimulation, low-intensity, high-frequency electrical current is applied through a pulse generator and electrodes at a specific level of the spinal cord or a specific peripheral nerve (see Chapter 8).[33,34] Neurostimulation techniques work by the principle of gate control theory, first proposed by Melzack and Wall in 1965.[35] According to the theory, the substantia gelatinosa within the dorsal horn of the spinal cord acts as a gate control system, modulating afferent signals to the brain. The more "open" the gate, the greater the flow of nerve impulses to the brain, and hence the greater the sensation of pain. Both peripheral and central input can influence the degree to which the gate is opened or closed. For example, the brain can increase gate opening (e.g., anxiety, fear) or increase gate closing (e.g., distraction, relaxed breathing).[36]

CONCLUSION

Post-traumatic neuralgia arises from a wide range of traumatic peripheral nerve injuries. While the pathophysiology of iatrogenic and noniatrogenic etiologies may be similar, each category presents unique risk factors and diagnostic challenges. Regardless of cause, early diagnosis and consultation with pain medicine, neurology, and neurosurgery is crucial for recovery. Management of post-traumatic neuralgia aims to restore nerve function and minimize chronic neuropathic pain.

GUIDING QUESTIONS

- Describe Seddon's classification of peripheral nerve damage.
- Describe the "double crush" phenomenon.
- Describe the diagnostic challenges of iatrogenic and noniatrogenic peripheral nerve injury.
- Describe the indications for obtaining a pain medicine, neurology, or neurosurgical consultation after peripheral nerve injury.
- Describe the treatment options for post-traumatic neuralgia.

KEY POINTS

- Peripheral nerve damage is classified into three categories based on severity: neurapraxia, axonotmesis, and neurotmesis. In neurapraxia, myelin dysfunction is transient without interruption of the nerve axon. Neurological impairment also is transient. In axonotmesis, continuity of the axon

is lost without damage to the connective tissue sheath. Preservation of the sheath framework provides a path for the regenerating axons to reach their target end-organ to reinnervate and to recover function. In neurotmesis, both the axon and the connective tissue sheath are interrupted. Loss of the sheath framework along with formation of scar tissue prevents the axons from regenerating along the correct path, disrupting reinnervation and functional recovery.
- In the American Society of Anesthesiologists' closed-claims database, peripheral nerve damage is the second most common category of claims, accounting for 16% of all cases. The top three most frequent sites affected are the ulnar nerve, the brachial plexus, and the lumbosacral nerve roots.
- Perioperative risk factors for iatrogenic peripheral nerve injury can be subdivided into anesthetic, surgical, or position related. Anesthetic risk factors come from placement of peripheral nerve blocks and vascular catheterization. Surgical risk factors are associated with surgical technique and implantation of foreign bodies. Inappropriate patient positioning can subject nerves to compression and stretch injuries.
- The "double-crush" phenomenon is a term used to describe preexisting neurological injury that limits the neurological reserve of affected nerves. The risk of clinical deficits from a subsequent nerve injury is increased with the double crush phenomenon. The underlying neurological disease may be subclinical: metabolic, ischemic, mechanical, toxic, or autoimmune. Electrophysiological studies of nerve damage in animal models have shown that the level of nerve function is lower than would be expected by simple additive damage of each injury.
- Noniatrogenic traumatic nerve injury is most common in young adult males. Sites of injury are peripheral nerves (63.5%; the top three nerves are the radial > ulnar > median), the brachial plexus (36%; with trunks > cords > roots), and lumbrosacral plexus (0.5%).

- Brachial plexus injuries are classified into three types based on their location relative to the dorsal root ganglion: stretch lesion, postganglionic lesion (rupture), and preganglionic lesion (avulsion). Stretch lesions weaken the nerve anywhere along its course. In postganglionic lesions traction results in discontinuity of the nerve. Finally, preganglionic lesions (avulsion) occur when the root is torn out of the spinal cord.
- Management of post-traumatic neuralgia often involves consultation with pain medicine, neurology, and neurosurgery. This multidisciplinary approach has two central goals, restoring nerve function and minimizing chronic neuropathic pain.
- Pharmacotherapy and procedural therapies are the treatments for neuropathic pain. Pharmacological agents include secondary amine tricyclic antidepressants (e.g., nortriptyline, desipramine), calcium channel α-2-δ ligand anticonvulsants (e.g., pregabalin, gabapentin), opioids, ketamine, and topical lidocaine. Procedural interventions may be indicated when pain remains refractory to multiple pharmacological therapies. Procedures include blocks, ablation, and neurostimulation, designed to interfere with, interrupt, or modulate pain pathways.

REFERENCES

1. Burnett MG, Zager EL. Pathophysiology of peripheral nerve injury: a brief review. *Neurosurg Focus.* 2004;16:1–7.
2. van Alfen N, Malessy M. Diagnosis of brachial and lumbosacral plexus lesions. In: Said G, Krarup C, ed. *Peripheral Nerve Disorders: Handbook of Clinical Neurology.* V. 115, series 3. New York: Elsevier B.V.; 2013:293–310.
3. Seddon HJ. Three types of nerve injury. *Brain.* 1943;66:237–288.
4. Neal JM, Barrington MJ, Brull R, et al. The second ASRA practice advisory on neurologic complications associated with regional anesthesia and pain medicine executive summary 2015. *Reg Anesth Pain Med.* 2015;40:401–430.
5. Cheney FW, Domino KB, Caplan RA, Posner KL. Nerve injury associated with anesthesia: a closed claims analysis. *Anesthesiology.* 1999;90:1062–1069.
6. Watson JC, Huntoon MA. Neurologic evaluation and management of perioperative nerve injury. *Reg Anesth Pain Med.* 2015;40:491–501.
7. Zhang J, Moore AE, Stringer MD. Iatrogenic upper limb nerve injuries; a systemic review. *ANZ J Surg.* 2011;81:227–236.
8. Hakeem A, Shanmugam V. Current trends in the diagnosis and management of post-herniorraphy chronic groin pain. *World J Gastrointest Surg.* 2011;3:73–81.
9. Demirer S, Kepenekci I, Evirgen O, et al. The effect of polypropylene mesh on ilioinguinal nerve in open mesh repair of groin hernia. *J Surg Res.* 2006;131:175–181.
10. Lundberg G, Rydevik B. Effects of stretching the tibial nerve of the rabbit. *J Bone Joint Surg Br.* 1973;55:390–401.
11. Rempel D, Dahlin L, Lundborg G. Pathophysiology of nerve compression syndromes: response of peripheral nerves to loading. *J Bone and Joint Surg.* 1999;81-A:1600–1610.
12. Coppieters MW, Van De Velde M, Stappaerts KH. Positioning in anesthesiology: Toward a better understanding of stretch-induced perioperative neuropathies. *Anesthesiology.* 2002;97:75–81.
13. Upton AR, McComas AJ. The double crush in nerve entrapment syndromes. Lancet. 1973;2:359–362.
14. Dyck PJ, Kratz KM, Karnes JL, et al. The prevalence by staged severity of various types of diabetic neuropathy, retinopathy and nephropathy in a population-based cohort: the Rochester Diabetic Neuropathy Study. *Neurology.* 1993;43:817–824.
15. Nemoto K, Matsumoto N, Tazaki K, Horiuchi Y, Uchinishi K, Mori Y. An experimental study on the "double crush" hypothesis. *J Hand Surg Am.* 1987;12:552–559.
16. Ciaramitaro P, Mondelli M, Logullo F, et al. Traumatic peripheral nerve injuries: epidemiological findings, neuropathic pain and quality of life in 158 patients. *Peripher Nerv Syst.* 2010;15:120–127.
17. Robinson LR. Traumatic injury to peripheral nerves. *Muscle Nerve.* 2000;23:863–873.
18. Noble J, Munro CA, Prasad VS, Midha R. Analysis of upper and lower extremity peripheral nerve injuries in a population of patients with multiple injuries. *J Trauma.* 1998;45:116–122.
19. Gin-shaw JL, Jorden RC. Multiple trauma. In: Marx R, ed. *Rosen's Emergency Medicine: Concepts and Clinical Practice.* New York: Mosby; 2002:242–254.

20. Eser F, Aktekin LA, Bodur H, Atan C. Etiological factors of traumatic peripheral nerve injuries. *Neurol India*. 2009;57:434–437.

21. van Dongen R, Cohen SP, van Kleef M, Mekhail N, Huygen F. Traumatic plexus lesion. *Pain Pract*. 2011;11:414–420.

22. Bowles AO, Graves DE, Chiou-Tan FY. Distribution and extent of involvement in brachial plexopathies caused by gunshot wounds, motor vehicle crashes and other etiologies: a 10-year electromyography study. *Arch Phys Med Rehabil*. 2004;85:1708–1710.

23. Midha R. Epidemiology of brachial plexus injuries in a multitrauma population. *Neurosurgery*. 1997;40:1182–1188.

24. Khadilkar SV, Khade SS. Brachial plexopathy. *Ann Indian Acad Neurol*. 2013;16:12–18.

25. Teixeira MJ, da Paz MG, Bina MT, et al. Neuropathic pain after brachial plexus avulsion—central and peripheral mechanisms. *BMC Neurol*. 2015;15:73.

26. Shin AY, Spinner RJ, Steinmann SP, Bishop AT. Adult traumatic brachial plexus injuries. *J Am Acad Orthop Surg*. 2005;13:382–396.

27. Foster M. Traumatic brachial plexus injuries. eMedicine.com http//emedicine.medscape.com/article/1268993-overview. Accessed June 2016.

28. Carvalho GA, Nikkhah G, Matthies C, et al. Diagnosis of root avulsions in traumatic brachial plexus injuries: value of computerized tomography myelography and magnetic resonance imaging. *J Neurosurg*. 1997;86:69–76.

29. Tharin BD, Kini JA, York GE, Ritter JL. Brachial plexopathy: a review of traumatic and nontraumatic causes. *Am J Roentgenol*. 2014;202:W67–W75.

30. Terzis JK, Vekris MD, Soucacos PN. Outcomes of brachial plexus reconstruction in 204 patients with devastating paralysis. *Plast Reconstr Surg*. 1999;104:1221–1240.

31. Sindou MP, Blondet E, Emery E, Mertens P. Microsurgical lesioning in the dorsal root entry zone for pain due to brachial plexus avulsion: a prospective series of 55 patients. *J Neurosurg*. 2005;102:1018–1028.

32. Ali M, Saitoh Y, Oshino S et al. Differential efficacy of electric motor cortex stimulation and lesioning of the dorsal root entry zone for continuous vs paroxysmal pain after brachial plexus avulsion. *Neurosurgery*. 2011;68:1252–1258.

33. Lai HY, Lee CY, Lee ST. High cervical spinal cord stimulation after failed dorsal root entry zone surgery for brachial plexus avulsion pain. *Surg Neurol*. 2009;72:286–289.

34. Stevanato G, Devigili G, Eleopra R, et al. Chronic post-traumatic neuropathic pain of brachial plexus and upper limb: a new technique of peripheral nerve stimulation. *Neurosurg Rev*. 2014;37:473–480.

35. Melzack R, Wall PD. Pain mechanisms: A new theory. *Science*. 1965;150:971–979.

36. LeFort S, Webster L, Lorig K, et al. *Living a Healthy Life with Chronic Pain*. Boulder, CO: Bull Publishing Company; 2015.

PART II

Focal or Multifocal Lesions of the Peripheral Nervous System

11

Herpes Zoster and Postherpetic Neuralgia

JIANGUO CHENG

CASE

A 67-year-old female presents with right-sided head and neck pain that she has had for 8 weeks. The pain is located in the right occiput, at the side of the head and radiates to the right neck; she describes it as itchiness, burning, and throbbing. Current pain intensity is 8/10. The onset was about 8 weeks ago. Skin rashes erupted a few days after the onset of pain. The rashes eventually healed in about 2 weeks, but the pain has continued and is getting worse. On examination, slight discoloration is noticed on the right side of the neck and behind the ear. The skin is extremely sensitive to light touch. Brushing her hair causes severe sharp and burning pain. Skin is tender to palpation at the base of her neck on the right. Her past medical history is significant for breast cancer and unspecified essential hypertension. She underwent right partial mastectomy and radiation therapy 11 years ago. She has recently been restarted on Exemestane to prevent recurrence of breast cancer. She was diagnosed with herpes zoster and prescribed acyclovir 500 mg QID and prednisone 40 mg daily, as well as acetaminophen-codeine and tramadol 50 mg q4h PRN for pain.

HERPES ZOSTER

Definition

Herpes zoster, also known as zoster and shingles, is caused by reactivation of the latent varicella zoster virus (VZV) that causes chicken pox. Once chicken pox resolves, VZV remains dormant in the dorsal root and cranial ganglia and can reactivate later in a person's life and cause herpes zoster. Approximately 95% of the US adult population has had varicella and thus can have herpes zoster. It appears predominantly among older adults but may also occur in those that are immunocompromised.

Pathophysiology

Primary infection begins with nasopharyngeal replication of VZV. Infection of the abundant memory $CD4^+$ T cells in nearby lymphoid tissue results in delivery of VZV to cutaneous epithelia within several days. Cell-to-cell spread of virus eventually overcomes innate defense and results in vesicles containing free viruses that can infect sensory nerve endings in the epithelia. VZV migrates along the sensory exons to reach the dorsal root or cranial ganglia, where the virus becomes dormant or latent.[1]

Herpes zoster results from reactivation of varicella virus from its latent state in the dorsal root and cranial nerve ganglia and spread through the afferent nerve to the skin to cause characteristic rashes in corresponding dermatomes.[1] The virus can also spread, in many cases, to the dorsal horn and cause manifestations of spinal cord infection. The reason the virus suddenly become active again is not clear. Declining cell-mediated immunity in advanced age has been associated with reactivation of VZV. Re-exposure to VZV can booster cell-mediated immunity against VZV in people who have previously had the virus. Often only one attack occurs, but second and even third episodes are possible.

Epidemiology

Herpes zoster (shingles) is a painful, blistering skin rash due to reactivation of VZV, the virus that causes chickenpox. As much as 95% of the US adult population is susceptible to herpes zoster because of previous exposure to and infection with varicella.[1,2] Herpes zoster occurs in approximately 1 million people in the United States annually. This represents a significant reduction from the annual incidence of as high as 4 million cases in the United States before the introduction of VZV vaccine (OKA strain). It is estimated that up to one-third of the population will have an episode of herpes zoster in their lifetime. Shingles may develop in any age group but is more likely in people with (1) advanced age (age >60 years), (2) chickenpox before age 1 year, or (3) immune compromise due to medications or disease. An adult or child who has not had chickenpox or the chickenpox vaccine may develop chickenpox, rather than shingles, after direct contact with the shingles rash.

Clinical Features and Diagnosis

The first symptom of acute herpes zoster is usually one-sided pain, tingling, or burning. The pain and burning may be severe and is usually present before any rash appears. Red patches on the skin form in most people, followed by small blisters. The blisters break, forming small ulcers that begin to dry and form crusts. The crusts fall off in 2 to 3 weeks. Scarring is rare. The rash usually involves a narrow area from the spine around to the front of the abdomen or chest in one dermatome. Thoracic dermatomes are the mostly commonly affected sites, accounting for 50%–70% of all cases (Figure 11.1). Other sites of herpes zoster include cranial, cervical, lumbar, and sacral dermatomes. The rash may involve the face, eyes (ophthalmic herpes), mouth, and ears. Other symptoms include paresthesia and motor deficits, usually within 2 weeks of zoster eruption and typically in the cervical and lumbosacral dermatomes (Figure 11.2). In addition to acute herpes zoster, there are a few clinical variations:

Subclinical disease: Asymptomatic viral replication is evidenced by a rise in VZV antibody titers and detection of VZV DNA in the cerebrospinal fluid (CSF) by polymerase chain reaction (PCR).

Preherpetic neuralgia: Pain, pruritus, and paresthesia are usually reported by patients 7–21 days before rash eruption. This phase can last more than 100 days.

Zoster sine herpete (ZSH): This refers to a condition in which a dermatomal distribution of pain and/or motor deficits occurs in the absence of an antecedent rash. ZSH later became a distinct disease entity when PCR provided definitive virological confirmation. Diagnosis is established by rising VZV titers, VZV DNA extraction from CSF, and viral isolation.

A diagnosis of herpes zoster can be made by looking at the skin and gathering a medical history. Complaints range from mild itching or tingling to severe pain in the involved dermatome. Fully developed herpes zoster is distinct and mimicked by few other diseases. When a clinical diagnosis of herpes zoster is not obvious, confirmatory laboratory tests may be needed. Blood tests may show an increase in white blood cells and antibodies to the chickenpox virus but cannot confirm that the rash is due to shingles.

Differential diagnoses include contact dermatitis and herpes simplex virus infection. Consultation with appropriate specialists may be necessary when the presentation of herpes zoster is atypical or complex. This is particularly true of active herpes zoster involving the V1 dermatome, which may result in corneal ulcers and loss of vision.

Treatment

An antiviral frequently helps to reduce pain and complications and shorten the course of the disease. Ideally, medications should be started within 24 hours of the person feeling the pain or burning and preferably before the blisters appear. The drugs are usually given orally within 72 hours of the onset of lesions. Acyclovir is prescribed only if neither famciclovir nor valacyclovir is available, because acyclovir's complicated dosing schedule reduces the likelihood of compliance. Its pharmacokinetic and pharmacodynamic characteristics are also inferior to

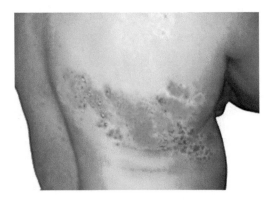

FIGURE 11.1. Skin lesions of acute herpes zoster.

Available from: http://www.bing.com/images/search?q=shingles+adam&qs=n&form=QBIR&pq=shingles+adam&sc=3-13&sp=-1&sk=.

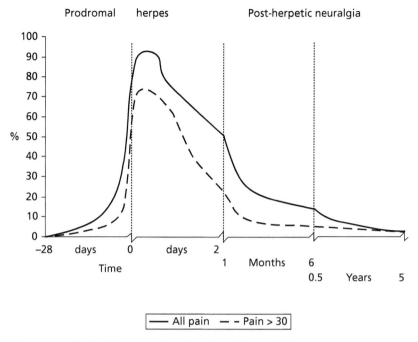

FIGURE 11.2. Time course of pain in herpes zoster and postherpetic neuralgia.

From van Wijck AJM et al. *Pain Practice* 2011;11:88–97.

those of famciclovir and valacyclovir. Following is the dosing regimen[1]:

- Famciclovir, 500 mg orally three times a day for 7 days
- Valacyclovir, 1 g orally three times a day for 7 days
- Acyclovir, 800 mg orally five times a day for 7 days

Intravenous acyclovir (10 to 15 mg/kg, IV, every 8 hours) should be administered in patients with herpes zoster that is complicated by central nervous system involvement, especially myelitis. For patients with severe herpes zoster ophthalmicus, intravenous acyclovir for initial therapy is also recommended.

Other medicines that are commonly used to treat herpes zoster include the following:

- Corticosteroids (such as prednisone) to reduce swelling and the risk of continued pain
- Antihistamines to reduce itching (oral or topical)
- Analgesics to relieve pain
- Zostrix, a cream containing capsaicin that may reduce the risk of postherpetic neuralgia (PHN).

- Early initiation of tricyclic antidepressants may reduce the risk of PHN.

Nonpharmacological interventions to consider include the following[1,2]:

- Cool, wet compresses can be used to reduce pain.
- Soothing baths and lotions may help to relieve itching and discomfort.
- The patient can rest in bed until the fever goes down.
- The skin should be kept clean, and contaminated items should not be reused.
- Nondisposables should be washed in boiling water or otherwise disinfected before reuse.
- The patient may need to be isolated while lesions are oozing to prevent infecting others who have never had chickenpox— especially pregnant women.

Interventional approaches to consider are as follows:

- Epidural injections or targeted nerve blocks may help to reduce pain
- Repeated paravertebral blocks may reduce not only pain but also the risk of developing PHN.[3]

Prevention

- Avoid touching the rash and blisters of persons with shingles or chickenpox.
- A herpes zoster vaccine is not the same as the chickenpox vaccine so should not be confused with it. Shingrix is a new non-live, subunit vaccine recently approved and recommended by the FDA.[4] In contrast to Zostavax, which consists of attenuated varicella virus at a concentration at least 14 times that found in chickenpox vaccine, Shingrix is 97% effective against shingles and 91% effective against PHN for people 50 and older.
- Adults older than 50 should receive the herpes zoster vaccine as part of routine medical care.
- A single shot of the herpes zoster vaccine, Zostavax, can cut the risk of getting shingles by about 50%. It may also help prevent PHN and ophthalmic herpes. Because the vaccine contains a live virus, it cannot be given to people with a weak immune system.

POSTHERPETIC NEURALGIA

Definition

Postherpetic neuralgia (PHN) is defined as pain in the affected dermatome that is still present 1 month after the development of herpes zoster vesicles.[1] Between 10% and 40% of patients with herpes zoster develop PHN. The incidence increases with age.

Pathophysiology

PHN occurs when nerve tissue has been damaged after an outbreak of herpes zoster. It is a common complication and is the result of damage that may involve the dorsal root and cranial nerve ganglia, spinal cord, and epidermis in discrete body segments. In PHN skin, there is a marked reduction in the density of epidermal nerve fibers that are predominantly unmyelinated C fibers with a small proportion of Aδ fibers. A nearly complete loss of the subepidermal nerve plexus has also been observed in immunostaining of skin biopsies.

Epidemiology

PHN develops in 10%–40% of patients with acute herpes zoster.[1,5] The probability of PHN increases with age and is more likely to occur in people over age 60. The estimated number of PHN cases in the United States is between 500,000 and 1 million. Age and severity of acute herpes zoster pain are the strongest predictors of PHN development.

Clinical Features and Diagnosis

PHN is zoster-related pain that is still present 1 month after the development of the skin lesions. The main symptom of PHN is pain in the area where shingles once occurred. The pain can range from mild to severe. It may be constant or come and go. The pain is often described as a deep aching, burning, stabbing, or an electric shock–like sensation. Skin discoloration along the affected dermatome is common. The affected area is often very sensitive to touch or temperature changes (allodynia), and often displays an increased painful response to pinpricks (hyperalgesia). In some cases, there is loss of peripheral sensation and the patient may experience anesthesia dolorosa. The diagnosis is based on a history of herpes zoster, typical dermatomal distribution of the pain, and hyperalgesia and/or allodynia on physical examination.

Treatment

Pharmacological treatment is the cornerstone of PHN therapy.[5,6,7] A large number of medications have been studied and commonly used clinically, although only lidocaine patch, pregabalin, gabapentin, and 8% capsaicin patch are approved by the Food and Drug Administration (FDA) for this indication.

- Anticonvulsant drugs may reduce the pain from damaged nerves. Gabapentin (1200–3600 mg in three divided doses) and pregabalin (300600 mg, in two divided doses) are those most often used (first line).
- Antidepressants such as amitriptyline (25–150 mg at bedtime, or in two divided doses) may help reduce pain and help with sleep (first line).
- Serotonin-noradrenaline reuptake inhibitors (SNRIs) such as duloxetine (60–120 mg, once daily) or venlafaxine (150–225 mg, once daily) may be used (first line).
- 5% Lidocaine patches to the painful area (one to three patches, once a day for up to

12 hours) may relieve some of the pain for a period of time (second line).

- 8% Capsaicin patch to the painful area (one to four patches for 30–60 minutes every 3 months) has been demonstrated to be effective (second line).
- Tramadol (200–400 mg in two or three divided doses) (second line)
- Strong opioids (third line).
- Botulinum toxin A (50–200 units) to the painful area every 3 months (third line).
- Combination therapies are often necessary.
- Interventional options such as epidural injections, paravertebral blocks, sympathetic nerve blocks, spinal cord stimulation, and intrathecal therapy may be considered in refractory cases.[5,8]
- Psychological support is often helpful in persistent cases because of the chronicity of pain.

GUIDING QUESTIONS

- Can you describe the pathophysiology of herpes zoster and postherpetic neuralgia (PHN)?
- How do you diagnose herpes zoster and PHN?
- How do you manage herpes zoster and PHN?
- Are there preventive measures for herpes zoster and PHN?

KEY POINTS

- Herpes zoster, also known as zoster and shingles, is caused by reactivation of the latent varicella zoster virus (VZV) that causes chicken pox. Once chicken pox resolves, VZV remains dormant in the dorsal root and cranial ganglia and can reactivate later in a person's life and cause herpes zoster. Approximately 95% of the US adult population has had varicella and thus can develop herpes zoster. It appears predominantly in older adults, but may also occur in those who are immunocompromised. Most people typically have only one episode of herpes zoster in their lifetime. However, second and even third episodes are possible.
- Postherpetic neuralgia (PHN) is defined as pain in the affected dermatome that is still present 1 month after the development of the vesicles. Between 10% and 40% of patients with herpes zoster develop PHN. The incidence increases with age.

- A herpes zoster vaccine is not the same as the chickenpox vaccine so should not be confused with it. Shingrix is a new non-live, subunit vaccine recently approved and recommended by the FDA.[4] In contrast to Zostavax, which consists of attenuated varicella virus at a concentration at least 14 times that found in chickenpox vaccine, Shingrix is 97% effective against shingles and 91% effective against PHN for people 50 and older. The diagnosis of herpes zoster can be made on the basis of characteristic skin lesions and pain and itching in the involved dermatome. Differential diagnoses include contact dermatitis and herpes simplex virus infection.
- During the acute phase, an antiviral helps to reduce pain and complications and shorten the course of the disease. Antiviral medications should be started as early as possible, usually given orally within 72 hours of the onset of lesions.
- The diagnosis of PHN is based on a history of herpes zoster, typical dermatomal distribution of the pain, and hyperalgesia and/or allodynia on physical examination.
- A large number of medications have been used to treat PHN, although only lidocaine patch, pregabalin, gabapentin, and 8% capsaicin patch are approved by the FDA for this indication. First-line pharmacotherapy includes gabapentin or pregabalin, tricyclic antidepressants, and SNRIs. Combination therapies are often necessary.
- Interventional options such as epidural injections, paravertebral blocks, selective nerve root blocks, sympathetic nerve blocks, intercostal nerve blocks, trigeminal nerve blocks, spinal cord stimulation, and intrathecal therapy may be considered in refractory cases.

REFERENCES

1. Cotton D, Taichman D, Williams S. Herpes zoster. *Ann Intern Med.* 2011;154:ITC31–15.
2. Baron R, Wasner G. Prevention and treatment of postherpetic neuralgia. *Lancet.* 2006;367:186–188.
3. Ji G, Niu J, Shi Y, Hou L, Lu Y, Xiong L. The effectiveness of repetitive paravertebral injections with

local anesthetics and steroids for the prevention of postherpetic neuralgia in patients with acute herpes zoster. *Anesth Analg.* 2009;109:1651–1655.

4. Center for Disease Control and Prevention. Shingles (herpes zoster). Available from: http://www.cdc.gov/shingles/hcp/clinical-overview.html.

5. van Wijck AJM, Wallace M, Mekhail N, van Kleef M. Evidence-based interventional pain medicine according to clinical diagnoses. 17. Herpes zoster and post-herpetic neuralgia. *Pain Pract.* 2011;11:88–97.

6. Dworkin RH, Schmader KE. Herpes zoster and postherpetic neuralgia. In Benson HT, Raja SN, Molloy RE, Liu SS, Fishman SM, eds. *Essentials of Pain Medicine and Regional Anesthesia.* St. Louis: Elsevier; 2005:386–393.

7. Finnerup NB, Attal N, Haroutounian S, et al. Pharmacotherapy for neuropathic pain in adults: a systematic review and meta-analysis. *Lancet Neurol.* 2015;14:162–173.

8. Dworkin RH, O'Connor AB, Kent J, et al; International Association for the Study of Pain Neuropathic Pain Special Interest Group. Interventional management of neuropathic pain: NeuPSIG recommendations. *Pain.* 2013;154:2249–2261.

12

Entrapment Syndromes

JONATHAN P. ESKANDER, ZEESHAN MALIK, AND RINOO V. SHAH

CASE

A 41-year-old woman presents with insidious onset of left-hand numbness and tingling sensation beginning less than 2 months ago. The patient endorses these symptoms mainly on the palmar surface of her index and pointer fingers, especially when she types on the computer and rides her bike. On examination her Phalen's sign test is positive. Her past medical history is unremarkable and her physical exam is negative for neck pain. She was diagnosed with carpal tunnel syndrome and prescribed ibuprofen, physical therapy, and a wrist splint. If these conservative measures fail, eventually she could be a candidate for interventions as well as an orthopedic surgery consult for possible carpal tunnel release.

CARPAL TUNNEL SYNDROME

Definition

Carpal tunnel syndrome (CTS) results from compression of the median nerve as it passes over the carpal bones of the wrist and alongside flexor tendons of the hand. It may be caused by repetitive movements over a long period of time (keyboard typing, playing certain instruments, biking, and more), fluid retention, pregnancy, or myxedema secondary to hypothyroidism among other factors. Typically, it is characterized by numbness, tingling, and burning pain along the median nerve distribution. This may occur in one or both arms.

Pathophysiology

CTS is the result of median nerve compression along the carpal tunnel at the wrist. The floor of the tunnel is formed by the carpal bones, the roof by the flexor retinaculum, and nine flexor tendons pass through this space.[1] This entrapment neuropathy is the result of compression and traction in a crowded space. In tandem, these phenomena may cause lesions in the nerve fibers, supporting connective tissue alterations, and abnormal intraneural microcirculation.[1] The two most common sites of compression are at the hook of the hamate and the proximal edge of the carpal tunnel caused by wrist flexion.

Epidemiology

In the general population, CTS may occur in about 3 in 1000 people.[2] This incidence is higher in groups with known risk factors. These risk factors include repetitive wrist motions, pregnancy, hypothyroidism, obesity, diabetes, lupus, and rheumatoid arthritis. Interestingly, epidemiological data show that this disease is more common in females, developed nations, and Caucasians.[3]

Clinical Features and Diagnosis

Numbness, tingling, and even pain can be experienced at the palmar surface and dorsal tips of the inner half of the ring finger, middle finger, index finger, and thumb. Diagnosis can be made via physical exam maneuvers that transiently increase pressure in the carpal tunnel, for example, Phalen's maneuver. Within 30–60 seconds, most patients report reproduction of CTS symptoms. If the physical exam is unremarkable an electromyogram (EMG) may be ordered. A positive EMG will demonstrate a delay in distal latency of the median nerve. This study can be helpful in ruling out other disease processes such as cervical radiculopathy, neuropathies of various origin, and thoracic outlet syndrome (TOS).

Treatment

Conservative measures are first-line. These include physical therapy, wrist splinting to maintain neutral wrist position, and nonsteroidal anti-inflammatory drugs (NSAIDs). If these measures fail, some patients may be candidates for steroid injections and, in severe cases, surgical decompression. Treatment regimens for CTS are summarized as follows:

- Ibuprofen 400–800 mg PO q6–8h; do not exceed 3.2 g/day (first-line).
- Prednisolone 20 mg PO daily for 2 weeks, followed by 10 mg PO daily for 2 weeks (second-line).
- Refractory cases may require corticosteroid injections into the flexor retinaculum, with or without a local anesthetic, to help reduce inflammation.
- If conservative measures fail, surgical decompression is indicated.

Prevention

Measures that patients can take to prevent CTS are as follows:

- Avoid repetitive wrist motion.
- Take frequent breaks from repetitive tasks.
- Reduce the force of extension and flexion of the wrist, relax grip.
- Weight loss
- Avoid sleeping on the hands.

In addition, the clinician should treat other comorbidities such as hypothyroidism, diabetes, lupus, and rheumatoid arthritis.

CASE

A 36-year-old man presents with onset of left fourth- and fifth-digit numbness and tingling beginning immediately after a hernia repair under general anesthesia. The patient has an unremarkable medical history other than bilateral inguinal hernias status post-repair. He was diagnosed with ulnar neuropathy at the elbow, likely due to poor positioning during surgery, and prescribed ibuprofen, gabapentin, vitamin B6, and an elbow pad.

ULNAR NEUROPATHY

Definition

Ulnar neuropathy (UN) is an entrapment of the ulnar nerve at the elbow region, most commonly at the epicondylar groove or at the cubital tunnel.

Pathophysiology

Pressure on or injury to the ulnar nerve may lead to denervation and possible paralysis of the muscles supplied by the nerve. The ulnar nerve is particularly vulnerable when the elbow is bent and the epicondylar groove disappears, making the ulnar nerve relatively superficial.[4] An acute blow to this area is colloquially known as "hitting the funny bone."

Epidemiology

Next to CTS, UN at the elbow is the second most common site of nerve entrapment in the upper extremity. Patients tend to be male and over 35 years of age.[5] Interestingly, men develop perioperative ulnar neuropathies at the elbow more frequently than women do. This may be attributed to women having a higher fat content than men and men having a larger coronoid process.

Clinical Features and Diagnosis

Symptoms typically present as numbness and tingling sensation along the distribution of the ulnar nerve, as well as loss of strength in the muscles supplied by the ulnar nerve. The most sensitive test for UN at the elbow, while the elbow is in flexion, is applying direct pressure to the ulnar nerve, located posterior to the medial epicondyle. Like in CTS, nerve conduction studies may help differentiate this process from brachial plexopathy or ulnar entrapment at the wrist.

Treatment

The mainstay of conservative therapy is the application of an elbow pad or night-splinting for a 3-month trial period, to reduce the trauma and ischemia time while the elbow is in flexion for long periods of time.[6] Depending on the exact location, severe cases of UN require surgical transposition of the ulnar nerve with or without a medial epicondylectomy or decompression at the aponeurosis. Treatment regimens for UN are summarized as follows:

Ibuprofen 400–800 mg PO q6–8h; do not exceed 3.2 g/day (first-line).

Gabapentin 300 mg PO TID, titrate upward of maximum 3600 mg daily (second-line).

Oral vitamin B6 supplementation for 6–12 weeks may be helpful.

If elbow pads fail, then a 3-week trial of daytime immobilization can be considered as the last type of conservative management.

CASE

A 42-year-old man presents with gradual onset of clumsiness in his left ulnar three digits, as well as numbness of the medial forearm and aching pain poorly localized to the upper arm and anterior chest. His medical history is unremarkable. On physical exam he denies neck pain. An electrodiagnostic study was negative. He was diagnosed with TOS, prescribed physical therapy with the goal of correcting shoulder posture, and given botulinum toxin injections into the scalene muscles. (Of note, early EMG studies in TOS can be negative. Later responses such as F-waves will become prolonged and conductions along the plexus will slow.)

THORACIC OUTLET SYNDROME

Definition

TOS is generally a group of disorders caused by compression of the brachial plexus and surrounding neurovascular structures. It is a progressive condition resulting from compression of nerves and blood vessels that feed the thoracic outlet.

Pathophysiology

Various structures can be the source responsible for the development of the constellation of symptoms known as TOS. A cervical rib, an anatomical variation present in 1 in 500 people that is easily spotted on X-ray, may be the cause of TOS for some. Other causes include entrapment by scalene, subclavius, or pectoralis muscles. Typically, the lower trunk of the brachial plexus exhibits symptoms in TOS if there is neurovascular compromise.

Epidemiology

There are three types of TOS: arterial, venous, and neurological. The majority of TOS cases are diagnosed between the ages of 20 and 50. Women are more likely to develop neurogenic TOS, whereas athletic men are more likely to develop vascular TOS.

Clinical Features and Diagnosis

Vascular TOS may be caused by repetitive limb motions that lead to claudication, whereas neurogenic TOS is usually the result of trauma to the shoulder girdle or neck. Since TOS is a diagnosis of exclusion, a careful history and thorough physical examination are critical to establishing a diagnosis. It is important to note that other entrapment neuropathies are often diagnosed simultaneously with TOS, so it is important to be suspicious of them as well.

Treatment

The mainstay of therapy is physical therapy, improved shoulder posture, and NSAIDs. Excellent results have been reported with botulism injections, whereas surgery is falling out of favor because of significant morbidity. Treatment regimens for TOS are summarized as follows:

> Ibuprofen 400–800 mg PO q6–8h; do not exceed 3.2 g/day (first-line).
>
> Correction of shoulder posture can completely eliminate symptoms of TOS in many cases. Focus should be on rhomboid and trapezius muscle strengthening.
>
> Clavicle straps may assist with maintaining correct shoulder posture.
>
> If other conservative measures fail, botulinum toxin injections into the scalene, subclavius, pectoralis minor, trapezius, and levator scapula may be effective.

CASE

An 18-year-old man presents with numbness of the lateral aspect of his thigh after being involved in motor vehicle collision. He was wearing a seatbelt. No injuries were noted. His medical history is unremarkable. On physical exam he endorses some soreness along his waist where the seatbelt was. He was diagnosed with meralgia paresthetica and advised to avoid wearing tight clothing and belts along the waistline. He was also advised that most symptoms might resolve within 6 months. He was also offered a lateral femoral cutaneous nerve block for symptomatic relief.

MERALGIA PARESTHETICA

Definition

Meralgia paresthetica (MP) is a lateral femoral cutaneous neuropathy. It is an entrapment of the purely sensory lateral femoral cutaneous nerve cause by trauma, pregnancy, or tight-fitting clothes.

Pathophysiology

The lateral femoral cutaneous nerve is usually trapped as it passes through or under the inguinal ligament. This phenomenon typically results from increased intra-abdominal pressure secondary to pregnancy, weight gain, and, rarely, from mass lesions. Additional causes of MP include blunt trauma, diabetic neuropathy, and tight-fitting clothes and belts.

Epidemiology

An incidence of 4 per 10,000 patient years has been reported in the general population; among diabetics, the incidence increases to 247 per 100,000 patient years.[7] Additionally, an increase in diagnoses has been noted among teenagers who wear tight-fitting jeans, which has led this disorder to be colloquially coined "skinny pants syndrome."

Clinical Features and Diagnosis

Pain or decreased sensitivity to touch is typically noted along the lateral portion of the thigh. There is no motor component to the lateral femoral cutaneous nerve, therefore, finding are purely sensory. History and physical exam are often essential to achieving a diagnosis. Electroconductive studies are not useful unless they are used to exclude lumbar radiculopathy.

Treatment

- Typically, this is a self-limiting disorder that resolves within 6 months. Nerve blocks are successful in some cases, as well as treatment with pulsed radiofrequency.
- Lidocaine patches may be useful if the condition is painful.

CASE

A 22-year-old track-and-field athlete presents with gradual onset of pain in his heel. His medical history is unremarkable and radiological imaging is negative for fractures, ligament, or tendon injury. He was diagnosed with tarsal tunnel syndrome due to entrapment of the lateral plantar nerve and was consulted to rest his foot, avoid ill-fitting footwear, and take anti-inflammatory medication. He was advised that surgical decompression may be effective if conservative measures are not.

ENTRAPMENT OF THE LATERAL PLANTAR NERVE AND ITS BRANCHES

Definition

Tarsal tunnel syndrome (TTS) is now a revised term to describe entrapment of the tibial nerve and one of its branches.

Pathophysiology

Compression of the tibial nerve or its branches along the tarsal tunnel or anterior to the calcaneus results in a constellation of symptoms known as TTS. This can be caused by poorly fitting footwear, trauma, pregnancy, diabetes, thyroid diseases, rheumatoid arthritis, and mass lesions.

Epidemiology

TTS occurs more dominantly in active adults, especially among those whose activities include jumping and landing on the heel of the foot.[6]

Clinical Features and Diagnosis

Typical features of TTS include numbness radiating from the heel to the toes, including the big toe. The symptoms may vary because there is great variability in the area of entrapment. Some authors divide TTS into proximal TTS and distal tunnel syndrome. However, the lateral plantar nerve and its branches are the most common site of entrapment.

Treatment

Rest, immobilization, and replace poorly fitting footwear.
NSAIDS, steroid injections, and lidocaine patches may be effective.
Surgical decompression may be effective.

OTHER PERIPHERAL NERVE INJURIES

Numerous peripheral nerve injuries have been described that are not necessarily considered entrapment syndromes but may result from similar pathology. Peripheral nerve injuries are relatively common during the perioperative period. Poor patient positioning under general anesthesia may result in injuries to the ulnar nerve, brachial plexus, obturator nerve, or common peritoneal nerve, among many others. Peripheral nerve blocks may contribute to nerve injury due to high speeds of local anesthetic injection. For example, the common peroneal nerve is sensitive to this mechanism of injury during a popliteal sciatic block even under ultrasound guidance. Neuraxial blockade is also associated with peripheral nerve injuries, particularly the obturator nerve during labor and delivery as well as gynecological procedures. Some less common peripheral nerve injuries may be associated with anatomical abnormalities or surgical procedures. These include anomalous vertebral arteries causing cervical nerve root compression or C5 nerve palsy, thought to be caused by preoperative spinal cord rotation and subsequent tethering during cervical spine surgery.[8,9] Much of the nerve injury described in this chapter relates to direct compression and stretching of nerves, which lead to local ischemia and, subsequently, focal demyelination with axonal damage and scarring if severe enough.[10-12]

GUIDING QUESTIONS

Can you describe the pathophysiology of carpal tunnel syndrome (CTS)?

How do you diagnose CTS, ulnar neuropathy (UN), thoracic outlet syndrome (TOS), and meralgia paresthetica (MP)?

How do you manage CTS, UN, TOS, MP, tarsal tunnel syndrome (TTS), and perioperative peripheral nerve injuries?

What are the preventive measures for the these entrapment syndromes?

KEY POINTS

- Carpal tunnel syndrome (CTS) results from compression of the median nerve as it passes over the carpal bones. CTS may be caused by repetitive movements of the wrist.
- Ulnar nerve entrapment, aka the "funny bone," is the second most common nerve entrapment due to the superficial location of the nerve at the bent elbow. Ulnar neuropathy is also the most common neuropathy during the perioperative period if general anesthesia is used.
- Surgery, particularly under general anesthesia, may result in many possible neuropathies due to malpositioning of the patient. These peripheral nerve injuries

commonly include the ulnar nerve, brachial plexus, and obturator nerve. Some neuropathies are not quite as common, including C5 nerve palsy, which may be secondary to spinal cord rotation and tethering during cervical spine surgery.

- Thoracic outlet syndrome (TOS) is a group of disorders causing brachial plexus and neurovascular compression. The three types are neurological, arterial, and venous.
- Arterial and venous TOS can be differentiated by a sudden onset of upper extremity pain and weakness with cold and pale fingers in the former, and abrupt spontaneous swelling of the arm in the latter.
- Meralgia paresthetica (MP) is due to entrapment of the lateral femoral cutaneous nerve, which is a pure sensory nerve. Causes include tight-fitting clothes and/or belts, blunt trauma, and diabetic neuropathy.
- Tarsal tunnel syndrome (TTS) may result from ankle trauma and entrapment of the tibial nerve or its branches at the ankle. TTS most commonly affects the lateral plantar nerve or one of its branches.

REFERENCES

1. Bland JDP. Carpal tunnel syndrome. *BMJ*. 2007;335(7615):343–346.
2. Padua L, Coraci D, Erra C, et al. Carpal tunnel syndrome: clinical features, diagnosis, and management. *Lancet Neurol*. 2016;15(12):1273–1284.
3. Rota E, Morelli N. Entrapment neuropathies in diabetes mellitus. *World J Diabetes*. 2016;7(17):342–353.
4. Robertson C, Saratsiotis J. A review of compressive ulnar neuropathy at the elbow. *J Manipulative Physiol Ther*. 2005;28(5):345.
5. Contreras MG, Warner MA, Charboneau WJ, Cahill DR. Anatomy of the ulnar nerve at the elbow: potential relationship of acute ulnar neuropathy to gender differences. *Clin Anat*. 1998;11(6):372–378.
6. Cheatham SW, Kolber MJ, Salamh PA. Meralgia paresthetica: a review of the literature. *Int J Sports Phys Ther*. 2013;8(6):883–893.
7. Freischlag J, Orion K. Understanding thoracic outlets Syndrome. *Scientifica*. 2014:248163.
8. Eskander MS, Howard CM, Connolly PJ, et al. Does the rotation of the spinal cord predict postoperative C5 nerve palsies? *J Bone and Joint Surg Am*. 2012;94(17):1605–1609.

9. Clark, T, Eskander JP, Eskander MS. Scapular pain caused by an anomalous vertebral artery. *J Spine Neurosurg* 2014;3:1–2.

10. Eversmann WW. Entrapment and compression neuropathies. In: Green DP, ed. *Operative Hand Surgery*. Vol. 2. New York: Churchill Livingstone; 1982:957–1009.

11. Lanzetta M, Foucher G. Entrapment of the superficial branch of the radial nerve (Wartenberg's syndrome): a report of 52 cases. *Int Orthop.* 1993;17:342–345.

12. Keith MW, Masear V, Amadio PC, et al. Treatment of carpal tunnel syndrome. *J Am Acad Orthop Surg.* 2009;17:397–405.

13

Neuroma

JOHN BLACKBURN AND ALEXANDER BAUTISTA

CASE

A 28-year-old right-handed woman presents with a chief complaint of sharp pain in the back of her left thigh. She had an above-the-knee amputation of her left leg due to a motor vehicle accident 3 years ago. The pain is localized in the back of her thigh about 15 cm above the stump. She describes the pain as electricity-like, sharp, burning, and throbbing. It is often spontaneous and is extremely sensitive to touch or pressure over a distinct area in the back of her left thigh. It makes it difficult for her to use the prosthetic leg. She is currently taking gabapentin 600 mg TID, amitriptyline 25 mg HS, and hydrocodone-acetaminophen 5–325 mg q8h PRN. An MRI was performed and showed a flattened nerve with T2 hyperintensity of the sciatic nerve proximal to the stump. She was diagnosed with formation of neuroma.

NEUROMA

Definition

The word *neuroma* originates from the Greek word *neuro*, which means "nerve," and *-oma*, which denotes swelling. Neuroma is a benign condition that is associated with growth or tumor of the nerve tissue. It is a disorganized fibroneural tissue mass that contains axons, connective tissue, and different type of Schwann's cells, macrophages, fibroblasts, and myofibroblasts.[1] *Neuroma* is also a term that refers to any swelling of the nerve in the absence of abnormal cell growth. Following a traumatic nerve injury and regeneration, development of neuromas can be painful with associated altered sensation along the distribution of the injured nerve. For the purpose of this chapter, we will focus on neuroma formation from abnormal nerve regeneration following a peripheral nerve lesion.

Epidemiology

The development of neuromas adversely affects the patient's quality of life. The incidence of symptomatic neuromas is estimated to be approximately 3%–5% of all patients involved in peripheral nerve injury.[2] Phantom limb pain is a type of neuropathic pain that may or may not be associated with neuromas. Neuromas have been reported to occur in 50%–80% of amputees.[3]

Pathophysiology

Axotomy leads to neuroma formation, where budding regenerative nerve sprouts devoid of growth guidance from denervated Schwann cells form an entangled mass. Many neuromas are painful, but for unclear reasons, some are not. Neuromas may be tethered to adjacent moving structures (e.g., tendons), such that otherwise normal movements, stretch, or pressure evokes an increase in pain. Neuromas can also form from peripheral nerves as a result of chronic irritation, pressure, stretch, poor repair of nerve lesions, and nerve trauma caused by laceration, blunt, or crush injury. After a traumatic nerve injury, a derangement in the neural architecture occurs involving degeneration of the proximal stump for a variable distance and Wallerian degeneration of the distal stump. Fascicular escape, another hallmark of neuroma formation, occurs when the regenerating axons escape into the surrounding epineural tissue in a disorganized fashion accompanied by blood vessels, Schwann cells, and proliferating fibroblasts. A functional deficit occurs due to inadequate regeneration and gapping of the nerve endings.

The mechanism of pain in neuroma is a result of persistent mechanical or chemical irritation of axons within the neuroma and development of spontaneous and disturbing nociceptive signals from neurons in the dorsal root ganglion to the dorsal horn of the spinal cord and from there forward.[4] The spontaneous activity and ectopic sensitivity to mechanical, thermal, and chemical stimuli that originate from the traumatic neuroma have been well documented. Both nociceptive neurons (C fibers and A-δ fibers) and non-nociceptive neurons (A-β) may contribute to the genesis of pain.[5] Spontaneous activity in "A-β" nociceptors has been documented in rodents and primates. The tissue damage from neuroma results in overall sensitization of the nociceptors, resulting in altered transduction and increased conduction of the nociceptive impulses toward the central nervous system, creating a hyperexcitable and hyperalgesic state.[6]

There is proliferation of abnormal potassium and sodium channels, which explains the hyperexcitability and spontaneous discharges from the injured nerves.[6] This has been supported by the use of antineuropathic agents that block sodium ion channels or membrane stabilizers that inhibit spontaneous activity and decrease conductance. Another part of the mechanism involves neuroanatomical and neurophysiological changes in the spinal cord and brain. These changes involve expansion of receptive field size and an increase in magnitude and duration of response to stimuli. Chronic activation of glial cells produces inflammatory cytokines, including interleukin 1, interleukin 6, and tumor necrosis factor-alpha, that activate dorsal horn neurons in the spinal cord responsible for pain transmission.[7]

Clinical Features and Diagnosis

The clinical hallmarks of neuroma include the presence of a scar in close proximity that causes substantial pain and altered sensibility in the distribution of the involved nerve. Each peripheral neuroma presents with distinct clinical characteristics (see Table 13.1). The evaluation begins with a detailed history of the inciting event. Understanding the characteristics of the pain and its psychological implications is important in determining the success of the treatment, especially

TABLE 13.1. COMMON PERIPHERAL NEUROMAS

Common Peripheral Neuromas	Distinguishing Characteristics
Ulnar digital nerve (bowler's thumb)	Common injury in baseball players and bowlers. Repetitive compression by insertion of thumb into bowling ball and baseball gloves leads to proliferation of fibrous tissue around the nerve.[9,10]
Superficial radial nerve	Purely sensory nerve that is commonly associated with neuroma formation and difficult to treat. In up to 10% of the population this nerve takes a subcutaneous course from the brachioradialis muscle, rendering the nerve susceptible to injury.[11]
Palmar cutaneous nerve	Branch from median nerve prone to neuroma formation, most often due to iatrogenic injury during carpal tunnel release. Surgical incision should be made on ulnar side of the ring finger to prevent injury.[12]
Amputation stump neuromas	Perhaps overlooked source of pain in patients following amputation, though present in up to 25% postoperatively.[13]
Neuromas from poor surgical repair	Technicalities related to surgical repair, including mismatched diameter between severed nerve and graft or scarring at suture line altering nerve regeneration, promote neuroma formation. Neuroma formation is the most frequent complication after nerve grafting in the upper extremities.[14]
Morton's neuroma (metatarsalagia)	Neuroma of intermetatarsal plantar nerve. Symptoms are reproduced with tight-fitting shoes or compression over metatarsal heads. It is more common in younger adults, long distance runners, and females, who are afflicted five times more frequently than males.[15]

if surgery is being contemplated. Determining the distribution of the pain assists in identifying the involved nerve. There are four types of pain descriptors that have been identified: (1) spontaneous pain, (2) pain on pressure over the neuroma, (3) pain on movement of the adjacent joints, and (4) painful hyperesthesia on light skin touch in the vicinity of the neuromas. The modified Hendler's back pain rating scale has been used to evaluate pain associated with neuroma. The scale consists of three components: a body diagram for indicating pain location, a numerical scale, and a list of pain descriptors.[7,8]

On physical examination, palpation of a discrete area of tenderness resulting in radiating pain in the distribution of the peripheral nerve supports the diagnosis of neuroma. One starts with gentle manipulation outside the area of the described discomfort, gradually moving toward the affected area to determine if there are multiple nerves contributing to the neuroma. Eliciting a Tinel-like response by percussion approximately 3 inches proximal to the site of neuroma formation along the course the nerve will aid in localization of the involved nerve.[6]

A diagnostic nerve block of the affected nerve(s), typically under ultrasound guidance, is usually employed after a thorough history and physical examination.[7] This will help determine if the patient is a good surgical candidate. The sensory change produced should block the pain from the neuroma. To eliminate a placebo response, the nerve block may be repeated on more than one occasion.

Treatment

Neuroma as a form of neuropathic pain is difficult and challenging to treat. Strategies for treatment begin with the least invasive option and progress toward more invasive approaches after failed conservative management trials. The acuity of pain, mechanism of injury, nerve involvement, and physiological and psychosocial factors affect treatment plans in patients with neuroma. The treatment plan should be individualized to meet each patient's needs. A proposed treatment approach is summarized in Figure 13.1.

Nonoperative Management

Nonoperative management is almost always the first step once the diagnosis is made. Pharmacotherapy runs the gamut of antineuropathic regimens that include antidepressants, anticonvulsants, and analgesics.

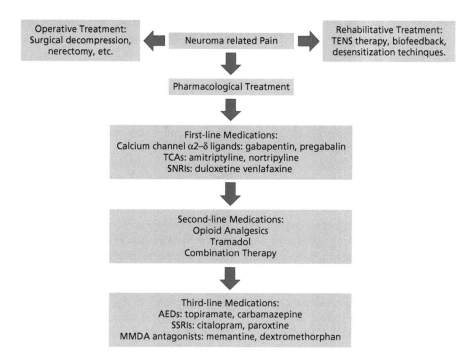

FIGURE 13.1. Summary of treatment approach for neuroma. AEDs, antiepileptic drugs; SNRIs, serotonin-noradrenaline reuptake inhibitors; SSRIs, selective serotonin reuptake inhibitors; TCAs, tricyclic antidepressants; TENS, transcutaneous electrical nerve stimulation.

Rehabilitation plays a vital role, including physical therapy massages and alternative holistic therapies such as acupuncture. In patients with significant psychosocial issues, mind–body interventions such as counseling, biofeedback, relaxation therapy, and support groups may prove to be beneficial. Painful neuromas have been found to respond to desensitization therapy and it is therefore recommended as part of the treatment plan.[6]

Anticonvulsants

This class of drugs exerts effect by binding to voltage-gated calcium channels, thereby reducing the influx of calcium channels into nerve terminals.[9] The reduction of calcium influx decreases neurotransmitter release, including glutamate, CGRP, ATP, and substance P. Pregabalin and gabapentin are the prototypes for this class. Both drugs share the same pharmacokinetics and pharmacodynamics. They are well absorbed orally and are not bound to plasma proteins. Their main route of elimination is renal, so the dose must be adjusted accordingly. Side effects commonly reported include dizziness, somnolence, peripheral edema, nausea, and gastrointestinal upset. The advantages of pregabalin over gabapentin are its linear pharmacokinetics, narrow dosing range, and easy dose titration.

Antidepressants

These medications are traditionally approved to treat major depressive disorders. However, studies have shown their utility in providing effective pain relief in neuropathic conditions. The analgesic effects of antidepressants are evident at a lower dose than the antidepressant effects. The tricyclic antidepressants (TCAs) and serotonin-norepinephrine reuptake inhibitors (SNRIs) possess stronger analgesic qualities than those of selective serotonin reuptake inhibitors (SSRIs). The mechanism of action of how they provide analgesia is uncertain, but it has been postulated that the analgesic property is associated with their action as serotonin and norepinephrine reuptake inhibitors and may also potentiate endogenous opioids. TCAs in particular may cause anticholinergic adverse effects that include dry mouth, orthostatic hypotension, constipation, and urinary retention. The most potent TCA is amitriptyline, which also comes with adverse effects. Secondary amines like nortriptyline and desipramine are well tolerated, especially in the elderly population, owing to their less anticholinergic effect.

Venlafaxine, dexvenlafaxine, duloxetine, and milnacipran are the four SNRIs that are available in the United States.

Analgesics

The choice of an appropriate initial therapeutic strategy varies among individuals. Nonopioid analgesics include acetaminophen, nonselective nonsteroidal anti-inflammatory drugs (NSAIDs), and cyclooxygenase 2 (COX-2) inhibitors. Whenever possible, the use of NSAIDs should be avoided in elderly patients because of the drug's renal effects. Use of opioids for managing neuropathic pain is controversial and should be reserved for select patients with moderate to severe chronic pain. An assessment of the risks and benefits should be undertaken before starting opioid therapy. Guidelines from World Health Organization can be used as a framework for pain control with opioids. Opioid treatment should be goal directed, and appropriate dosing should depend on the patient's improvement in function and quality of life.

Rehabilitation

The primary goal of this treatment is to enable patients to transition back into their normal activities as much as possible. Methods for rehabilitation include desensitization, massage, transcutaneous nerve stimulation, and vibration.[8] The use of vibration therapy aids in sensory re-education and desensitization of painful areas. The process involves stimulation of the periphery with gradual movement toward the center. Specific treatment is geared toward patients with deformities, weakness, loss of balance, loss of endurance, and neuropathic pain.

Operative Management

Patient selection is of utmost importance when considering any invasive approach. Surgical excision or decompression is commonly applied to many peripheral nerves. The aim is to free the nerves by releasing the compressive structure, or giving the nerve clearance from a compressive ligament. Mobilization of the nerves involves dissection outside the epineurium to free the nerves from compression, strangulation, or tethering.

Neurolysis of a nerve from a scarring is applied to nerves that have experienced injury and altered signaling caused by focal changes in the environment.[6,10] In patients who have pain in purely sensory nerves, neurectomy can be considered a treatment option. The goal is to abate painful dysesthesias for numbness in the distribution of the nerves. The numbness may last as long as 1 year but diminishes over time because other overlapping or neighboring nerves fill in at the edges of the area. Diagnostic blocks are helpful in predicting the response and allow the patient to experience the odd sensation in advance. This technique is usually employed after a failed neurolysis or nerve reconstruction. Often, if the original neurectomy was suboptimally performed, a repeat neurectomy can be considered. Nerves amenable to neurectomy include the saphenous nerve, sural nerve, superficial radial nerve, and most cutaneous nerves of the arm, forearm, thigh, leg, and trunk. If neurectomy is contemplated for mixed nerves, it should be taken into account whether or not function of the nerve can be sacrificed.

When intractable pain is an issue, nerve repair and reconstruction can be considered. If a focal neuroma-in-continuity exists or when proximal and distal stumps are in close proximity, direct repair of the nerve can be accomplished surgically. On occasion, nerve grafts or biological or synthetic nerve conduit can be used for longer gaps.[7] For painful neuromas, favorable outcomes range between 64% and 75% with traditional resection and reimplantation techniques.[8] The long-term outcome of nerve repair focuses only on motor recovery. There is still a paucity of data examining whether these interventions provide long-term pain relief in patients with neuroma.

Neuromodulation may play a role in management of neuroma as the technology continues to advance. The hyperexcitable and hypersensitive state of the injured nerve may be controlled by continuous electrical stimulation produced by nerve stimulation.[6] By overriding stimulation of the proximal large afferent fibers, modulation of distal painful stimuli can be achieved. Still, proper patient selection is vital for a successful outcome.

Prevention

Theoretically, peripheral nerves have the capability to be repaired and to restore their function after an injury. However, complete recovery after peripheral nerve lesioning rarely occurs in the clinical setting. Prevention is the key to neuroma management, but is easier said than done. Painful neuroma following a peripheral nerve injury are recalcitrant to pharmacological treatment and may require surgical intervention. Following surgical removal of the neuroma, an extrasurgical procedure is often required, and the outcome is rarely satisfactory, owing to induction of further neuroma formation. To date, there is no widely accepted standard management to prevent neuroma formation. Special care should be taken to minimize scar formation, such as use of the laser or scissor transection method instead of electrocoagulation or cryoneurolysis.[10] The most effective method of prevention is implantation of the nerve into the muscle or capping the nerve stump with an epineural graft after surgical resection of the neuroma.

GUIDING QUESTIONS
- Can you describe the pathophysiology of neuroma formation?
- How do you diagnose neuroma?
- How do you manage patients with neuroma?

KEY POINTS
- Neuroma is a benign condition that is associated with growth or tumor of nerve tissue.
- Neuromas can form from cutaneous nerves as a result of chronic irritation, pressure, stretch, poor repair of nerve lesions, nerve trauma caused by laceration, or blunt or crush injury.
- The clinical hallmarks of neuroma include presence of a scar that is associated with substantial pain and altered sensibility in the distribution of the involved nerve.
- The initial treatment for neuroma includes physical therapy and antineuropathic pain medications.
- More invasive treatment involves primary nerve ablative procedures, including neurolysis, neurectomy, and nerve repair/ reconstruction.
- Neuromodulation with either dorsal column stimulation or peripheral nerve stimulation may play a role in the treatment of neuromas.

REFERENCES
1. Mavrogenis AF, Pavlakis K, Stamatoukou A, et al. Current treatment concepts for neuromas-in-continuity. *Injury.* 2008;39(Suppl 3):S43–S48.
2. Atherton DD, Taherzadeh O, Facer P, Elliot D, Anad P. The potential role of nerve growth factor (NGF) in painful neuromas and the mechanism of pain relief by their relocation to muscle. *J Hand Surg Br.* 2006;31(6):652–656.

3. Flor H. Phantom-limb pain: characteristics, causes, and treatment. *Lancet Neurol.* 2002;1(3):182–189.

4. von Hehn CA, Baron R, Woolf CJ. Deconstructing the neuropathic pain phenotype to reveal neural mechanisms. *Neuron.* 2012;73(4):638–652.

5. Campbell JN, Meyer RA. Mechanisms of neuropathic pain. *Neuron.* 2006;52(1):77–92.

6. Vernadakis AJ, Koch H, Mackinnon SE. Management of neuromas. *Clin Plast Surg.* 2003;30(2):247–268, vii.

7. Stokvis A, van der Avoort DJ, van Neck JW, Hovius SE, Coert JH. Surgical management of neuroma pain: a prospective follow-up study. *Pain.* 2010;151(3):862–869.

8. Watson J, Gonzalez M, Romero A, Kerns J. Neuromas of the hand and upper extremity. *J Hand Surg Am.* 2010;35(3):499–510.

9. Gidal BE. New and emerging treatment options for neuropathic pain. *Am J Manag Care.* 2006;12(9 Suppl):S269–S278.

10. Lewin-Kowalik J, Marcol W, Kotulska K, Mandera M, Klimczak A. Prevention and management of painful neuroma. *Neurol Med Chir (Tokyo).* 2006;46(2):62–67; discussion 67-8.

11. Dellon AL, Mackinnon, SE. Susceptibility of the superficial sensory branch of the radial nerve to form painful neuromas. *J Hand Surg Br.* 1984;9(1):42–45.

12. Evans GR, Dellon AL. Implantation of the palmar cutaneous branch of the median nerve into the pronator quadratus for treatment of painful neuroma. *J Hand Surg Am.* 1994;19(2):203–206.

13. Ducic I, et al. The role of peripheral nerve surgery in the treatment of chronic pain associated with amputation stumps. *Plast Reconstr Surg.* 2008;121(3):908–914; discussion 915–917.

14. Meek MF, Coert JH, Robinson PH. Poor results after nerve grafting in the upper extremity: Quo vadis? *Microsurgery.* 2005;25(5):396–402.

15. O'Connor FG, Wilder RP, Nirschl R. Foot injuries in the runner. In: *Textbook of Running Medicine.* New York: McGraw-Hill; 2001:258–260.

14

Stump Pain

JAGAN DEVARAJAN AND BETH H. MINZTER

CASE

A 65-year-old man was referred to the pain clinic for pain in the right leg at the level of his amputation. He had undergone a below-knee amputation 3 weeks ago because of development of gangrene of his foot as a result of peripheral vascular insufficiency. His pain has been present since the amputation. He was prescribed oxycodone and ibuprofen. Initially, the analgesics kept him comfortable, but for the past 1 week the pain has not been responsive to the analgesics. He denies any injury to the leg or any fever suggestive of infection. He does not have any back pain or radicular pain. On examination, the wound appears to be slowly healing and there is redness in a couple of areas at the incision. There is tenderness at the incisional sites. Staples have been removed. There is a small, clear exudate seeping from the incisional site. His pulses were palpable at femoral and popliteal regions.

DEFINITIONS

In a 16th century tractate, French military surgeon Ambroise Pare described the sensation felt in an amputated leg.[1] The term "phantom limb" was coined by American neurologist Silas Weir Mitchell during the American Civil War, in 1871.[2] The pathogenesis is complex and involves not only sensitization of nerve endings at the local tissue level but also central sensitization.[3] This is one of the most difficult conditions to treat.

Stump pain or residual limb pain is pain localized in the stump where the amputation was performed. The persistent stump pain is also called residual limb pain (RLP) and about 80% of amputees suffer from this condition in the short term. Fortunately, it resolves in the majority of patients, but can persist for years in some cases.[4] Amputees may also suffer from phantom pain, which is a sensation that is perceived as pain related to an organ or limb which is not present

in the body.[5] Phantom sensations are sensations other than pain in the absent body part, including sensations that the body part is still present.

In this chapter we discuss stump pain. The success and outcomes from amputation depend not only on the adequacy of removal of the diseased part of the body but also on the ability to rehabilitate the patient with a painless stump. Residual limb pain is the most common impediment to a successful outcome following lower limb amputation. Residual stump pain occurs in 80% of patients following amputation in the short term.[4] Fortunately, this pain resolves in most patients, although a significant number of patients have persistent stump pain, which interferes with fitting and use of prosthesis. Stump pain worsens the disability index and may exacerbate depression.[6]

EPIDEMIOLOGY OF STUMP PAIN

There are about 30,000–40,000 amputations performed every year in the United States. The most common etiology leading to amputation is peripheral vascular disease (82%), followed by trauma (16.4%), cancer (0.9%), and congenital anomalies (0.8%).[7] It has been estimated that around 12–50 persons per 100,000 undergo major amputations due to peripheral arterial disease. The most common etiologies for the development of peripheral vascular disease are diabetes mellitus, atherosclerosis, and smoking.[8] Given the rising age of baby boomers, this number is expected to increase by 50% over the next 15 years or so. Patients with diabetes mellitus have a 10-fold greater risk of requiring an amputation compared to non-diabetics. It is expected that there will be 3.6 million amputees surviving by 2050.[9]

There are many risk factors for stump pain. Preoperative anxiety has been associated with the incidences of both postoperative stump pain and phantom limb pain. Among patients with preoperative anxiety, about 30% to 50% reported stump pain and 25% reported phantom pain more than 2 years after the surgery.[10] Both the incidence and intensity of preoperative pain have been associated with significantly higher incidences of postoperative and chronic stump pain. In addition, the amount of preoperative opioids taken was associated with increased incidence of residual limb pain.

Any amputations above the ankle are referred to as major amputations,[9] whereas amputations below the ankle are categorized as minor and termed foot amputation. Major etiologies for amputation are as follows:

1. Peripheral arterial disease
2. Acute and chronic thromboembolic phenomena
3. Trauma
4. Severe infections
5. Malignant tumors
6. Failed management of frostbite
7. Severe untreatable Charcot's degenerative osteoarthropathy
8. Painful or infectious flared paralyzed extremity

PATHOPHYSIOLOGY OF STUMP PAIN

Pain is a complex phenomenon which arises from the interactions between cellular communication, receptor sensitization and a wide array of inflammatory mediators. Stump pain is often elicited by the stimulation of nociceptors located at the sites of amputation such as joints, tendons, ligaments, and viscera. Multiple nociceptors have been identified to initiate the neural transmission of pain signals, including mechanoreceptors, thermoreceptors, and specific chemoreceptors. The chemoreceptors respond to bradykinin, histamine, and prostaglandins. The mediators are released into extracellular fluid following tissue injury; this release initiates the pain response.

Action potentials generated from the pain stimuli are conducted to the dorsal horn of the spinal cord through C fibers and A-δ fibers that terminate in a complex array of synaptic arrangements[11] The small myelinated fibers proceed to the Lissauer tract. They ascend or descend one or two segments and synapse with marginal neurons and substantia gelatinosa cells. From the spinal cord, the signals are transmitted through neo- and paleospinothalamic tracts.[12]

The neospinothalamic tract is projected to ventrolateral and posterior parts of thalamus. The third-order neurons are then relayed to the postcentral gyrus, which is the primary somatosensory cortex of the brain. This system not only transmits the signals faster but also provides accurate location and intensity. The paleothalamic tract projects to the reticular formation, pons, and the midbrain. The fibers then travel to medial intralaminar thalamic nuclei and then to the limbic formation, hypothalamus, and diffuse areas of brain. The paleothalamic tract conducts through slow pain fibers and transmits nondiscrete and deep unpleasant sensations.[13] The supraspinal descending neural system from the periaqueductal gray and rostral ventral medulla influences synaptic transmission in the dorsal horn and along the course of ascending somatosensory tracts. Thus, the pain is mediated by a complex interaction between ascending and descending neurons, as well as immune cells and glial cells in the peripheral nervous system (PNS) and central nervous system (CNS). The degree of modulation is influenced by the relative activity of nociceptors and descending fibers in the CNS. Sympathetic post ganglionic neurons may also be involved in the generation of pain. This explains the difficulty and complexity involved in control of stump and phantom pain.

Stump pain is usually nociceptive in the initial postoperative period. It then becomes inflammatory pain in the next 2 to 6 weeks as the stump begins to heal. Any pain after this initial 6-week period is either neuropathic or secondary to a specific etiology such as infection or trauma. Depending on the nature of origin and type of stump pain, it can be nociceptive, neuropathic, inflammatory, arthrogenic, neurogenic, myogenic, prosthogenic, ischemic, or miscellaneous.[14]

Nociceptive pain arises as a result of nonneural tissue damage. A-delta and C fibers are involved, and the stimuli are mechanical (surgery), chemical (local chemokines), or thermal. Pain is the normal adaptive manifestation of the somatosensory system to injury. Multiple peripheral receptors like ion channels and G protein–coupled receptors are involved.

Inflammatory pain is due to a response to tissue injury and inflammation. Inflammatory mediators such as chemokines and cytokines sensitize local peripheral receptors and lower their threshold to responsiveness. Inflammatory pain should resolve as the tissue heals from injury; however, inadequate resolution of inflammation at the peripheral receptor level due to poor tissue repair or maladaptation in healing can lead to sensitization.

Neuropathic pain arises as a result of injury to the somatosensory nervous system. Tissue injuries result not only in sensory loss but also in elevated responsiveness to both innocuous and noxious stimuli. This is known as peripheral sensitization.[15] Much of the chronic pain in patients after amputation is explained by neuropathic pain. The characteristic changes in neuropathic pain include alterations in ion channels, G protein–coupled receptors, neurotransmitters, and central sensitization.

The autonomic nervous system may be related to chronic stump pain. Though the sensory nervous system and autonomic nervous system produce integrated responses, there is no cross-communication between their afferent fibers in normal conditions. Both systems are coordinated independently and become integrated at the CNS. However, an injury to the peripheral nerve generates plastic changes in both of its afferent sensory and sympathetic components. The plastic changes depend on whether there is complete or partial injury to the nerves. Both sensory and post ganglionic sympathetic fibers exhibit degenerative and regenerative changes and allow collateral sprouting which causes coupling between them in the periphery. This same phenomenon occurs in the dorsal root ganglion as well. This reorganization leads to chemical coupling between sympathetic and sensory neurons which is responsible for sensitization of peripheral nerve endings. The mediator most commonly involbed is norepinephrine. This is called "sympathetic-afferent coupling," which may result in the development of chronic pain.[16] The underlying molecular mechanisms may be related to expression and activation of adrenergic receptors on afferent nociceptive neurons as a result of increased concentration of local inflammatory mediators such as interleukin-8. The sprouting of sympathetic nerve fibers into dorsal root ganglia contributes as well. These processes are initiated and maintained by locally-induced vasoconstriction, which further causes sympathetic nerve stimulation and accentuates nociceptor activation and sensitization.[17] Sympathetic-afferent coupling plays a major role in central sensitization and causes heightened activity in the brain and spinal cord in response to both normal and subthreshold afferent input.

CLINICAL PRESENTATION OF STUMP PAIN

Residual limb pain is common following amputation. It is more common in the early postoperative period. Stump pain generally diminishes as healing occurs. In 5%–10% of cases, stump pain persists or even worsens.[18] Stump pain is an important risk factor for and prelude to phantom limb pain. Early detection and effective management may reduce subsequent development of phantom pain and disability. Stump pain is classified into acute and chronic forms. Acute stump pain is pain arising from the amputated limb at the level of the stump, which is of 1- to 6-week duration. Any pain at the site of the amputation beyond 6 weeks is referred to as chronic stump pain. It is important to distinguish between these two types of stump pain, as management and outcomes are different between the two.

Acute stump pain occurs in the immediate postoperative period. If it lasts beyond 6 weeks, it is termed chronic stump pain. The higher the level of amputation, the greater the incidence and severity of pain would be. Pain also depends on the severity of dissections during surgery. The presence and duration of preoperative pain can play a minor role in the development of acute stump pain, but preoperative pain is one of the main determinants of phantom pain.[19] The presence of preoperative pain is a risk factor for the subsequent development of severe postoperative pain and its evolution into chronic stump pain.

History and physical examination are critical to the diagnosis of residual limb pain and stump pain. It is important to rule out the existence of infection. Infection is characterized by the presence of redness, swelling, and tenderness and usually is accompanied by systemic symptoms of fever and chills and malaise. The infection could be related to decreased blood flow, which makes the stump further prone to infection or could be related to wounds caused by ill-fitting prostheses. A thorough physical exam of the stump and prosthesis can help make the diagnosis. Soft tissues, bone structures, and neural tissues should be examined for integrity. Infection needs to be treated promptly by systemic antibiotics in combination with localized dressing changes and debridement as necessary.

Ongoing ischemia should be ruled out, as it causes persistent pain in the stump. Transcutaneous oxygen tension can be measured at the distal part of the stump. If it is less than 20 mmHg, this would indicate decrease in blood flow and oxygen supply to the tissues.[20] It can be due to localized blood flow limitation or chronic occlusive disease or embolic events. It can be related to systemic and generalized decrease in blood flow. The treatment should be directed to the underlying causes.

Back pain with radicular component can also manifest as stump pain. Patients with amputation are at greater risk of developing chronic arthritis of the lumbar zygapophyseal joints and sacroiliac joints that subsequently leads to the development of back pain.[21] Patients with amputation had a 71% incidence of back pain compared to 41% in the general population.[21] Hence it is important to rule out back pain and radiating radicular pain as etiologies of the pain symptoms.[14]

The other more common cause of stump pain is the formation of a neuroma, which can be either diagnosed by examination or other physical means. Tinel's test is simple and can be done at the bedside. The presence of tingling and pain upon tapping of the tissue over the nerve usually indicates the presence of a neuroma.

An ill-fitting prosthesis or a prosthesis-related pressure sore can also cause pain. Frequent visits to physical therapy to assess the appropriateness of the prosthesis may be required as the residual limb undergoes atrophy. A malaligned pressure point can cause ulceration or chronic irritation of the underlying bone, and this can cause either formation of bone spurs or heterotopic ossification, both of which can be very painful and difficult to reverse.[21]

Osteomyelitis and residual graft infection should also be ruled out as etiologies of the pain.

MANAGEMENT OF STUMP PAIN

Management of acute stump pain should be initiated early and may include the following multimodal approaches:

1. Regional neuraxial blocks
2. Peripheral extremity blocks
3. NSAIDs
4. Antidepressants
5. Anticonvulsants
6. Opioids

Amputation of extremities causes moderate to severe pain.[22,23] Patients undergoing amputation are usually ill and have multiple comorbid conditions. Poorly treated postoperative pain can increase stress on the compromised myocardium in vascular patients and potentially cause complications such as myocardial infarction and pneumonia. Hence management of pain is essential for these patients in order to prevent postoperative complications. Pain management options can be influenced by the presence of anticoagulation and chronic pain in these patients.

Regional conduction blockade with continuous epidural analgesia is an established method of providing analgesia.[24] This has been shown to be effective and may also help prevent development of phantom pain,[25] although subsequent studies have not been able to confirm the beneficial preventive effects of preoperative regional block.

Over the most recent decade, peripheral nerve blocks have become more common and have been used extensively as one of the most effective methods of providing postoperative analgesia.[26] Peripheral nerve blocks give better pain relief than epidural blocks and are devoid of the more common side effects associated with continuous epidural analgesia, such as hypotension and urinary retention.[27] Moreover, peripheral nerve blocks allow ambulation more readily than epidural blocks.

Parenteral analgesics are usually used as the primary analgesic or at least as an adjuvant to provide pain relief.[28] Patients undergoing amputation are at risk of developing depression, which can further worsen pain and contribute to subsequent development of chronic pain.[17] Antidepressants often form a main component of medical therapy for the majority of patients undergoing amputation.

No specific intraoperative or postoperative pain management strategy has been shown to prevent or decrease the incidence of phantom limb pain or chronic stump pain. However, there is weak evidence that adequate perioperative management of pain beginning in the preoperative period and transitioning through several days postoperatively may prevent the development of chronic neuropathic pain.[29] Though studies provide evidence that both epidural and perineural catheters provide excellent analgesia in the immediate postoperative period, long-term outcomes are not different compared to traditional methods of analgesia.[30] The most common reasons for lower extremity amputation are ischemia and infection, whereas trauma is the prime cause of upper extremity amputation.[31] There are certain surgical modalities that may serve greatly to reduce long-term residual limb pain and improve function. Gentle handling of delicate tissues and clean and proximal transection of nerves without retracting them can help to reduce the degree of postoperative residual limb pain and future stump pain. The proximal clean transection of the nerve facilitates retraction of nerves into muscular tissue and thereby prevents development of neuroma at the distal site of the junction of the prosthesis and stump.[32] The procedure of myodesis or myoplasty, by which the muscular tissues are appropriately engaged with bones to seal the severed nerve, also serves to reduce stump pain.[33] However, this procedure may be technically challenging and may require staged operations.

Management of Coexisting Conditions

Patients with vascular disease have multiple comorbidities, including cognitive impairment, cerebral vascular disease, coronary artery disease and/or congestive heart failure, and neuropathy, all of which complicate pain management.[34] Comprehensive pain management should be multidisciplinary and multimodal, as no one modality alone has been shown to be effective. Patients may have to be followed by an acute pain consultant for days to weeks. The higher incidence of ischemia of limbs in vascular patients would dictate that appropriate measures be taken to ensure adequate blood flow and oxygen supply to the stump, which would improve healing response and decrease ischemic pain and infection.[35] Adequate blood flow, appropriate healing and regular scar formation, and avoidance of infection are some of the key factors which play significant roles in managing postoperative pain and reducing the incidence of chronic stump pain.

Since amputees have a higher incidence of comorbidities, special attention and adequate management of comorbid conditions are required in the postoperative period.[36] For example, ill-managed congestive heart failure may contribute to decreased blood flow to the tissues due to low cardiac output. If chronic obstructive pulmonary disease (COPD) is not managed well, the patients may continue to have decreased oxygen supply to the stump. Both low cardiac output and reduced oxygenation would delay wound healing and hence make pain management more challenging.

Patients undergoing amputation often suffer from depression and anxiety as a result of potential future functional disability.[37] Appropriate mental health management is crucial for successful pain management in these patients. The impaired functional abilities should be simultaneously addressed by physical therapists and occupational therapists.[38] Poor social support necessitates social work involvement and psychological counseling. This underscores the importance of coordinated and integrative collaboration with multidisciplinary specialties to improve overall patient satisfaction and long-term functional rehabilitation.[39] Physical therapists facilitate improved range of motion early on in the postoperative period, which can further improve blood flow and healing to the tissues. In fact, multidisciplinary management not only improved pain scores but also facilitated early discharge and improved 1-year survival rates.[40]

Management of Chronic Stump Pain
Pharmacological Management

The residual limb pain is composed of a combination of nociceptive and neuropathic pain components. Nociceptive pain is managed best with regional nerve blocks, opioids, and nonsteroidal anti-inflammatory drugs (NSAIDs).[41] However, neuropathic pain requires treatment with adjuvant medications such as membrane stabilizers and antidepressants.

Membrane stabilizers include gabapentin and pregabalin.[42] The effectiveness of gabapentin has not been studied in the immediate postoperative period exclusively in patients following amputations. However, its use has been extensively investigated for the management of postoperative pain and phantom limb pain. Few studies have shown an improvement of pain scores, although reduction in opioid requirements with the use of gabapentin has also been reported.[43]

Despite the lack of studies of gabapentin on stump pain, we can extrapolate the findings from orthopedic and general surgery literature. In other surgical specialties, gabapentin has been shown to be effective in reducing pain scores. The side effects of gabapentin include dizziness, depression, and sedative effects. So caution should be exercised when gabapentin is instituted in high-risk patients. The usual starting dose is 100 mg orally once daily and can be increased gradually up to 600 mg orally three times daily. These higher doses, however, may be associated with intolerable side effects.[105] Pregabalin is an alternative for gabapentin and may confer fewer side effects. Its most common side effects are dizziness and sedation. The usual loading dose is 300 mg orally followed by 150 mg twice daily.[44]

NMDA receptor antagonists include ketamine and memantine. They both have been utilized in the treatment of post-amputation pain. Ketamine is administered intravenously and memantine orally.[45] Though ketamine has also been administered epidurally,[23] its administration in epidural route is not recommended given the limited number of studies that exist, as well as the unproven, yet postulated, neurotoxic nature of ketamine. For immediate postoperative pain, low-dose ketamine infusion at 1.2 mg/kg/hr maintained for 48 hours reduced opioid requirements by 40%.[46] Even a single dose of ketamine was shown to reduce opioid requirement and pain scores up to 12–24 hours following surgery. Ketamine has been administered orally 50 mg three times daily to reduce phantom limb pain.[47] Similarly, oral memantine has been shown to significantly reduce analgesic requirements and improve pain scores in patients undergoing upper extremity amputation. Although the incidence and prevalence of phantom pain was reduced at 1 and 6 months, the beneficial effect has been reported to fade away at 12 months.

Ketamine usually not only produces short-term benefits for stump pain but is also associated with reduction of long-term phantom pain. Although there is a lack of conclusive evidence about whether ketamine is effective for post-amputation pain and phantom pain, the relative absence of side effects and their efficacy in other surgical settings make ketamine and memantine attractive medications to include in a multimodal regimen.

In a randomized study, the effect of calcitonin on phantom limb pain has been shown to be marginally beneficial.[48] It decreased the incidence and severity of both stump pain and phantom pain. For stump pain, the effect was no longer evident after 6 weeks. For phantom limb pain, however, the relief lasted up to 12 months in more than 50% of patients, though relapse occurred eventually after 12 months. Calcitonin is relatively devoid of any major side effects and is an effective therapeutic agent. The dosage used was 200 IU intravenously once or twice daily. It can also be administered intranasally without any side effects. It was effective in patients with stump pain due to heterotopic ossification[49] and in pregnant patients with phantom and stump pain.

Anti-inflammatory medications may be used. An inflammatory component contributes to a significant part of pain in post-amputation and phantom pains. Etanercept is a tumor necrosis factor alpha (TNF-α) inhibitor[50] and has been shown to be effective after perineural injection for management of both stump pain and phantom pain in case series reports. It also improved functional capacity and psychological well-being.

NSAIDs and acetaminophen are useful for the treatment of stump pain. NSAIDs not only serve as an adjunct to treatment of acute pain but can also inhibit heterotopic ossification. Inhibition of heterotopic ossification helps reduce long-term stump pain. NSAIDs has been shown to be effective for residual limb pain and stump pain.[21]

Role of Epidural Analgesia

Epidural analgesia is an effective management solution for immediate postoperative pain and phantom limb pain. However, it was not effective in reducing late-onset stump pain or residual limb pain in 6 months. This is confirmed by a landmark study, which further raised doubts about the beneficial effects of preoperative epidural placement and subsequent anesthesia on the incidence phantom pain.[51] It is necessary that epidural infusion of medication be started in the preoperative period and continued for 48 to 72 hours postoperatively. Comparison of the effectiveness of epidural versus an intraoperatively placed perineural catheter for prevention of phantom pain did not show any difference. Furthermore, effective analgesia produced by either epidural or patient-controlled analgesia (PCA) had similar effects on the reduction of incidence or severity of phantom pain.

Peripheral Nerve Blocks

Peripheral nerve blocks are becoming an increasingly popular option for providing analgesia following amputation. The advantages are that they provide profound postoperative analgesia, prevent a wind-up phenomenon, cause less hemodynamic instability, and result in fewer pulmonary complications. They can be continued postoperatively for a prolonged period of time. The effect on stump pain was present while the infusion was maintained and disappeared after discontinuation of the infusion.[52] Peripheral nerve blocks can be performed at a site either distal[25] or proximal. Proximal nerve catheters are more effective than distal catheters for providing analgesia. Distal catheters are usually placed perineurally during surgery by the surgeons.

The following peripheral nerve blocks can be considered for different procedures. The main disadvantage of nerve blocks when treating stump pain is that they only last for a maximum of approximately 24 hours. Continuous nerve block is an option. It can be performed before surgery and maintained for 30 days to reduce the risk of developing phantom pain. Infection with these indwelling catheters is a risk, albeit one that is very low.

Upper Extremities

Shoulder disarticulation: C1–C6 roots are involved, and the superficial cervical plexus and axillary, suprascapular, and lateral pectoral nerves are involved. Interscalene brachial plexus blockade with or without superficial cervical plexus blocks can be utilized.

Amputation above the elbow: Musculocutaneous, radial, medial cutaneous nerves of the arm and axillary nerves are involved. Adequate coverage can be obtained from either interscalene block or the supraclavicular approach to brachial plexus block. Infraclavicular blocks may not provide adequate coverage for amputations at the level of the proximal humerus.

Elbow disarticulation or below-elbow amputation: Median, radial, and ulnar nerves are involved in addition to the musculocutaneous nerve and medial cutaneous nerve of forearm. Reliable coverage can be obtained from either the supraclavicular, infraclavicular approaches or axillary approach to brachial plexus.

Wrist and finger level: Radial, median, and ulnar nerves are involved, and axillary or infraclavicular approach to brachial plexus block is the recommended technique, as supraclavicular blockade tends to miss the ulnar territory. However, if a continuous prolonged infusion is required, an infraclavicular approach is preferable to an axillary approach, as an axillary catheter is more at risk of getting dislodged and/or infected. Infraclavicular catheters provide reliable analgesia and patients often tolerate infraclavicular catheters better than those placed via other approaches due to their strategic position.

Lower Extremities

Hemipelvectomy or hip disarticulation: The lumbar plexus and sacral plexus are involved, and reliable analgesia can be obtained via either epidural neuraxial block or combined lumbar and sacral plexus blocks.

Above-knee amputation: Femoral, sciatic, obturator, and lateral cutaneous nerves innervate the region. In addition to epidural and combined lumbar and sciatic plexus blocks, individual femoral and transgluteal sciatic nerve blocks provide adequate analgesia. Occasionally, obturator nerve block may be required.

Below-knee amputation: Two distal components of the sciatic nerve, the lateral peroneal and common tibial nerves, are involved in addition to the saphenous nerve, which is a sensory division of the femoral nerve. Popliteal approach to sciatic nerve block and adductor canal block would be sufficient to provide effective analgesia.

Below the ankle: Ankle block is a relatively simple block to perform and involves the saphenous, sural, and posterior tibial nerves. Deep and superficial peroneal nerves, which are divisions of common peroneal nerves, are also blocked through the ankle block.

Management of Neuroma Pain

Different modalities for the management of neuroma pain at the stump site have been reported. A neuroma is one of the major causes of stump pain. It can be diagnosed via visual inspection and can be confirmed by ultrasonogram.[53] The various management strategies are as follows:

1. Local injection
2. Perineuromal injection
3. Peripheral nerve block
4. Radiofrequency ablation
5. Coblation
6. Spinal cord stimulation
7. Peripheral nerve stimulation
8. Transcutaneous electrical nerve stimulation (TENS)
9. Sympathetic blockade

The less effective managements of neuroma pain are transcutaneous electrical nerve stimulation, spinal cord stimulation, peripheral nerve stimulation, deep brain stimulation,[54] and desensitization. These stimulation techniques are effective only in 10% of patients with stump pain. However, they are more effective for phantom pain.

Local injection can be used to diagnose the presence of pain due to neuroma and the responsiveness of treatment. The analgesic effect usually lasts for 30 minutes. Perineuromal injection can provide approximately 2–3 hours of pain relief. Peripheral nerve blocks confined to the territory of the neuroma can confer long-lasting analgesia up to a period of 10–24 hours depending on the type of local anesthetic used. Injection of dexamethasone into the neuroma has been reported to prolong the analgesia. Pulsed radiofrequency may be useful to prolong analgesia once the administration of lidocaine reproducibly provides pain relief. Alcohol and phenol have been used to obtain long-term pain relief.[55] Focal injection of botulinum type-A has also been tried with success.[56] This was as effective as local injection of lidocaine and Depo-Medrol, with prolonged effect up to a period of 6 months. In the same way, botulinum toxin-B has also been used with variable success. Injection of botulinum toxin did not prevent development of phantom pain, however.

The two long-term analgesia modalities that have been used in treatment are radiofrequency ablation and coblation. Radiofrequency ablation utilizes heat from medium-frequency alternating current to ablate nerve fibers of the neuroma. It uses thermal energy to interrupt neuronal conduction by the process of Wallerian degeneration of neuronal tissues. It should be noted that, due to this disruption, Wallerian degeneration also poses the risk of regeneration and recurrence of neuroma and subsequent reappearance of pain.

Coblation is a newer technique used to treat neuropathic pain. Coblation uses low thermal energy. Radiofrequency energy is applied through conductive solution and causes disintegration of tissues. It uses radiofrequency energy and excites the electrolytes in conductive medium resulting in energized plasma. Energized plasma produces chemically reactive radical species, which interact with organic tissue and possess sufficient energy to break molecular bonds, thus effecting tissue dissolution at a low temperature (approximately 40° to 70°C). Recurrence is rare, and damage to surrounding tissues is avoided as it uses low temperature. In addition to decreasing ectopic afferent input from neuroma, coblation also suppresses dorsal root ganglion activity, which serves to reduce the input to the CNS. Cryoablation was also used to destroy a neuroma successfully.[57]

Surgery

Surgery should be the last resort to address stump pain.[58] Revision surgery may be considered if the stump produces prosthetic dysfunction. It may be effective if the pain is due to heterotopic bone formation. If the pain is due to neuroma, however, the results of surgery are usually disappointing. For any stump-related abscess and infection, drainage and debridement should be considered.

GUIDING QUESTIONS
- What are the differences between stump pain and phantom pain?
- What are the risk factors associated with stump pain?
- What is the pathophysiology of development of stump pain?
- What are the different modalities of management of acute stump pain?
- What is the significance of managing stump pain in high-risk patients?
- What is the role of gabapentinoids in managing stump pain?
- What are the advantages of selective peripheral nerve block over epidural block in managing stump pain?
- What are the different modalities of treatment of neuroma associated with amputation?
- Name the two modalities of long-term management of stump pain associated with neuroma.

KEY POINTS
- Stump pain or residual limb pain is pain localized in the stump where the amputation was performed and occurs in 80% of patients in the short term.
- Phantom pain is a sensation perceived as pain related to an organ or limb which is not present in the body.
- In terms of etiology, 82% of amputations are caused by peripheral vascular disease, followed by trauma in 16.4% of patients.
- Preoperative anxiety and pain and the nature of surgery and site of amputation constitute significant risk factors for stump pain.
- The nature of stump pain can be nociceptive, neuropathic, inflammatory, arthrogenic, neurogenic, myogenic, prosthogenic, ischemic, or miscellaneous depending on the pathophysiology of origin of pain.

- Stump pain lasting less than 6 weeks is termed acute and more than 6 weeks, chronic pain.
- History and physical examination findings are the hallmarks for the diagnosis of residual limb pain and stump pain, and it is essential to rule out infection and ischemia.
- Both regional and peripheral nerve blocks form the mainstay of treatment of acute stump pain, and NSAIDs, membrane stabilizers, and opioids form adjuvants.
- Comprehensive pain management should be multidisciplinary and multimodal and should address underlying comorbid conditions, including depression.
- Pharmacological management with membrane stabilizers and NMDA receptor antagonists form the mainstay of treatment of chronic stump pain.
- Prolonged peripheral nerve blocks using catheters have been reported to manage chronic stump pain.
- Neuromas must be looked for in chronic stump pain.
- TENS, sympathetic block, spinal cord stimulation, and peripheral nerve stimulation are the modes commonly used for treating chronic neuropathic pain associated with stump pain.
- Surgery is useful for heterotopic bone formation and to address stump-related abscess and infection, drainage, and debridement.
- Radiofrequency ablation and coblation are other noninvasive methods used for treatment of neuroma.

REFERENCES

1. Hernigou P. Ambroise Pare II: Pare's contributions to amputation and ligature. *Int Orthop.* 2013;37(4):769–772. doi:10.1007/s00264-013-1857-x [doi]
2. Louis ED, York GK. Weir Mitchell's observations on sensory localization and their influence on Jacksonian neurology. *Neurology.* 2006;66(8):1241–1244. doi:66/8/1241 [pii]
3. Weeks SR, Anderson-Barnes VC, Tsao JW. Phantom limb pain: theories and therapies. *Neurologist.* 2010;16(5):277–286. doi:10.1097/NRL.0b013e3181edf128 [doi]
4. Ehde DM, Czerniecki JM, Smith DG, et al. Chronic phantom sensations, phantom pain, residual limb pain, and other regional pain after lower limb amputation. *Arch Phys Med Rehabil.* 2000;81(8):1039–1044. doi:S0003-9993(00)67766-3 [pii]
5. Jensen TS, Krebs B, Nielsen J, Rasmussen P. Phantom limb, phantom pain and stump pain in amputees during the first 6 months following limb amputation. *Pain.* 1983;17(3):243–256.
6. Sahu A, Sagar R, Sarkar S, Sagar S. Psychological effects of amputation: A review of studies from India. *Ind Psychiatry J.* 2016;25(1):4–10. doi:10.4103/0972-6748.196041 [doi]
7. Dillingham TR, Pezzin LE, MacKenzie EJ. Limb amputation and limb deficiency: epidemiology and recent trends in the United States. *South Med J.* 2002;95(8):875–883.
8. Setacci F, Sirignano P, De Donato G, et al. Primary amputation: is there still a place for it? *J Cardiovasc Surg (Torino).* 2012;53(1):53–59. doi:R37127003 [pii]
9. Tseng CL, Rajan M, Miller DR, Lafrance JP, Pogach L. Trends in initial lower extremity amputation rates among Veterans Health Administration health care System users from 2000 to 2004. *Diabetes Care.* 2011;34(5):1157–1163. doi:10.2337/dc10-1775 [doi]
10. Raichle KA, Osborne TL, Jensen MP, Ehde DM, Smith DG, Robinson LR. Preoperative state anxiety, acute postoperative pain, and analgesic use in persons undergoing lower limb amputation. *Clin J Pain.* 2015;31(8):699–706. doi:10.1097/AJP.0000000000000150 [doi]
11. Melzack R. Pain--an overview. *Acta Anaesthesiol Scand.* 1999;43(9):880–884.
12. Wilson ME. The neurological mechanisms of pain. A review. *Anaesthesia.* 1974;29(4):407–421.
13. Nikolajsen L. Postamputation pain: studies on mechanisms. *Dan Med J.* 2012;59(10):B4527. doi:A527 [pii]
14. Hsu E, Cohen SP. Postamputation pain: epidemiology, mechanisms, and treatment. *J Pain Res.* 2013;6:121–136. doi:10.2147/JPR.S32299 [doi]
15. Flor H. Phantom-limb pain: characteristics, causes, and treatment. *Lancet Neurol.* 2002;1(3):182–189.
16. Chen Y, Michaelis M, Janig W, Devor M. Adrenoreceptor subtype mediating sympathetic-sensory coupling in injured sensory neurons. *J Neurophysiol.* 1996;76(6):3721–3730.
17. Subedi B, Grossberg GT. Phantom limb pain: mechanisms and treatment approaches. *Pain Res Treat.* 2011;2011:864605. doi:10.1155/2011/864605 [doi]
18. Behr J, Friedly J, Molton I, Morgenroth D, Jensen MP, Smith DG. Pain and pain-related interference in adults with lower-limb amputation: comparison of knee-disarticulation, transtibial, and transfemoral surgical sites. *J Rehabil Res Dev.* 2009;46(7):963–972.

19. Bosmans JC, Geertzen JH, Post WJ, van der Schans CP, Dijkstra PU. Factors associated with phantom limb pain: a 31/2-year prospective study. *Clin Rehabil.* 2010;24(5):444–453. doi:10.1177/0269215509360645 [doi]

20. Claeys LG, Horsch S. Transcutaneous oxygen pressure as predictive parameter for ulcer healing in endstage vascular patients treated with spinal cord stimulation. *Int Angiol.* 1996;15(4):344–349.

21. Smith DG, Ehde DM, Legro MW, Reiber GE, del Aguila M, Boone DA. Phantom limb, residual limb, and back pain after lower extremity amputations. *Clin Orthop Relat Res.* 1999;(361)(361):29–38.

22. Ephraim PL, Wegener ST, MacKenzie EJ, Dillingham TR, Pezzin LE. Phantom pain, residual limb pain, and back pain in amputees: results of a national survey. *Arch Phys Med Rehabil.* 2005;86(10):1910–1919. doi:S0003-9993(05)00358-8 [pii]

23. Schley MT, Wilms P, Toepfner S, et al. Painful and nonpainful phantom and stump sensations in acute traumatic amputees. *J Trauma.* 2008;65(4):858–864. doi:10.1097/TA.0b013e31812eed9e [doi]

24. Wilson JA, Nimmo AF, Fleetwood-Walker SM, Colvin LA. A randomised double blind trial of the effect of pre-emptive epidural ketamine on persistent pain after lower limb amputation. *Pain.* 2008;135(1–2):108–118. doi:S0304-3959(07)00268-0 [pii]

25. Borghi B, D'Addabbo M, White PF, et al. The use of prolonged peripheral neural blockade after lower extremity amputation: the effect on symptoms associated with phantom limb syndrome. *Anesth Analg.* 2010;111(5):1308–1315. doi:10.1213/ANE.0b013e3181f4e848 [doi]

26. Borghi B, D'Addabbo M, Borghi R. Can neural blocks prevent phantom limb pain? *Pain Manag.* 2014;4(4):261–266. doi:10.2217/pmt.14.17 [doi]

27. Hakim M, Burrier C, Bhalla T, et al. Regional anesthesia for an upper extremity amputation for palliative care in a patient with end-stage osteosarcoma complicated by a large anterior mediastinal mass. *J Pain Res.* 2015;8:641–645. doi:10.2147/JPR.S92941 [doi]

28. Humble SR, Dalton AJ, Li L. A systematic review of therapeutic interventions to reduce acute and chronic post-surgical pain after amputation, thoracotomy or mastectomy. *Eur J Pain.* 2015;19(4):451–465. doi:10.1002/ejp.567 [doi]

29. Bosanquet DC, Glasbey JC, Stimpson A, Williams IM, Twine CP. Systematic review and meta-analysis of the efficacy of perineural local anaesthetic catheters after major lower limb amputation. *Eur J Vasc Endovasc Surg.* 2015;50(2):241–249. doi:10.1016/j.ejvs.2015.04.030 [doi]

30. Ayling OG, Montbriand J, Jiang J, et al. Continuous regional anaesthesia provides effective pain management and reduces opioid requirement following major lower limb amputation. *Eur J Vasc Endovasc Surg.* 2014;48(5):559–564. doi:10.1016/j.ejvs.2014.07.002 [doi]

31. Marchessault JA, McKay PL, Hammert WC. Management of upper limb amputations. *J Hand Surg Am.* 2011;36(10):1718–1726. doi:10.1016/j.jhsa.2011.07.025 [doi]

32. Souza JM, Cheesborough JE, Ko JH, Cho MS, Kuiken TA, Dumanian GA. Targeted muscle reinnervation: a novel approach to postamputation neuroma pain. *Clin Orthop Relat Res.* 2014;472(10):2984–2990. doi:10.1007/s11999-014-3528-7 [doi]

33. Shenaq SM, Krouskop T, Stal S, Spira M. Salvage of amputation stumps by secondary reconstruction utilizing microsurgical free-tissue transfer. *Plast Reconstr Surg.* 1987;79(6):861–870.

34. Davenport DL, Ritchie JD, Xenos ES. Incidence and risk factors for 30-day postdischarge mortality in patients with vascular disease undergoing major lower extremity amputation. *Ann Vasc Surg.* 2012;26(2):219–224. doi:10.1016/j.avsg.2011.05.012 [doi]

35. Richardson C, Glenn S, Nurmikko T, Horgan M. Incidence of phantom phenomena including phantom limb pain 6 months after major lower limb amputation in patients with peripheral vascular disease. *Clin J Pain.* 2006;22(4):353–358. doi:10.1097/01.ajp.0000177793.01415.bd [doi]

36. van Netten JJ, Fortington L V, Hinchliffe RJ, Hijmans JM. Early Post-operative Mortality After Major Lower Limb Amputation: A Systematic Review of Population and Regional Based Studies. *Eur J Vasc Endovasc Surg.* 2016;51(2):248–257. doi:10.1016/j.ejvs.2015.10.001 [doi]

37. Horgan O, MacLachlan M. Psychosocial adjustment to lower-limb amputation: a review. *Disabil Rehabil.* 2004;26(14–15):837–850.

38. Coffey L, Gallagher P, Horgan O, Desmond D, MacLachlan M. Psychosocial adjustment to diabetes-related lower limb amputation. *Diabet Med.* 2009;26(10):1063–1067. doi:10.1111/j.1464-5491.2009.02802.x [doi]

39. Burger H, Marincek C. Return to work after lower limb amputation. *Disabil Rehabil.* 2007;29(17):1323–1329. doi:779651423 [pii]

40. Stineman MG, Kwong PL, Kurichi JE, et al. The effectiveness of inpatient rehabilitation in the acute postoperative phase of care after transtibial or transfemoral amputation: study of an integrated health care delivery system. *Arch Phys Med Rehabil.* 2008;89(10):1863–1872. doi:10.1016/j.apmr.2008.03.013 [doi]

41. Alviar MJ, Hale T, Dungca M. Pharmacologic interventions for treating phantom limb pain. *Cochrane database Syst Rev.* 2016;10:CD006380. doi:10.1002/14651858.CD006380.pub3 [doi]

42. Schmidt PC, Ruchelli G, Mackey SC, Carroll IR. Perioperative gabapentinoids: choice of agent, dose, timing, and effects on chronic postsurgical pain. *Anesthesiology.* 2013;119(5):1215–1221. doi:10.1097/ALN.0b013e3182a9a896 [doi]

43. Tiippana EM, Hamunen K, Kontinen VK, Kalso E. Do surgical patients benefit from perioperative gabapentin/pregabalin? A systematic review of efficacy and safety. *Anesth Analg.* 2007;104(6):1545–1556, table of contents. doi:104/6/1545 [pii]

44. Zhang J, Ho KY, Wang Y. Efficacy of pregabalin in acute postoperative pain: a meta-analysis. *Br J Anaesth.* 2011;106(4):454–462. doi:10.1093/bja/aer027 [doi]

45. Schley M, Topfner S, Wiech K, et al. Continuous brachial plexus blockade in combination with the NMDA receptor antagonist memantine prevents phantom pain in acute traumatic upper limb amputees. *Eur J Pain.* 2007;11(3):299–308. doi:S1090-3801(06)00053-X [pii]

46. Jouguelet-Lacoste J, La Colla L, Schilling D, Chelly JE. The use of intravenous infusion or single dose of low-dose ketamine for postoperative analgesia: a review of the current literature. *Pain Med.* 2015;16(2):383–403. doi:10.1111/pme.12619 [doi]

47. Nikolajsen L, Hansen PO, Jensen TS. Oral ketamine therapy in the treatment of postamputation stump pain. *Acta Anaesthesiol Scand.* 1997;41(3):427–429.

48. Jaeger H, Maier C. Calcitonin in phantom limb pain: a double-blind study. *Pain.* 1992;48(1):21–27. doi:0304-3959(92)90127-W [pii]

49. Viana R, Payne MWC. Use of calcitonin in recalcitrant phantom limb pain complicated by heterotopic ossification. *Pain Res Manag.* 2015;20(5):229–233.

50. Dahl E, Cohen SP. Perineural injection of etanercept as a treatment for postamputation pain. *Clin J Pain.* 2008;24(2):172–175. doi:10.1097/AJP.0b013e31815b32c8 [doi]

51. Nikolajsen L, Ilkjaer S, Jensen TS. Effect of preoperative extradural bupivacaine and morphine on stump sensation in lower limb amputees. *Br J Anaesth.* 1998;81(3):348–354.

52. Sahin SH, Colak A, Arar C, et al. A retrospective trial comparing the effects of different anesthetic techniques on phantom pain after lower limb amputation. *Curr Ther Res Clin Exp.* 2011;72(3):127–137. doi:10.1016/j.curtheres.2011.06.001 [doi]

53. Brogan DM, Kakar S. Management of neuromas of the upper extremity. *Hand Clin.* 2013;29(3):409–420. doi:10.1016/j.hcl.2013.04.007 [doi]

54. Pereira EA, Boccard SG, Linhares P, et al. Thalamic deep brain stimulation for neuropathic pain after amputation or brachial plexus avulsion. *Neurosurg Focus.* 2013;35(3):E7. doi:10.3171/2013.7.FOCUS1346 [doi]

55. Gruber H, Glodny B, Kopf H, et al. Practical experience with sonographically guided phenol instillation of stump neuroma: predictors of effects, success, and outcome. *AJR American J Roentgenol.* 2008;190(5):1263–1269. doi:10.2214/AJR.07.2050 [doi]

56. Jin L, Kollewe K, Krampfl K, Dengler R, Mohammadi B. Treatment of phantom limb pain with botulinum toxin type A. *Pain Med.* 2009;10(2):300–303. doi:10.1111/j.1526-4637.2008.00554.x [doi]

57. Neumann V, O'Connor RJ, Bush D. Cryoprobe treatment: an alternative to phenol injections for painful neuromas after amputation. *AJR American J Roentgenol.* 2008;191(6):W313; author reply W314. doi:10.2214/AJR.08.1371 [doi]

58. Stokvis A, van der Avoort DJ, van Neck JW, Hovius SE, Coert JH. Surgical management of neuroma pain: a prospective follow-up study. *Pain.* 2010;151(3):862–869. doi:10.1016/j.pain.2010.09.032 [doi]

15

Ischemic Neuropathy

JAGAN DEVARAJAN AND BETH H. MINZTER

CASE

A 55-year-old man is referred to the pain clinic by his primary care provider for evaluation of his leg pain. The pain is present in both legs and is located in the calf and feet. It starts in the buttock and radiates along the back of the thigh and then spreads to the legs and feet. The pain is described as hot, burning pain, worsened by walking and exercise, and reduced with rest. The pain is also alleviated by keeping the legs in a dependent position so he always sleeps in sitting posture. He also describes some numbness and tingling in the feet that are associated with pain. The past medical history includes diabetes treated with insulin, and coronary artery disease treated with anti-angina medications. He also mentions an ulcer present in his great toe.

INTRODUCTION

Peripheral arterial disease (PAD) consists of a range of non–coronary arterial syndromes that are caused by altered structure and function of the arteries that supply the brain, visceral organs, and the limbs.[1] The importance of recognition and management of peripheral vascular disease can not be overemphasized. The predominant arteries involved are in the legs. About 200 million individuals worldwide are affected by this condition.[2] The two most important pathophysiological divisions of the disease[3] include atherosclerosis, which mainly affects the legs,[4] and autoimmune disease, which predominantly affects the arms.[5] Atherosclerotic claudication arising primarily as a result of smoking is typically known as *thromboangitis obliterans*,[6] and occlusion due to arteritis of autoimmune origin is known as *Raynaud's disease*.[7] These conditions are also called peripheral arterial occlusive disease, as their main pathophysiology involves narrowing of the arterioles.

Narrowing of the arteries causes ischemia and subsequent ischemic pain in the limbs. When there is a severe compromise of blood flow to the extent of depriving the tissues of their basal metabolic demand, there is critical limb ischemia and pain.[8] *Critical limb ischemia* is defined by the following criteria: condition with persistently recurring ischemic rest pain requiring regular adequate analgesia for more than 2 weeks, with an ankle systolic pressure ≤50 mmHg and/or toe systolic pressure ≤30 mmHg; and patient's ulceration or gangrene of the foot or toes, with an ankle systolic pressure ≤50 mmHg or toe systolic pressure ≤30 mmHg. This stage usually implies pending limb loss and amputation.

EPIDEMIOLOGY

The incidence of PAD varies between 0.25 and 0.45 per 1000 population/year.[9] It commonly occurs in adults over 55 years of age and ultimately ends in tissue necrosis resulting in amputation in the majority of patients within 6 months of disease. The incidence of Raynaud's phenomenon is 3% to 21%.[10] The wide variation in incidence is due to the varied manifestations included in the description of Raynaud's phenomenon. Moreover, prevalence strongly depends on the population surveyed and the climate conditions prevailing in the region.[11] Raynaud's phenomenon can be due to primary Raynaud's disease or secondarily to a known pathophysiology such as rheumatic disease, systemic sclerosis,[12] or scleroderma.[13] Thromboangitis obliterans, or Buerger's disease, is vasculitis of inflammatory origin predominantly caused by smoking and is characterized by a prothrombotic state and vaso-occlusive phenomena.[6]

Up to 5% of men and 2.5% of women suffer from "intermittent claudication pain" due to arterial occlusive disease.[14] However, the incidence increases threefold if the condition includes asymptomatic individuals identified by sensitive noninvasive testing.[15] About 20% of men and 15% of women older than 65 years of age are affected by peripheral vascular disease.[16] For symptomatic patients, the progression depends on the risk factors involved.[17] Approximately 70% of symptomatic patients do not have any progression of disease and instead show some interval of improvement of symptoms.[18] About 20%–30% of patients will experience progression to intolerable symptoms requiring intervention. Unfortunately, the condition worsens in 10% of those patients to a stage that requires amputation. Approximately 7 million patients who are older than 40 years old will suffer from peripheral vascular disease by 2020.[19] It affects 1 in 10 adults over 70 years of age. It is estimated that 150–200 people per million will progress from intermittent claudication pain to critical limb ischemia that will require major surgical intervention. Revascularization procedures are successful in 70% of patients but do not help in the remainder, hence leading to amputation in about 30% of patients. About half of the patients with peripheral vascular disease have either symptomatic or asymptomatic occlusive coronary and cerebral arterial circulation.[20] This explains the threefold increase in mortality among these patients compared to age-matched controls.[21,22] Peripheral vascular disease constitutes 20% of hospital admissions in the United States.[23]

CLINICAL PRESENTATION AND CLASSIFICATION

The symptoms of ischemic neuropathy may range from intermittent claudication to rest pain. Intermittent claudication consists of pain particularly in the calf muscles and rarely in the buttocks that is associated with exercise and walking and relieved by rest.[3] Peripheral arterial occlusive disease causes alterations in skin sensibility owing to progressive ischemia of the peripheral nerves. Subsequent muscle damage, weakness, and atrophy can occur from selective loss of motor nerve fibers and atrophy of muscles. The Fontaine classification for PAD is commonly used in clinical practice.

The Fontaine Classification for PAD

Fontaine classification	Definition
I	Asymptomatic
IIa	Compensated intermittent claudication
IIb	Decompensated intermittent claudication
III	Rest pain
IV	Nonhealing ulceration

Pain usually occurs at the region supplied by occluded arterial vessels. Popliteal and superficial femoral arteries are commonly involved, resulting in pain in legs and feet. The distal aorta and bifurcation of the femoral vessels are occasionally involved, giving rise to pain in the buttocks and thighs. Pain physicians should have a high index of suspicion of ischemic-related pain in the legs because of its high prevalence.[1,24] Pain physicians should also consider concomitant presence of ischemic coronary artery disease and make appropriate referrals for evaluation. Identification and management of chronic ischemic pain not only improve symptoms and quality of life but also can increase patients' longevity.

PATHOPHYSIOLOGY

The risk factors contributing to development of peripheral occlusive vascular disease are similar to those of coronary and cerebral vascular diseases: age, male sex, family history, smoking, diabetes mellitus, hypertension, and hyperlipidemia (increased low-density lipoprotein [LDL] and low high-density lipoprotein [HDL]).[25,26] Lack of physical activity may lead to other risk factors such as obesity and diabetes and atherosclerosis of the peripheral arterial system. An unhealthy diet creates a risk for development of arterial disease.[27,28] Unbalanced elevated lipid levels cause arterial wall injury, which in turn elicits inflammation and angiogenesis, causing gradual obstruction to distal blood flow. There is an emerging role of inflammation as evidenced by the presence of high levels of C-reactive protein (CRP), which may contribute to the development of this disease.[28] Sleep apnea, stress, and heavy alcohol intake are also associated with peripheral vascular disease. Age plays a critical role in its development[1]; the prevalence of intermittent claudication is 1%–2% in patients less than

40 years of age and increases to 5% over the age of 50. The prevalence is lower in women under 50 years of age and is the same for both sexes after age 70. Diabetes is one of the most important contributors to peripheral vascular disease. Diabetics have a sevenfold increased risk of development of lower extremity vascular disease; about 25% of patients undergoing lower extremity revascularization are diabetics.[29] In addition to producing diffuse and distal vascular disease in diabetics, the concomitant presence of peripheral sensory neuropathy can lead to traumatic ulceration with an increased risk of amputation. Cigarette smoking is also a strong risk factor with a relative risk ratio of 1.7–7.5. There is convincing evidence connecting hypertension with PAD and fasting cholesterol level with intermittent claudication (270 mg% or more doubles the risk). Other risk factors are renal failure, hypothyroidism, congestive heart failure, and autoimmune disorders such as Raynaud's disease.[30]

Chronic ischemia in the legs often results in ischemic neuropathy. There are no definitive studies on the effects of chronic ischemia on neuropathological changes, which are always accompanied by effects of concomitant risk factors such as aging, diabetes, and other vasculitides.[31] Sensory and motor impairment and pain are often associated with peripheral ischemic neuropathy. There is still controversy over whether ischemia results predominantly in sensory or motor neuropathies. Histopathological changes reveal both axonal loss and demyelination and remyelination.[31,32] Microscopic pathological changes are seen in distal parts of axons of nerve fibers of all sizes. However, large and myelinated fibers are more vulnerable to ischemia than are small and nonmyelinated fibers. The neuropathic changes are due to chronic ischemia, acute ischemia during exercise, and injury caused by subsequent reperfusion to the nerves during rest.[33]

Blood-flow limitation caused by atheroscelerotic obstruction forms the mainstay of intermittent claudication and subsequent functional disability caused by PAD. Inadequate augmentation of skeletal muscle blood flow as required by walking and exercise leads to claudication pain, which is relieved by rest.[1] In addition to reduced blood flow, other pathophysiological mechanisms associated with PAD include vascular dysfunction, altered muscle metabolism and mitochondrial dysfunction, impaired angiogenesis, and inflammatory activation. The

underlying pathophysiological mechanisms causing arterial occlusion are atherosclerosis and arteriosclerosis. Ischemia of the lower limbs can be functional or critical.[34] Functional ischemia presents as intermittent claudication due to failure to improve blood flow in response to exercise. The blood flow at rest is adequate and there is no pain at rest. In fact, pain is relieved by rest. Critical ischemia results when there is decrease in blood flow and the flow cannot meet the demands of basal metabolism even at rest. It is characterized by pain at rest and is usually accompanied by trophic changes and ulceration.

These two categories are determined by the rapidity of progression of atherosclerotic disease, localization of obstruction, and extension of the disease. Arterial insufficiency develops owing to the presence of atherosclerotic thrombus, which gradually extends inside the wall and results in complete occlusion of arteries. Arteriosclerosis is commonly present at the bifurcation of vessels where turbulence of blood flow occurs. Lower limb vessels are involved more often than upper limb vessels. The femoropopliteal segment is affected in 60% of patients. As narrowing of vessels is caused by progressive atherosclerosis, velocity of blood flow increases to maintain blood flow. Vessel size may increase and collaterals may also develop to maintain the blood flow. However, when more than 70% of the lumen becomes narrowed and collaterals are not sufficient, patients start to manifest symptoms. Initially, symptoms occur only when there is an increase in demand, such as with exercise or walking. As the disease progresses, however, resting blood flow is also compromised, resulting in critical limb ischemia. This may result in development of collateral blood vessels. Collateral blood flow depends on the chronicity of the process.[35] When there is an imbalance between the need for blood flow and supply by original and collateral vessels, ischemia results in ischemic pain and, if persistent, leads to trophic changes reflecting chronic blood-flow deprivation to the tissues.

When there is decreased blood flow to the lower limb the nerves can become compromised. This results in abnormal metabolic pathway intraneuronally, which leads to abnormal activation of degenerative neurons. When the unmyelinated and small myelinated fibers regenerate, there is aberration of nociceptive neuronal impulse activation and transmission. This gets transmitted through the dorsal horn of the spinal cord. Any local nerve injury due to ischemia spreads to distal parts of the nerves as well as to the central nervous system (CNS). Repeated and prolonged ischemia and reperfusion result in abnormal intracellular second-messenger transport, causing abnormal conduction to the spinal cord.[36] Abnormal protein synthesis occurs, which progresses to escalated nervous excitability. Release of inflammatory cytokines from endothelial cells and macrophages is implicated in this pain model. Endothelial dysfunction due to ischemia also generates chemical mediators responsible for pain. The ectopic discharges cause abnormal spontaneous activation of uninjured nerves by "cross-talk" and cause them to transmit pain signals; this in turn results in peripheral sensitization. The hyperexcitability leads to increased neurotransmitter release from spinal cord neurons and the CNS, causing "wind-up" and central sensitization. Neurons of both the peripheral and central nervous system continue to transmit pain signals even in the absence of persistent stimulus. Hypoxia triggers altered calcium signaling inside vascular smooth muscle cells.[36] It also induces gene transcription and release of chemical substances like interleukin (IL)-1 and IL-10, tumor necrosis factor (TNF), and other cytokine factors promoting cell growth. Endothelial dysfunction is associated with release of nitric oxide (NO), endothelium derived relaxing factor, endothelin, and angiotensin-II. Inflammatory mediators activate the coagulation cascade to increase the release of plasminogen activator inhibitor and decrease plasminogen activator. Imbalance between NO and endothelin causes vessel activation and causes vasoconstriction and release of thromboxane.[37] All inflammatory and procoagulatory mediators either directly or indirectly activate C-fiber nociceptor barrage into the spinal cord and CNS and cause the perception of pain.[38]

SYMPTOMS AND SIGNS

Claudication pain is the hallmark of pain due to vascular disease.[39] Pain in the calf and, less commonly, inside the thigh and buttock is exacerbated by walking and exercise and relieved by rest. As the disease progresses, the walking distance becomes shorter until patients develop rest pain. Sometimes it is difficult to elicit the history of claudication pain as many of these patients are elderly and suffer from arthritis. Hence, 50% of patients with peripheral vascular disease have asymptomatic occult coronary artery disease.

The site of pain gives an approximate idea about the location of obstruction of the vessels. Femoropopliteal artery blockade results in pain in the calf. This type of claudication pain should be differentiated from neurogenic claudication. Popliteal artery and tibial and common peroneal arterial obstruction cause pain in the sole and foot. The presence of atherosclerotic blockade in the aortoiliac region causes pain in the buttocks. Thigh pain is usually associated with blockage in the common femoral arterial region. As ischemia progresses, patients develop rest pain and nocturnal pain. Patients often feel better sleeping in a sitting position as limb dependency relieves pain. Patients often complain about fatigue and numbness in the legs. Subsequently, patients develop trophic changes, including loss of skin texture, ulceration, and ultimately gangrene. Distal hair loss and hypertrophic nails can occur. There is delay or nonhealing of wounds. A wound is considered nonhealing if it fails to respond to conservative management of 4–12 weeks' duration. Conservative management includes rest, dressing changes, avoidance of trauma, and treatment of infection with or without debridement of necrotic wounds. Tissue necrosis and gangrene of toes can occur, leading to amputation. The same process could affect mesenteric arteries, causing intestinal ischemia, characterized by postprandial abdominal pain and loss of appetite and loss of weight.

The sites and characteristics of pain should be differentiated from neurogenic claudication. In patients with spinal canal stenosis, walking or standing causes narrowing of the canal and compression of the cauda equina and causes pain that goes along the buttock to the legs, mimicking claudication pain. This pain is exacerbated by extension of the spine and relieved by forward bending or flexion. A family history of arterial disease is often present in vascular claudication syndromes.[40]

PAD is associated with several comorbidities. Concomitant smoking can result in symptoms and signs of chronic obstructive pulmonary disease (COPD). Coronary and cerebral vascular diseases often accompany peripheral vascular disease, resulting in exertional angina and dyspnea. Carotid obstruction can cause carotid bruit, transient ischemic attacks (TIAs), and cerebrovascular accidents (CVAs). About 25% of diabetics develop peripheral vascular disease, so in diabetes and patients with renal failure, associated neuropathies have to be excluded. Absence of proprioception and two-point tactile discrimination suggest early signs of neuropathy.

Lower extremities may feel cold and can be clammy due to poor circulation. Physical examination should include palpation of pulses and measurement of blood pressure in both the upper arms and legs. PAD is characterized by presence of feeble or absent pulses in feet and presence of smooth and shiny skin over the affected parts. There will be muscle wasting over the calves and legs.

Ankle-brachial index (ABI) measurements are commonly used in the diagnosis of PAD. This is defined as the ratio of the systolic pressures of dorsalis pedis or posterior tibial arteries relative to that of the brachial artery.[41] An ABI of 0.9–1.3 is considered normal. Patients with PAD have less than 0.8 ABI. When the index falls to 0.5–0.8, claudication pain develops. In patients with critical limb ischemia, the index is less than 0.4. Simple measurement of systolic pressures at the ankle or toe can also be used to make the diagnosis. Systolic pressures less than 50 mmHg in the ankle and less than 30 mmHg in the toe signify presence of critical limb ischemia.[42] An exercise ABI and toe-brachial index are the more sensitive measurements used to identify asymptomatic peripheral vascular disease when ABI is normal. The toe-brachial index measures digital perfusion to identify small-vessel arterial disease. Segmental pressure examination and pulse volume recording are used to predict limb survival and nature of wound healing. Continuous-wave Doppler and duplex ultrasound are the other noninvasive methods used to assess the location and severity of obstruction.

A Doppler probe can also be used to measure blood flow and pressures in the lower limb.[43] Pulse volume waveforms can be obtained from Doppler measurements. A progressive change in waveform from triphasic to biphasic to monophasic and then stenotic waveforms indicates worsening of obstruction at the arteries. Highly sensitive MRI angiography can be used to measure the degree of obstruction noninvasively. The other methods available are CT angiography and arteriography. Digital subtraction angiography and arteriography are occasionally used to assess the presence and extent of obstruction.

MANAGEMENT OF PERIPHERAL ARTERIAL DISEASE

In this section we outline the principles of managing arterial occlusive disease; management of the pain component is described in detail. The mainstay of treating pain due to ischemic neuropathy is to address the underlying issue: restoration of blood flow. Blood flow may be restored by the following treatment methods: medical management, percutaneous minimally invasive management, and surgical management.

Risk factor modification and antiplatelet therapy should accompany all forms of treatment. Risk factor management includes cessation of smoking, normalization of blood pressure, and improved control of diabetes and cholesterol levels.

Antiplatelet therapy with aspirin not only improves blood flow by preventing platelet aggregation but also decreases mortality due to coronary artery disease and cerebral vascular disease. Aspirin at 75–325 mg PO is recommended.[44] For patients who cannot tolerate aspirin, clopidogrel 75 mg PO is recommended. Cilostazol is a phosphodiesterase type III inhibitor and a vasodilator and platelet inhibitor. Cilostazol is effective at improving symptoms of pain and discomfort and can increase walking distance.[45] Pentoxifylline is a methylxanthine derivative and is reported to decrease blood and plasma viscosity and lower procoagulant fibrinogen concentrations. It is used as a second-line agent as an alternative to cilostazol to improve walking distance in patients with claudication.[46]

NO acts as a vasodilator, thus drugs increasing intracellular NO have been tried to improve vasodilatation and blood flow. L-arginine improves endothelial dependent vasodilatation, but it does not improve walking distance. In patients with PAD, abnormal skeletal muscle metabolism occurs and the muscles accumulate abnormal levels of acyl-coenzyme-A and acyl carnitine. L-Carnitine and related propionyl-L-carnitine increase the availability of carnitine in skeletal muscles and improve muscle metabolism and facilitate an increase in walking distance.

Ginkgo biloba is used as vasodilator. It acts through a decrease in red blood cell aggregation and blood viscosity and inhibits platelet-activating factor; its use is marginally beneficial.

Prostaglandins are useful for maintaining patency of blood vessels. Arachidonic acid derivatives of cell membrane get converted into thromboxane and prostacyclin by endoperoxidase. Thromboxane is a vasoconstrictor and platelet aggregator, whereas prostacyclin is a vasodilator and inhibitor of platelet aggregation. Both intra-arterial and intravenous administration of prostaglandins have been shown to be useful in healing and relieving rest pain in a small group of patients. Prostaglandin I2 is a vasodilator and platelet inhibitor and has been used both intravenously (Iloprost) and orally (Beraprost) with encouraging results.

Treatment with HMG Co-A reductase inhibitor to lower LDL levels to less than 70 mg% is commonly used. Patients with low HDL may benefit from a fibric acid derivative. Patients with hypertension should be aggressively treated to achieve a target of less than 140/90 mmHg in nondiabetics and less than 130/80 mmHg in diabetics. Previously, beta blockers were contraindicated in patients with PAD, but this is no longer the case and they can be safely used. Smoking cessation and enrollment in programs to prevent relapse are equally important.[47]

Management of diabetes involves not only lowering blood glucose values but also proper care of the leg and foot to prevent diabetic foot problems. The American Diabetes Association (ADA) recommends aggressive management of elevated blood glucose levels in diabetics with PAD to obtain an HbA1c level of less than 7%. Daily foot examination, appropriate footwear, and skin cleansing are strongly encouraged. Any skin lesions or ulcers should be immediately addressed and treated with antibiotics, dressing changes, and debridement as appropriate. In patients with elevated homocysteine levels, vitamin B12 and folic acid supplements can be considered although their efficacy is not yet proven. Better management of congestive heart failure increases peripheral perfusion, and management of COPD improves oxygen supply to the tissues.

A supervised exercise regimen is the first therapy recommended for patients who suffer from claudication and limited walking due to PAD. It is usually advised that patients do 30–45 minutes of supervised exercise a day three times a week for 12 weeks. Exercise therapy increases the time to claudication and increases peak walking capabilities. Endothelial function has also been improved. Although exercise in general is known to increase NO in patients with PAD, a paradoxical decrease in NO may occur. Dietary supplements of precursors of NO, such as nitrates, may be beneficial.

Vasodilator therapy has been suggested to improve blood flow. Calcium channel blockers and serotonin receptor antagonists have been tried with lower success rates. The systemic effects of vasodilators cause hypotension and thus the local effect of vasodilated normal vessels steals blood away from ischemic regions.

Fibrinogen gets converted into fibrin by activated thrombin. Fibrinolysis can be achieved using streptokinase, urokinase, and tissue plasminogen activator (tPA). These medications are useful for acute embolism and acute obstruction rather than for treatment of the chronic process. They will not affect atheroma, and restenosis is common after cessation of their use; hence their usage is always followed by administration of thrombolytics to maintain patency of the vessels.

Gene therapy has been trialed to restore blood flow to ischemic extremities. Genetic engineering was used to manufacture vascular endothelium-derived growth factor (VEGF). VEGF injection causes edema of skeletal muscles and swelling. However, with time it increased blood vessel formation, increased blood flow, and led to improved healing and exercise tolerance. It is still in the experimental stage, but there is promise that local intramuscular injection of VEGF may produce therapeutic angiogenesis.

If a patient does not respond to conservative management or medical therapy, either percutaneous interventional procedures or open surgical methods are used to relieve the obstruction or bypass obstruction to improve blood flow. If the lesions are isolated and located in major blood vessels like iliac or femoral arteries, percutaneous angioplasty is very effective. Stenting can also be used to bypass obstruction. Percutaneous procedures are minimally invasive and pose lower risk than open surgical procedures.[48] However, if the lesions are confined to smaller arteries not amenable to dilatation or stenting, open surgical procedures may be an option.

MANAGEMENT OF ISCHEMIC NEUROPATHY PAIN
Interventional measures include sympatholysis (lumbar sympathectomy) and intravenous regional block.

Lumbar Sympathectomy
Medical management alone may not be sufficient or possible in certain patients with rest pain, and either an interventional procedure or surgery may be indicated. Around one in five patients fall into this category. There are options to improve blood flow to prevent amputation and decrease pain, such as lumbar sympathectomy, which can be performed at L2–L4 regions.

Sympathetic efferents to the lower extremities originate from T10 to L3. Preganglionic fibers form extensive synapses with postganglionic neurons in the paravertebral ganglia in front of L1–S3. The foot and lower leg areas are primarily innervated from L2, and the proximal leg and thigh by L1–L2. There are mainly three ganglia at L2–L4 that are targeted by a lumbar sympathectomy.[49] L1 is often fused with L2. However, L1 is spared, as L1 ganglion blockade may result in impotence. Lumbar sympathectomy can be carried out through an invasive permanent surgical approach or percutaneous methods. It can also be performed by chemical injection. It can be performed percutaneously under either CT or fluoroscopy guidance.

Lumbar sympathectomy may improve blood flow by causing vasodilatation of small peripheral arterial vessels which in turn may improve wound healing and increase walking distance. Hence this can result in decreased symptoms of pain and claudication. If the popliteal flow index is less than 0.7, as measured by blood pressure in the popliteal artery to brachial artery, a significant response can be predicted from sympathectomy. If the ABI is less than 0.35, it may not be beneficial. Arteriolar-venous anastamoses have a rich plexus of sympathetic nerves, so sympathectomy causes vasodilatation and relieves ischemic pain. However, when rest pain occurs from critical impairment of blood flow, sympathectomy not only helps vasodilatation but also addresses pain by interrupting transmission of sympathetic afferent fibers carrying neuropathic and/or ischemic pain.

Chemical percutaneous sympathectomy is as effective as an open surgical procedure to relieve rest pain and improve claudication distance. Chemical sympathectomy can be temporary and used as a trial for successful relief of pain when performed with local anesthetic, which has a relatively short duration of action. More "permanent" blockade can be achieved when performed with neurolytic agents, which can last up to 1–2 years, although duration of the effect is unpredictable. The most common causes of failure of sympathectomy are poor patient selection, and sprouting and regeneration of sympathetic nerves. Post-sympathectomy neuralgia is defined as pain in distribution of the femoral nerve. This is an uncommon complication following lumbar sympathectomy that may resolve in a period of 6–8 weeks. Chemical sympathectomy has the potential to damage a motor nerve such as the femoral nerve if the neurolytic chemical is injected near or reaches the prevertebral region through the psoas fascia.

Intravenous Regional Sympathetic Block (IVRA or Bier Block)

Intravenous administration of drugs that affect postganglionic adrenergic neurons resulting in sympathetic block has been studied. But these techniques are marginally beneficial and hence seldom used because of their short duration of action and the adverse effects of tourniquet application during intravenous regional anesthesia (IVRA) in patients with PAD. They have a very limited role in the rare circumstance when operative lumbar sympathectomy is "wearing off" in a patient who requires temporary prolongation of sympathetic block and in whom percutaneous methods are contraindicated.

Guanethidine for IVRA has been used successfully; it inhibits reuptake of norepinephrine and hence causes sympatholysis. While this was effective, the manufacture of the drug was discontinued. Other drugs used as an adjuvant for IVRA techniques are clonidine, ketorolac, phenoxybenzamine, bretylium, and steroids.

Spinal Cord Stimulation

Spinal cord stimulation (SCS) is based on the gate control theory.[50] When dorsal column of the spinal cord is stimulated, large-diameter fibers are stimulated, leading to inhibition of transmission of pain impulses via small fibers. SCS increases GABA levels in the posterior columns and subsequent reduction in excitatory amino acids. Also, when a peripheral nerve is stimulated, this may simultaneously decrease the velocity of afferent conduction (frequency-related conduction block). The main mechanism of action for SCS in peripheral vascular disease may be activation of descending inhibitory pathways, which decreases sympathetic outflow and inflow and thereby not only improves blood flow but also decreases pain and improves claudication.[51] Descending inhibition also decreases the release of substance P, which is a nociceptive peptide. SCS enhances release of NO, which acts as a vasodilator. SCS also inhibits nicotinic transmission at the level of the ganglion, thereby inhibiting sympathetic outflow. It also enhances release of endogenous opioid peptides. By producing analgesia, it decreases pain-induced vasoconstriction. Antidromic stimulation of the dorsal horn of the spinal cord enhances prostaglandin-mediated vasodilatation in the periphery. Thus there are several mechanisms of SCS that act simultaneously, causing both neural and peptide-mediated inhibition of sympathetic outflow. These postulated mechanisms all serve to result in improved blood flow.[52]

SCS involves insertion of electrodes into the epidural space. The electrodes are more commonly inserted via a percutaneous approach and occasionally by open surgical procedure. The electrodes are then connected to an impulse generator. The procedure consists of inserting one to two electrodes, which cover a segmental space between T8 and T11. The electrodes are inserted at the paralaminar level between L1 and L2. They are placed in the midline or just off midline depending on the location of pain and response to stimulation. Patients often undergo a trial procedure, and during the trial period (approximately a week) they are observed for pain relief and improvement of circulation and quality of life. If this improvement is achieved, the trial is considered a success and treatment can proceed to permanent lead placement and generator implantation.

Patient selection is crucial to attain good success rates with SCS. SCS is considered for patients who have rest pain that is unresponsive to conventional medical therapy and who have severe nonoperable or nonreconstructive arterial obstruction. Usually the ABI index is less than 0.4 and toe pressure less than 30 mmHg in these patients. Patients should not have any active infective ulcers or deep ulcers that penetrate into subcutaneous tissues in the legs. Usually patients with ulcer size less than 3 cm are selected for implantation techniques. SCS is also useful for refractory pain in patients whose pain does not respond to a revascularization procedure. Patients with vasospastic disorders and frostbite and distal arterial embolization may also benefit from SCS therapy.[51]

SCS is currently considered the treatment of choice for patients with microcirculatory disease. It aids in reducing pain and healing ulcers owing to improved circulation and decreases the risk of amputation. In a randomized controlled trial outcomes with SCS were improved in patients with critical leg ischemia and intermediate microcirculation alone.

$TcPO_2$ is used as a guide to determine the need for SCS. It is also used as a prognostic indicator. Determinants of long-term success with

SCS are patients who experience significant pain relief ("successful trial"), peak flow velocity that increases by 10mm/s, and $TcPO_2$ more than 10 mmHg. The European Peripheral Vascular Disease Outcome Study (SCS-EPOS) showed that a trial screening with $TcPO_2$ predicted better outcomes with respect to limb survival following SCS. They recommend an increase of at least 10 mmHg of $TcPO_2$ during the trial period, which would predict success with SCS. It has been recommended that SCS be implanted in patients with a baseline $TcPO_2$ of less than 10–30 mmHg. SCS has been shown through Xenon-133 clearance experiments to improve both muscle and cutaneous blood flow. Jivegard has shown successful outcomes with SCS lasting longer than 18 months. Amputation rates were lower in patients receiving SCS than in those who received medical management. Reig et al. had an 88% success rate in their 20 years of experience of inserting SCS for PAD. SCS has been successfully used in patients with chronic renal failure with peripheral vascular disease. Usually patients with end-stage renal disease are not good candidates for revascularization; SCS has been shown to be very useful in providing good pain relief with improved quality of life in these patients. The long-term success rate of SCS is much better for patients with PAD (70%–90%) than for patients with neuropathic pain (50%–70%).[53]

Similarly, SCS has been successfully used in patients with anginal pain who are refractory to conventional medical and surgical methods. Often these patients have poor quality of life and have frequent hospitalizations and limited physical activities. European Society of Cardiology recommends SCS as first line of treatment for patients who are not candidates for revascularization. SCS reduces anginal symptoms as well as the number of anginal attacks. It also decreased the frequency of required treatments with short-acting vasodilator nitrates. It improved the overall angina classification of patients by facilitating improved activity level. Treatment with SCS increased the functional capacity of these patients and their walking time and capacity, thus improving their functional status and quality of life. SCS does not prevent patients from perceiving severe pain during acute attacks of angina nor their development of myocardial infarction symptoms and thus does not interfere with early medical intervention. While the effect on mortality has not been fully studied, one study showed a reduction in mortality with SCS compared to that with CABG. Similarly, its efficacy compared to that of percutaneous myocardial revascularization is not well known. One study showed that SCS resulted in longer time to development of angina and less severe anginal pain.[50]

SCS is a relatively safe procedure, albeit with an overall complication rate of 17%. The complications include hardware failure, such as lead migration and displacement, and generator failure and infection. Infection can occur at the site of epidural catheter entry or at the site of the generator. Kinfe and colleagues reported a complication rate of 2.5% with lead migration requiring revision.[54] The common location of infection risk is at the site of the generator pocket and its purported rate is less than 3%.

In summary, SCS is a valuable therapeutic option for patients with refractory and rest pain due to peripheral vascular disease. It results in significant reduction of pain and improves walking distance in most patients and improvement in circulatory parameters and blood flow in more than half of patients. Limb salvage and amputation rate reductions are variable.

RAYNAUD'S DISEASE

Case

A 33-year-old female presents to the pain clinic with pain and a bluish tinge in her fingertips. Her pain is stabbing and starts from the arm and radiates to the fingertips. The pain occurs with exposure to cold and gets worse during the winter. She also mentions that she has been suffering from systemic lupus erythematosus for the past 3 years and is being treated with immunosuppressants.

Introduction

Peripheral vascular disease is mainly due to atherosclerosis and frequently affects the legs. In contrast, Raynaud's phenomenon predominantly affects the upper extremities. Raynaud's disease is different from atherosclerotic occlusive arterial disease in terms of etiology, manifestations, and therapeutic approach.

Raynaud's phenomenon was originally described by Maurice Raynaud as early as 1862. Primary Raynaud's phenomenon occurs as a result of Raynaud's disease.[55] Raynaud's disease is an autoimmune disease, which is a diagnosis of exclusion. Secondary Raynaud's phenomenon is seen in patients diagnosed with pathological conditions such as systemic lupus erythematosis, systemic sclerosis, rheumatoid arthritis, occupational vibrating tool disease, and cryoglobulinemia. Drugs can produce symptoms which can mimic Raynaud's; e.g., some beta blockers and certain cytotoxic drugs. Females around the age of 40 are affected more often than males and other age cohorts.

Raynaud's disease affects fingers, toes, and the tip of the nose. These areas are affected owing to the presence of specialized functional and structural features of dense arteriovenous anastamoses. The areas affected undergo typical color change from pallor to cyanosis to rubor. Episodic color change is exacerbated by exposure to cold, stress, and anxiety. All three color changes may not be present in all cases. More often, patients note either pallor or cyanosis. The hands and fingertips should be examined for the presence of any ulcer, hypertrophic changes, or hyperkeratotic areas. Splinter hemorrhages under the nail bed are common. Axillary, brachial, and radial pulses will be palpable. Sometimes examination of the subclavian area may reveal the presence of a cervical rib, which may cause stenosis of the subclavian artery, producing a thrill on palpation over the area. On auscultation, there may be a bruit heard over the sternoclavicular area.

Segmental blood pressure measurement in the upper extremities is an important assessment used to diagnose Raynaud's disease. A pressure difference of 10 mmHg between brachial, upper elbow, and wrist level signifies the presence of underlying Raynaud's phenomenon. Finger systolic pressure measurements can also be taken using finger cuff, strain gauge plethysmography, or photoplethysmography. Pulse volume recording of finger blood flow can also be measured. A difference of 15 mmHg between fingers or an absolute finger blood pressure less than 70 mmHg indicates occlusive disease. The normal finger-brachial index is 0.9–1.3. Analysis of digital plethysmography may reveal blunted waveform due to Raynaud's, or "peaked pulse" due to vasospasm.

Management
Patient Education and General Measures
Patients should avoid exposure to cold and in case of exposure to cold, use of hand warming is highly recommended. They should also avoid hand trauma and closely inspect their hands

everyday. Such measures are sufficient to prevent 80–90% of attacks of Raynaud's disease. Smoking cessation should be strongly advised.

Pharmacological Measures

Patients who have symptoms despite conservative measures can be managed with pharmacological regimens.[56] Calcium channel blockers belonging to the dihydropyridine group, such as nifedipine and nicardipine, are efficacious and are considered the first drugs of choice. Nifedipine was shown to reduce the frequency of attacks by 66%. Other calcium channel blockers have also been shown to reduce the frequency and severity of attacks. Alpha-1-adrenergic blockers like prazosin inhibit postganglionic alpha-adrenergic receptors and cause vasodilatation and are thus found useful. In a double-blind, randomized trial, prazosin was shown to reduce the number and severity of attacks in two-thirds of patients and significantly improved finger blood flow as demonstrated by finger-cooling test.

Angiotensin II receptor blockers such as losartan and selective serotonin reuptake inhibitors such as fluoxetine have been shown to reduce the frequency of attacks. Phosphodiesterase-5-inhibitors such as sildenafil and tadalafil have been shown to improve the condition of Raynaud's disease by improving blood flow. These agents decrease the frequency and severity of attacks and improve ulcer healing and tissue blood flow. The endothelin-inhibitor bosentan has been shown to reduce the appearance of new ulcers in patients with Raynaud's disease. Prostaglandins and prostacyclins are potent vasodilators. Iloprost was shown to reduce the severity, frequency, and duration of Raynaud's attacks. Epoprostenol has been shown to increase fingertip temperature and laser blood flow and hence prevents new attacks of Raynaud's disease.

Sympathectomy

Pharmacological management remains the mainstay of managing Raynaud's disease. Stellate ganglion block has been shown to be beneficial in drug-resistant Raynaud's disease. Stellate ganglion block improves blood flow and neuropathy pain, but the response to sympathetic block is short-lived and thus not useful for long-term management.

GUIDING QUESTIONS

- What are the risk factors associated with peripheral vascular disease?
- Describe the pathophysiology of chronic ischemia associated with peripheral vascular disease.
- What are the symptoms of chronic ischemic neuropathy?
- How do you differentiate ischemic neuropathy from compressive myelopathy?
- How do you treat ischemic leg pain conservatively?
- What interventions are available to manage ischemic neuropathic pain?
- What are the advantages of spinal cord stimulator for patients with ischemic neuropathy in addition to pain relief?
- Differentiate between primary and secondary Raynaud's phenomenon.
- Enumerate the conditions associated with secondary Reynaud's phenomenon.

KEY POINTS

- Peripheral vascular disease involves progressive narrowing of non-coronary arteries. It affects 5% of men and 2.5% of women.
- The two main pathophysiological mechanisms underlying peripheral arterial disease (PAD) include atherosclerosis and autoimmune disease.
- Atherosclerosis predominantly affects lower extremity blood supply, and autoimmune diseases affect upper extremities.
- The risk factors associated with PAD are coronary and cerebral vascular diseases, age, male sex, family history, smoking, diabetes mellitus, hypertension, and hyperlipidemia (increased LDL and low HDL).
- Ischemic neuropathy arises as a result of chronic ischemia due to PAD-associated decreased blood flow to the tissues and peripheral nerves.
- Ischemic neuropathy consists of altered skin sensibility owing to progressive ischemia of the peripheral nerves.
- Subsequent muscle damage, weakness, and atrophy can occur from selective loss of motor nerve fibers and atrophy of muscles.
- Claudication pain is the hallmark of PAD.
- When more than 70% of the lumen becomes narrowed and collaterals are not sufficient, patients start to manifest symptoms of claudication.

- Progressive narrowing and ischemia subsequently result in rest pain.
- The involvement of specific arteries determines the site of origin of symptoms.
- The ankle-brachial index (ABI) and toe-brachial index are the most common measurements used to confirm PAD.
- An ABI of 0.9–1.3 is considered normal. Patients with PAD have less than 0.8 ABI. When the index falls to 0.5–0.8, claudication pain develops. In patients with resting pain and critical limb ischemia, the index is less than 0.4
- Conservative medical management includes risk factor management and use of antiplatelet agents and analgesics.
- Lumbar sympathectomy and spinal cord stimulation are the most common interventions used to improve symptoms and blood flow.
- Raynaud's phenomenon is managed primarily with medical conservative management, and acute exacerbations can be alleviated with sympathetic blocks.

REFERENCES

1. Hamburg NM, Creager MA. Pathophysiology of Intermittent Claudication in Peripheral Artery Disease. *Circ J*. 2017;81(3):281–289. doi:10.1253/circj.CJ-16-1286 [doi]
2. Sampson UK, Fowkes FG, McDermott MM, et al. Global and regional burden of death and disability from peripheral artery disease: 21 world regions, 1990 to 2010. *Glob Heart*. 2014;9(1):145–158.e21. doi:10.1016/j.gheart.2013.12.008 [doi]
3. Hiatt WR, Armstrong EJ, Larson CJ, Brass EP. Pathogenesis of the limb manifestations and exercise limitations in peripheral artery disease. *Circ Res*. 2015;116(9):1527–1539. doi:10.1161/CIRCRESAHA.116.303566 [doi]
4. Malgor RD, Alahdab F, Elraiyah TA, et al. A systematic review of treatment of intermittent claudication in the lower extremities. *J Vasc Surg*. 2015;61(3 Suppl):54S-73S. doi:10.1016/j.jvs.2014.12.007 [doi]
5. Linnemann B, Erbe M. Raynauds phenomenon - assessment and differential diagnoses. *VASAZeitschrift fur Gefasskrankheiten*. 2015;44(3):166–177. doi:10.1024/0301-1526/a000426 [doi]
6. Wu W, Chaer RA. Nonarteriosclerotic vascular disease. *Surg Clin North Am*. 2013;93(4):833–875, viii. doi:10.1016/j.suc.2013.04.003 [doi]
7. Bolster MB, Maricq HR, Leff RL. Office evaluation and treatment of Raynaud's phenomenon. *Cleve Clin J Med*. 1995;62(1):51–61.
8. Mangiafico RA, Mangiafico M. Medical treatment of critical limb ischemia: current state and future directions. *Curr Vasc Pharmacol*. 2011;9(6):658–676. doi:BSP/CVP/E-Pub/0000157 [pii]
9. Davies MG. Criticial limb ischemia: epidemiology. *Methodist Debakey Cardiovasc J*. 2012;8(4):10–14.
10. Bartelink ML, Wollersheim H, van de Lisdonk E, Spruijt R, van Weel C. Prevalence of Raynaud's phenomenon. *Neth J Med*. 1992;41(3–4):149–152.
11. Wigley FM. Raynaud's phenomenon. *Curr Opin Rheumatol*. 1993;5(6):773–784.
12. Generini S, Kahaleh B, Matucci-Cerinic M, Pignone A, Lombardi A, Ohtsuka T. Raynaud's phenomenon and systemic sclerosis. *Ann Ital Med Int*. 1996;11(2):125–131.
13. Valdovinos ST, Landry GJ. Raynaud syndrome. *Tech Vasc Interv Radiol*. 2014;17(4):241–246. doi:10.1053/j.tvir.2014.11.004 [doi]
14. Criqui MH, Aboyans V. Epidemiology of peripheral artery disease. *Circ Res*. 2015;116(9):1509–1526. doi:10.1161/CIRCRESAHA.116.303849 [doi]
15. Kannel WB, Skinner Jr JJ, Schwartz MJ, Shurtleff D. Intermittent claudication. Incidence in the Framingham Study. *Circulation*. 1970;41(5):875–883.
16. Hennion DR, Siano KA. Diagnosis and treatment of peripheral arterial disease. *Am Fam Physician*. 2013;88(5):306–310. doi:d11003 [pii]
17. Cimminiello C. PAD. Epidemiology and pathophysiology. *Thromb Res*. 2002;106(6):V295–301. doi:S0049384801004005 [pii]
18. Diehm C, Kareem S, Lawall H. Epidemiology of peripheral arterial disease. *VASAZeitschrift fur Gefasskrankheiten*. 2004;33(4):183–189. doi:10.1024/0301-1526.33.4.183 [doi]
19. Rooke TW, Hirsch AT, Misra S, et al. 2011 ACCF/AHA Focused Update of the Guideline for the Management of Patients With Peripheral Artery Disease (updating the 2005 guideline): a report of the American College of Cardiology Foundation/American Heart Association Task Force on Practice Guidelin. *J Am Coll Cardiol*. 2011;58(19):2020–2045. doi:10.1016/j.jacc.2011.08.023 [doi]
20. Jelnes R, Gaardsting O, Hougaard Jensen K, Baekgaard N, Tonnesen KH, Schroeder T. Fate in intermittent claudication: outcome and risk factors. *Br Med J (Clin Res Ed)*. 1986;293(6555):1137–1140.
21. Criqui MH, Langer RD, Fronek A, et al. Mortality over a period of 10 years in patients with peripheral arterial disease. *N Engl J*

Med. 1992;326(6):381–386. doi:10.1056/NEJM199202063260605 [doi]

22. Sayers RD, Thompson MM, Dunlop P, London NJ, Bell PR. The fate of infrainguinal PTFE grafts and an analysis of factors affecting outcome. *Eur J Vasc Surg.* 1994;8(5):607–610.

23. Hughson WG, Mann JI, Garrod A. Intermittent claudication: prevalence and risk factors. *Br Med J.* 1978;1(6124):1379–1381.

24. McDermott MM. Lower extremity manifestations of peripheral artery disease: the pathophysiologic and functional implications of leg ischemia. *Circ Res.* 2015;116(9):1540–1550. doi:10.1161/CIRCRESAHA.114.303517 [doi]

25. Ness J, Aronow WS, Ahn C. Risk factors for symptomatic peripheral arterial disease in older persons in an academic hospital-based geriatrics practice. *J Am Geriatr Soc.* 2000;48(3):312–314.

26. Aboyans V, Criqui MH, Denenberg JO, Knoke JD, Ridker PM, Fronek A. Risk factors for progression of peripheral arterial disease in large and small vessels. *Circulation.* 2006;113(22):2623–2629. doi:CIRCULATIONAHA.105.608679 [pii]

27. White PL. Peripheral vascular disease: diet, exercise, or both? *Jama.* 1983;249(24):3355–3356.

28. Taleb S. Inflammation in atherosclerosis. *Arch Cardiovasc Dis.* 2016;109(12):708–715. doi:S1875-2136(16)30112-7 [pii]

29. Hinchliffe RJ, Brownrigg JR, Apelqvist J, et al. IWGDF guidance on the diagnosis, prognosis and management of peripheral artery disease in patients with foot ulcers in diabetes. *Diabetes Metab Res Rev.* 2016;32 Suppl 1:37–44. doi:10.1002/dmrr.2698 [doi]

30. Mya MM, Aronow WS. Increased prevalence of peripheral arterial disease in older men and women with subclinical hypothyroidism. *journals Gerontol A, Biol Sci Med Sci.* 2003;58(1):68–69.

31. Weinberg DH, Simovic D, Isner J, Ropper AH. Chronic ischemic monomelic neuropathy from critical limb ischemia. *Neurology.* 2001;57(6):1008–1012.

32. Rodriguez-Sanchez C, Medina Sanchez M, Malik RA, Ah-See AK, Sharma AK. Morphological abnormalities in the sural nerve from patients with peripheral vascular disease. *Histol Histopathol.* 1991;6(1):63–71.

33. Wang Y, Schmelzer JD, Schmeichel A, Iida H, Low PA. Ischemia-reperfusion injury of peripheral nerve in experimental diabetic neuropathy. *J Neurol Sci.* 2004;227(1):101–107. doi:S0022-510X(04)00280-1 [pii]

34. Gernigon M, Marchand J, Ouedraogo N, Leftheriotis G, Piquet JM, Abraham P. Proximal ischemia is a frequent cause of exercise-induced pain in patients with a normal ankle to brachial index at rest. *Pain Physician.* 2013;16(1):57–64.

35. Slovut DP, Sullivan TM. Critical limb ischemia: medical and surgical management. *Vasc Med.* 2008;13(3):281–291. doi:10.1177/1358863X08091485 [doi]

36. Sayeed MM. Signaling mechanisms of altered cellular responses in trauma, burn, and sepsis: role of Ca2+. *Arch Surg (Chicago, Ill 1960).* 2000;135(12):1432–1442. doi:sbs0001 [pii]

37. Carnemolla R, Villa CH, Greineder CF, et al. Targeting thrombomodulin to circulating red blood cells augments its protective effects in models of endotoxemia and ischemia-reperfusion injury. *FASEB J.* 2017;31(2):761–770. doi:10.1096/fj.201600912R [doi]

38. Opal S, Thijs L, Cavaillon JM, Cohen J, Fourrier F. Roundtable I: relationships between coagulation and inflammatory processes. *Crit Care Med.* 2000;28(9 Suppl):S81–82.

39. Khan NA, Rahim SA, Anand SS, Simel DL, Panju A. Does the clinical examination predict lower extremity peripheral arterial disease? *Jama.* 2006;295(5):536–546. doi:295/5/536 [pii]

40. Arain FA, Cooper Jr LT. Peripheral arterial disease: diagnosis and management. *Mayo Clin Proc.* 2008;83(8):944–950. doi:10.4065/83.8.944 [doi]

41. Crawford F, Welch K, Andras A, Chappell FM. Ankle brachial index for the diagnosis of lower limb peripheral arterial disease. *Cochrane database Syst Rev.* 2016;9:CD010680. doi:10.1002/14651858.CD010680.pub2 [doi]

42. Khurana A, Stoner JA, Whitsett TL, Rathbun S, Montgomery PS, Gardner AW. Clinical significance of ankle systolic blood pressure following exercise in assessing calf muscle tissue ischemia in peripheral artery disease. *Angiology.* 2013;64(5):364–370. doi:10.1177/0003319712446797 [doi]

43. Tang GL, Chin J, Kibbe MR. Advances in diagnostic imaging for peripheral arterial disease. *Expert Rev Cardiovasc Ther.* 2010;8(10):1447–1455. doi:10.1586/erc.10.134 [doi]

44. Fowkes FG, Price JF, Stewart MC, et al. Aspirin for prevention of cardiovascular events in a general population screened for a low ankle brachial index: a randomized controlled trial. *Jama.* 2010;303(9):841–848. doi:10.1001/jama.2010.221 [doi]

45. Stevens JW, Simpson E, Harnan S, et al. Systematic review of the efficacy of cilostazol, naftidrofuryl oxalate and pentoxifylline for the treatment of intermittent claudication. *Br J Surg.* 2012;99(12):1630–1638. doi:10.1002/bjs.8895 [doi]

46. Bedenis R, Lethaby A, Maxwell H, Acosta S, Prins MH. Antiplatelet agents for preventing thrombosis after peripheral arterial bypass surgery. *Cochrane database Syst Rev*. 2015;(2):CD0005(2):CD000535. doi:10.1002/14651858.CD000535.pub3 [doi]

47. Wakabayashi I. Smoking and lipid-related indices in patients with diabetes mellitus. *Diabet Med*. 2014;31(7):868–878. doi:10.1111/dme.12430 [doi]

48. Lumsden AB, Davies MG, Peden EK. Medical and endovascular management of critical limb ischemia. *J Endovasc Ther*. 2009;16(2 Suppl 2):II31–62. doi:10.1583/08-2657.1 [doi]

49. Karanth VK, Karanth TK, Karanth L. Lumbar sympathectomy techniques for critical lower limb ischaemia due to non-reconstructable peripheral arterial disease. *Cochrane database Syst Rev*. 2016;12:CD011519. doi:10.1002/14651858.CD011519.pub2 [doi]

50. De Vries J, De Jongste MJ, Spincemaille G, Staal MJ. Spinal cord stimulation for ischemic heart disease and peripheral vascular disease. *Adv Tech Stand Neurosurg*. 2007;32:63–89.

51. Deogaonkar M, Zibly Z, Slavin K V. Spinal cord stimulation for the treatment of vascular pathology. *Neurosurg Clin N Am*. 2014;25(1):25–31. doi:10.1016/j.nec.2013.08.013 [doi]

52. Jitta DJ, DeJongste MJ, Kliphuis CM, Staal MJ. Multimorbidity, the predominant predictor of quality-of-life, following successful spinal cord stimulation for angina pectoris. *Neuromodulation*. 2011;14(1):13–19. doi:10.1111/j.1525-1403.2010.00321.x [doi]

53. Ubbink DT, Vermeulen H, Spincemaille GH, Gersbach PA, Berg P, Amann W. Systematic review and meta-analysis of controlled trials assessing spinal cord stimulation for inoperable critical leg ischaemia. *Br J Surg*. 2004;91(8):948–955. doi:10.1002/bjs.4629 [doi]

54. Kinfe TM, Schu S, Quack FJ, Wille C, Vesper J. Percutaneous implanted paddle lead for spinal cord stimulation: technical considerations and long-term follow-up. *Neuromodulation*. 2012;15(4):402–407. doi:10.1111/j.1525-1403.2012.00473.x

55. Hughes M, Herrick AL. Raynaud's phenomenon. *Best Pract Res Rheumatol*. 2016;30(1):112–132. doi:10.1016/j.berh.2016.04.001 [doi]

56. Prete M, Fatone MC, Favoino E, Perosa F. Raynaud's phenomenon: from molecular pathogenesis to therapy. *Autoimmun Rev*. 2014;13(6):655–667. doi:10.1016/j.autrev.2013.12.001 [doi]

PART III

Generalized Lesions of the Peripheral Nervous System

16

Diabetic Peripheral Neuropathy

MAXIMILIAN HSIA-KIUNG

CASE

A 72-year-old woman with newly diagnosed type 2 diabetes mellitus is seen in the office for pain in both feet. She says she cannot recall when the pain started but she describes it as a burning pain sensation on the bottom and top of both feet, extending just above her ankles. She was diagnosed with diabetes about 8 months ago and was recently started on insulin. She is very frustrated by the pain because she says her diabetes has been very well controlled over the course of the past few months and her endocrinologist has been very pleased with her progress. Touching her feet makes the burning worse and she has difficulty wearing socks or shoes. She also says she feels like the tips of all of her toes are numb to the touch and feel like they are "asleep." Upon examination, there is no discoloration, swelling, or skin breakdown and all of her toes look normal.

DIABETIC PERIPHERAL NEUROPATHY

Definition

Diabetic peripheral neuropathy (DPN), sometimes referred to as diabetic polyneuropathy, diabetic sensorimotor polyneuropathy, or simply diabetic neuropathy, is defined as symptoms or signs of peripheral nerve dysfunction in people with primary diabetes (type 1 or type 2) or secondary diabetes that is not due to other causes.[1] It typically manifests as a progressive, symmetrical loss of sensation affecting the distal extremities, most often the feet and legs and less commonly the hands, and may also be associated with a burning pain about the affected areas. Between 25% and 50% of patients with DPN develop neuropathic pain. It is important to note that while this is the most commonly seen presentation of diabetic neuropathy, dysfunction of peripheral nerves caused by impaired glucose metabolism

has been shown to affect nearly every part of the body and includes sensory, motor, and autonomic nerve dysfunction. Furthermore, it has been estimated that 5% of peripheral neuropathies diagnosed as diabetic neuropathy are attributable to other causes.[2] This makes the exclusion of other causes in the diagnosis of DPN critical to proper treatment and to delay or prevention of progression of the disease. This chapter will focus on the diagnosis and treatment of painful diabetic neuropathy affecting the distal limbs.

Pathophysiology

While the role of chronic hyperglycemia and its effects on the demyelination and axonal degeneration of peripheral nerves has often been attributed to DPN, the exact cause of peripheral nerve damage in diabetes has never been proven.[3] Furthermore, symptoms of loss of sensation to light touch and allodynia—the perception of a nonpainful stimulus as painful—may occur as multiple separate and distinct pathological processes throughout the course of diabetes onset and progression. A peripheral sensory neuropathy caused by hyperglycemia without structural changes that is rapidly and completely reversible with reduction in serum glucose levels has been long described.[4,5] Often seen in patients with newly diagnosed or poorly controlled diabetes, this often uncomfortable condition is associated with a reduced nerve conduction velocity which rapidly improves with establishment of euglycemia. While the mechanism for this conduction defect is unknown, nerve ischemia due to anaerobic glycolysis in the setting of hyperglycemia has been proposed.[6]

An irreversible, distal and symmetrical sensory polyneuropathy occurs in the setting of long-standing hyperglycemia. Proposed mechanisms for this nerve dysfunction have included increased water flux through the polyol pathway, a two-step metabolic pathway in which glucose is reduced to sorbitol, which is then converted to fructose, creating an osmotic swelling of nerve cells and subsequent conduction dysfunction,[7] the formation of advanced glycation end products leading to segmental demyelination of peripheral nerves,[8] and oxidative stress leading to the formation of free radicals causing cellular damage.[9] Glucose-induced activation of protein kinase C isoforms has also been suggested as a common intracellular mediator of each of these mechanisms of nerve dysfunction in the setting of long-standing hyperglycemia.[10]

The loss of sensation in the distal limbs associated with DPN is accompanied by a painful neuropathy in 25%–50% of diabetic patients. Painful diabetic neuropathy may also occur without loss of sensation and is sometimes considered a distinct syndrome, often associated with rapid control of serum glucose levels due to treatment (also known as insulin neuritis or treatment-induced neuropathy of diabetes), treatment-associated weight loss (diabetic cachexia neuritis), or unintentional weight loss (diabetic anorexia neuritis).[5] The precise mechanism of this pain is unknown, but it has been suggested that axonal regeneration occurring with rapid glycemic control causes ectopic action potential generation in previously damaged neurons.[11]

Epidemiology

Diabetic peripheral neuropathy is likely the most common cause of peripheral neuropathy in the developed world. However, precise measurement of the prevalence of DPN is difficult given current evidence. Accurate data are difficult to collect as they are plagued by variability in definition of the disease, inconsistency in diagnostic criteria, and the failure to exclude other causes of neuropathy. Furthermore, DPN is frequently present at the time of diagnosis of type 2 diabetes.[12] Given the fact that type 2 diabetes itself is often undiagnosed even in the face of comorbid disease, the actual annual incidence of DPN may be severely underestimated.

The largest recent population-based study performed in the United States, the Rochester Diabetic Neuropathy Study, estimated DPN to occur in 54% of insulin-dependent diabetics, and in 45% of non-insulin-dependent diabetics, with a total prevalence of 47.6% in patients diagnosed with type 1 or type 2 diabetes.[2] Studies assessing prevalence in a clinic-based setting report significantly lower figures, between 22.7% and 28.5%,[13,14] again suggesting DPN is significantly underdiagnosed. The prevalence of painful DPN is even less well studied. A clinic-based study from the UK suggested an overall prevalence of painful neuropathic symptoms in 34% of diabetics surveyed, a cohort which included both type 1 and type 2 diabetic patients.[15] Another study showed a 26% prevalence of painful diabetic polyneuropathy in type 2 diabetics, and found a positive association between severity of polyneuropathy and the concomitant occurrence of a painful neuropathy.[16]

Finally, therapy to reduce daily hyperglycemia has been shown to reduce incidence of diabetic neuropathy, in addition to slowing its progression and maybe reversing long-standing nerve injury.[17] This evidence serves to emphasize the fact that glycemic control is the key to prevention and treatment of complications associated with diabetes.

Clinical Features and Diagnosis of Diabetic Peripheral Neuropathy

Diabetic peripheral neuropathy affecting the distal extremities is the most common diabetic neuropathy and also the most common form of distal neuropathy seen in developed countries. Therefore, a high degree of clinical suspicion is prudent in the treatment of all diabetic patients. Any clinician who is considering a diagnosis of DPN should also be aware that a variety of focal and nonfocal neuropathies are often mistaken for DPN and must be ruled out.[3] Approximately 5% of patients with type 1 and type 2 diabetes who have been diagnosed with peripheral polyneuropathy have been shown to have a peripheral neuropathy of other origin,[2] obviating the need to rule out other causes.

The most common clinical presentation is a symmetrical loss of sensation to touch that begins in the feet and extends proximally up the legs as the disease progresses. As symptoms extend into the calves, the hands may become affected, a distribution commonly referred to as "stocking-glove." Symptoms in affected areas can range in severity from diminished sensation to light touch to complete loss of sensation to light and deep palpation, vibration, and proprioception (commonly described as "negative symptoms"). These areas may also be severely painful with or without stimuli (described as "positive symptoms") or be completely painless. Patients frequently describe symptoms of burning, shooting, and hypersensitivity. The severity and characteristics of these symptoms often change depending on activity. Patients may not be able to wear shoes or socks because of the allodynia they produce. Symptoms are often reported to be worse at night, although this is probably due to lack of distracting stimuli rather than a physiological circadian change.

Despite this classic clinical presentation, reporting of symptoms of peripheral polyneuropathy in diabetic patients is a poor surveillance and diagnostic tool. Patients with type 2 diabetes have been found to have a 28% sensitivity in recognizing symptoms of numbness in the feet,[18] indicating an annual exam by a clinician is critical.

Several tools have been developed and verified for diagnosing DPN, beginning with the San Antonio Conference in 1988, which called for a standardization of clinical tests and questionnaires to diagnose diabetic neuropathy of all kinds, including peripheral polyneuropathy.[1] Experts at the Mayo Clinic and the University of Toronto developed criteria for identification of four categories of diabetic sensorimotor peripheral neuropathy: possible clinical neuropathy, probable clinical neuropathy, confirmed clinical neuropathy, and subclinical neuropathy.[19] While very comprehensive, the criteria require the use of a nerve conduction study and are therefore difficult to employ broadly or to be used as an annual screening tool.

The Semmes Weinstein monofilament examination (SWME) was developed in the 1960s in an attempt to use a low-cost, noninvasive and rapid test that was standardized. In the exam, a monofilament of precise specifications is used to deliver a force of 10 g to pinpoint areas of the skin at various sites of the foot. Studies comparing the SWME to nerve conduction studies have varied greatly, however, in reported sensitivity of the test.[20]

At this time, the most validated and practical screening tool studied is the Michigan Neuropathy Screening Instrument (MNSI).[21] Developed in 1994, the MNSI has been validated several times by independent groups and remains the most reliable screening tool that is readily employed in the outpatient setting for patients with an established diagnosis of either type 1 or type 2 diabetes.[22,23] The instrument uses four criteria: appearance of feet, presence of ulceration, ankle reflexes, and vibration perception. Each foot is scored from 0 to 4 for a total score range from 0 to 8. A score greater than 2 has been shown to be diagnostic of DPN with 65% sensitivity and 83% specificity[24] and is positively correlated with pathological findings on nerve conduction studies.[21]

While the establishment of a validated tool for diabetic peripheral polyneuropathy has been well studied, little evidence supports a tool which incorporates symptoms of pain or discomfort associated with such nerve dysfunction in diabetes. Pain caused by existing nerve damage is only attributed to diabetic polyneuropathy if it occurs in areas that have already been found to be affected by the disease. Similarly, treatment-induced neuropathy of diabetes (also known as "insulin neuritis") has been correlated with acute onset of pain in the distal extremities within 8 weeks of a decrease in glycosylated hemoglobin A1C (HbA1C) of ≥2% points over a period no more than 3 months, even though no validated diagnostic criteria have been established.[25]

Differential Diagnosis

Other etiologies for peripheral sensory neuropathy must be considered when making the diagnosis of diabetic peripheral polyneuropathy. These include peripheral vascular disease, thyroid disease, and vitamin B12 deficiency. Extensive testing is not needed to differentiate these conditions, and misdiagnosis can often be avoided with consideration of a broad differential and a simple history and exam. Invasive and expensive electrodiagnostic and magnetic resonance imaging is rarely necessary and has been shown to be inferior to simple screening of HbA1C, thyroid function tests, and vitamin B12 levels in addition to a complete neurological exam in finding a diagnosis for new-onset distal, symmetrical polyneuropathy.[26]

An uncommon but potentially devastating disorder that is associated with DPN is Charcot's neuroarthropathy, sometimes referred to as Charcot's foot, although it can affect any joint in the body. Features of the disease are swelling, warmth, and erythema in a distal extremity that is sometimes associated with minor trauma. Onset is usually sudden, although a more insidious and progressive form has been described. Left untreated, Charcot neuroarthropathy can lead to ulceration and severe joint deformity.[27] Any patient with a history of diabetic neuropathy who presents with unilateral swelling in a distal extremity should warrant a diagnostic evaluation.

Treatment

Treatment of symptomatic diabetic peripheral polyneuropathy is focused broadly on prevention or slowing of the progressive extension of the affected areas from distal to proximal, and therapies to provide symptom relief.

Prevention

Good glycemic control is clearly important both in the primary prevention of diabetic peripheral polyneuropathy and in the prevention of its progression. Strangely, while the establishment of good glycemic control has been shown to reduce the risk of diabetic polyneuropathy in type 1 diabetics,[23,28] there is a paucity of data regarding type 2 diabetes. The American Diabetes Association has suggested, however, that glycemic control is a target in any patient with type 2 diabetes in avoiding all complications.[29] Patients with large fluctuations in serum glucose levels have been found to have a higher prevalence of painful DPN.[30]

Foot care is critical in prevention of trauma and ulceration of the skin and soft tissues in patients with diabetic peripheral polyneuropathy. Secondary pain due to chronic nonhealing ulcers or even osteomyelitis can be severe. In addition to good glycemic control, feet should be examined daily for the presence of skin abrasions, breakdown, cracking, or open wounds.

As the polyol pathway has been implicated as a mechanism of nerve injury with states of chronic hyperglycemia, there has been much interest in aldose reductase inhibitors as preventative pharmacotherapy for diabetic peripheral polyneuropathy. Aldose reductase is the enzyme thought to be responsible for the metabolism of intracellular glucose to sorbitol, which causes a rise in osmolarity leading to cell damage. Inhibitors of this enzyme have been successfully used in animal models in correcting nerve conduction defects. Data in human trials, however, have been equivocal.[31,32] We therefore do not recommend the use of an aldose reductase inhibitor at this time until further investigation can support its use in the setting of treatment or prevention of diabetic peripheral polyneuropathy.

Pharmacological Treatment of Pain

While diabetic peripheral polyneuropathy is most often characterized by negative symptoms and primarily a loss of sensation, a proportion of patients experience painful diabetic neuropathy. Although the etiology of such pain may include treatment-induced neuropathy, diabetic cachexia neuritis, diabetic anorexia neuritis, or long-standing peripheral polyneuropathy that has become uncomfortable or painful, the treatment of painful symptoms is often the same.

Among the most-studied oral medications used for symptomatic treatment of diabetic peripheral polyneuropathy are the tricyclic antidepressants. While side effects have often limited their use, they remain first-line agents, as several randomized, placebo-controlled clinical trials have proven their efficacy.[33] Amitriptyline was first described,[34] but desipramine has been shown to be equally effective with fewer side effects.[35] Newer dual serotonin and norepinephrine reuptake inhibitors have also been used,[36] and comparison trial between duloxetine and amitriptyline has shown similar efficacy.[37] We recommend beginning desipramine at a low dose of 25 mg to be taken at bedtime and titrated up by 25 mg once every 3 days for a target dose of 150 mg as tolerated. This may be substituted with duloxetine if the patient does not tolerate side effects.

Gabapentin has not been well studied for treatment of diabetic peripheral polyneuropathy, and evidence for its use in neuropathic pain of all types is not adequate to support routine use.[38] Nevertheless, it is frequently prescribed by physicians for the treatment of diabetic neuropathy. Pregabalin is structurally related to gabapentin and has been shown to have a significant and dose-dependent improvement in painful symptoms in patients with diabetic peripheral polyneuropathy.[39] We recommend beginning pregabalin at a dose of 50 mg taken twice daily, titrated up to 150–600 mg in two or three divided daily doses as tolerated.

Of the topical formulations, capsaicin cream has been the only medication with evidence to support its use in diabetic peripheral polyneuropathy. Capsaicin is a naturally occurring alkaloid found in many chili pepper varieties thought to cause a reduction in substance P found at nerve terminals in the skin. While modest, a statistically significant effect has been shown with use of 0.075% capsaicin cream in reducing pain and improving walking and sleeping.[40] We recommend its use in patients who have not responded to or do not tolerate standard oral pharmacotherapy.

Nonpharmacological Treatment of Pain

Transcutaneous electric nerve stimulation (TENS) is the use of a low electrical current applied across surface electrodes placed over the skin and has been studied for treatment of several painful conditions. Noninvasive, safe, and low-cost, TENS offers an alternative to pharmacotherapy that has few side effects. Evidence regarding the use of TENS in painful diabetic neuropathy has been modest, suggesting TENS is probably useful in reducing painful symptoms while being used.[41] We recommend use of TENS for painful diabetic neuropathy in patients who do not respond adequately or cannot use conventional pharmacotherapy.

Spinal cord stimulation (SCS) is a surgical procedure that has been used for a wide array of painful syndromes in the distal extremities.[42] The treatment consists of an implanted electrode that is placed in the posterior epidural space to produce electrical stimulation of the dorsal columns of the spinal cord. The mechanism of action of stimulation in alleviating pain is not completely understood, although modulation of both central and peripheral nervous systems has been suggested.[43,44] The use of SCS for painful diabetic neuropathy was first studied in 1996 and found to significantly reduce background pain and acute exacerbations of pain, as well as increase exercise tolerance.[45] The results have been replicated and shown to have long-term effects in reducing painful symptoms.[46,47] As the procedure is invasive and requires surgical implant of a device, careful patient selection is critical for successful use of SCS for treatment of painful diabetic peripheral polyneuropathy. We recommend consideration of an SCS trial for those patients who are severely limited in their physical activity due to pain from DPN who have failed to respond adequately to pharmacological and conservative therapy.

GUIDING QUESTIONS

- Can you describe the pathophysiology of painful diabetic polyneuropathy?
- How do you diagnose painful diabetic polyneuropathy?
- How do you manage patients with painful diabetic polyneuropathy?

KEY POINTS

- Diabetic peripheral neuropathy (DPN), sometimes referred to as diabetic polyneuropathy or diabetic sensorimotor polyneuropathy, is a disease marked by loss of sensation to touch and vibration, sometimes accompanied by pain, in patients with type 1 or type 2 diabetes. It is one of a constellation of neuropathies that can occur with diabetes.
- DPN affects about 50% of patients with type 1 or type 2 diabetes and may be present at diagnosis. Painful symptoms in affected areas may also occur with treatment, sometimes termed "insulin neuritis," usually when glucose control is rapid or when significant weight loss occurs.
- Many mechanisms of DPN have been proposed, including cell damage resulting from osmotic swelling due to high intracellular sorbitol, oxidative stress, and activation of protein kinase C.
- Diagnosis of DPN is often made when diabetic patients self-report symptoms, although this has shown to be ineffective. Patients with diabetes should be screened annually using a validated diagnostic tool such as the Michigan Neuropathy Screening Instrument (MNSI). Other causes for peripheral neuropathy must also be ruled out.
- Treatment of DPN and pain associated with the disease consists of prevention of progression and treatment of uncomfortable or painful symptoms. Prevention of the disease is achieved primarily through glycemic control, although aldose reductase inhibitors may offer benefit in the future.
- Medications used to treat uncomfortable or painful symptoms associated with DPN include tricyclic antidepressants, serotonin-norepinephrine reuptake inhibitors, and pregabalin. Topical medications may provide adjunctive treatment to those who do not adequately respond to oral therapy.
- Nonpharmacological therapies include transcutaneous electric nerve stimulation (TENS) and spinal cord stimulation (SCS), and may be useful in patient who are refractory or cannot tolerate conventional treatment. TENS therapy is relatively simple and easy, and benefit may be marginal. SCS is invasive but may be very effective in appropriately selected patients.

REFERENCES

1. American Diabetes Association & American Academy of Neurology. Consensus statement: report and recommendations of the San Antonio Conference on Diabetic Neuropathy. *Diabetes Care.* 1988;11:592–597.

2. Dyck PJ, Kratz KM, Karnes JL, et al. The prevalence by staged severity of various types of diabetic neuropathy, retinopathy, and nephropathy in a population-based cohort: the Rochester Diabetic Neuropathy Study. *Neurology.* 1993;43:817–824.

3. Powers A. Diabetes mellitus. In: Kasper DL, Harrison TR, eds. *Harrison's Principles of Internal Medicine.* 16th ed. New York: McGraw-Hill; 2005.

4. Boulton AJM, Malik RA, Arezzo JC, Sosenko JM. Diabetic somatic neuropathies. *Diabetes Care.* 2004;27:1458–1486.

5. Thomas PH. Classification, differential diagnosis, and staging of diabetic peripheral neuropathy. *Diabetes.* 1997;46(Suppl 2):S54–S57.

6. Schneider U, Niedermeier W, Grafe P. The paradox between resistance to hypoxia and liability to hypoxic damage in hyperglycemic peripheral nerves: evidence for glycolysis involvement. *Diabetes.* 1993;42:981–987.

7. Oates PJ. Aldose reductase, still a compelling target for diabetic neuropathy. *Curr Drug Targets.* 2008;9:14–36.

8. Sugimoto K, Yasujima M, Yagihashi S. Role of advanced glycation end products in diabetic neuropathy. *Curr Pharm Des.* 2008;14:953–961.

9. Henry WL. Perspectives in diabetes. *J Natl Med Assoc.* 1962;54:476–478.

10. Nishikawa T, Edelstein D, Du XL, et al. Normalizing mitochondrial superoxide production blocks three pathways of hyperglycaemic damage. *Nature.* 2000;404:787–790.

11. Hwang YT, Davies G. "Insulin neuritis" to "treatment-induced neuropathy of diabetes": new name, same mystery. *Pract Neurol.* 2016;16:53–55.

12. UK Prospective Diabetes Study Group. Effect of intensive blood glucose control with metformin on complications in overweight patients with type 2 diabetes (UKPDS 34). *Lancet.* 1998;352:854–865.

13. Cabezas-Cerrato J. The prevalence of clinical diabetic polyneuropathy in Spain: a study in primary care and hospital clinic groups. Neuropathy Spanish Study Group of the Spanish Diabetes Society (SDS). *Diabetologia.* 1998;41:1263–1269.

14. Young MJ, Boulton AJM, Macleod AF, Williams DRR, Sonksen PH. A multicentre study of the prevalence of diabetic peripheral neuropathy in the United Kingdom hospital clinic population. *Diabetologia.* 1993;36:150–154.

15. Abbott CA, Malik RA, Van Ross ERE, Kulkarni J, Boulton AJM. Prevalence and characteristics of painful diabetic neuropathy in a large community-based diabetic population in the UK. *Diabetes Care.* 2011;34:2220–2224.

16. Davies M, Brophy S, Williams R, Taylor A. The prevalence, severity, and impact of painful diabetic peripheral neuropathy in type 2 diabetes. *Diabetes Care.* 2006;29:1518–1522.

17. The Diabetes Control and Complications Trial Research Group. The effect of intensive diabetes therapy on the development and progression of neuropathy. *Ann Intern Med.* 1995;122:561–568.

18. Franse LV, Valk GD, Dekker JH, Heine RJ, Van Eijk JTM. "Numbness of the feet" is a poor indicator for polyneuropathy in type 2 diabetic patients. *Diabet Med.* 2000;17:105–110.

19. Dyck PJ, Albers JW, Andersen H, et al. Diabetic polyneuropathies: update on research definition, diagnostic criteria and estimation of severity. *Diabetes Metab Res Rev.* 2011;27:620–628.

20. Feng Y, Schlösser FJ, Sumpio BE. The Semmes Weinstein monofilament examination as a screening tool for diabetic peripheral neuropathy. *J Vasc Surg.* 2009;50:675–682.

21. Feldman EL, Stevens MJ, Thomas PK, Brown MB, Canal N, Greene DA. A practical two-step quantitative clinical and electrophysiological assessment for the diagnosis and staging of diabetic neuropathy. *Diabetes Care.* 1994;17:1281–1289.

22. Lunetta M, Le Moli R, Grasso G, Sangiorgio L. A simplified diagnostic test for ambulatory screening of peripheral diabetic neuropathy. *Diabetes Res Clin Pract.* 1998;39:165–172.

23. Pop-Busui R, Herman WH, Feldman EL, et al. DCCT and EDIC studies in type 1 diabetes: lessons for diabetic neuropathy regarding metabolic memory and natural history. *Curr Diab Rep.* 2010;10:276–282.

24. Moghtaderi A, Bakhshipour A, Rashidi H. Validation of Michigan Neuropathy Screening Instrument for diabetic peripheral neuropathy. *Clin Neurol Neurosurg.* 2006;108:477–481.

25. Gibbons CH, Freeman R. Treatment-induced neuropathy of diabetes: an acute, iatrogenic complication of diabetes. *Brain* 2015;138:43–52.

26. Callaghan BC, Kerber KA, Lisabeth LL, et al. Role of neurologists and diagnostic tests on the management of distal symmetric polyneuropathy. *JAMA Neurol.* 2014;71:1143–1149.

27. Wukich DK, Sung W, Wipf SAM, Armstrong DG. The consequences of complacency: managing the effects of unrecognized Charcot feet. *Diabet Med.* 2011;28:195–198.

28. Diabetes Control and Complications Trial Research Group. The effect of intensive treatment of diabetes on the development and progression of

long-term complications in insulin-dependent diabetes mellitus. *N Engl J Med.* 1993;329:977–986.

29. Boulton AJM, Vinik AI, Arezzo JC, et al. Diabetic neuropathies: a statement by the American Diabetes Association. *Diabetes Care.* 2005;28:956–962.

30. Oyibo SO, Prasad YDM, Jackson NJ, Jude EB, Boulton AJM. The relationship between blood glucose excursions and painful diabetic peripheral neuropathy: a pilot study. *Diabet Med.* 2002;19:870–873.

31. Bril V, Hirose T, Tomioka S, Buchanan R. Ranirestat for the management of diabetic sensorimotor polyneuropathy. *Diabetes Care.* 2009;32:1256–1260.

32. Hotta N, Toyota T, Matsuoka K, et al. Clinical efficacy of fidarestat, a novel aldose reductase inhibitor, for diabetic peripheral neuropathy: a 52-week multicenter placebo-controlled double-blind parallel group study. *Diabetes Care.* 2001;24:1776–1782.

33. Saarto T, Wiffen PJ. Antidepressants for neuropathic pain (review). *Cochrane Database Syst Rev.* 2007;4:CD005454.

34. Max MB, Culnane M, Schafer SC, et al. Amitriptyline relieves diabetic neuropathy pain in patients with normal or depressed mood. *Neurology* 1987;37:589–596.

35. Max MB, Lynch SA, Muir J, Shoaf SE, Smoller B, Dubner R. Effects of desipramine, amitriptyline, and fluoxetine on pain in diabetic neuropathy. *N Engl J Med.* 1992;326:1250–1256.

36. Lunn MPT, Hughes RAC, Wiffen PJ. Duloxetine for treating painful neuropathy or chronic pain. *Cochrane Database Syst Rev.* 2009;4:CD007115.

37. Kaur H, Hota D, Bhansali A, et al. A comparative evaluation of amitriptyline and duloxetine in painful diabetic neuropathy: a randomized, double-blind, cross-over clinical trial. *Diabetes Care.* 2011;34:818–822.

38. Moore RA, Wiffen PJ, Derry S, Toelle T, Rice ASC. Gabapentin for chronic neuropathic pain and fibromyalgia in adults. *Cochrane Database Syst Rev.* 2014;4:CD007938.

39. Freeman R, Durso-DeCruz E, Emir B. Efficacy, safety, and tolerability of pregabalin treatment for painful diabetic peripheral neuropathy: findings from seven randomized, controlled trials across a range of doses. *Diabetes Care.* 2008;31:1448–1454.

40. Capsaicin Study Group. Effect of treatment with capsaicin on daily activities of patients with painful diabetic neuropathy. *Diabetes Care.* 1992;15:159–165.

41. Dubinsky RM, Miyasaki J. Assessment: efficacy of transcutaneous electric nerve stimulation in the treatment of pain in neurologic disorders (an evidence-based review). *Neurology.* 2010;74:173–176.

42. Mekhail NA, Mathews M, Nageeb F, Guirguis M, Mekhail MN, Cheng J. Retrospective review of 707 cases of spinal cord stimulation: indications and complications. *Pain Pract.* 2011;11:148–153.

43. Compton AK, Shah B, Hayek SM. Spinal cord stimulation: a review. *Curr Pain Headache Rep.* 2012;16:35–42.

44. Linderoth B, Foreman RD. Mechanisms of spinal cord stimulation in painful syndromes: role of animal models. *Pain Med.* 2006;7(Suppl 1):S14–S26.

45. Tesfaye S, Watt J, Benbow SJ, Pang KA, Miles J, MacFarlane IA. Electrical spinal-cord stimulation for painful diabetic peripheral neuropathy. *Lancet.* 1996;348:1698–1701.

46. Slangen R, Schaper NC, Faber CG, et al. Spinal cord stimulation and pain relief in painful diabetic peripheral neuropathy: a prospective two-center randomized controlled trial. *Diabetes Care.* 2014;37:3016–3024.

47. van Beek M, Slangen R, Schaper NC, et al. Sustained treatment effect of spinal cord stimulation in painful diabetic peripheral neuropathy: 24-month follow-up of a prospective two-center randomized controlled trial. *Diabetes Care.* 2015;38:e132–e134.

17

HIV Polyneuropathy

HERSIMREN BASI

CASE

A 34-year-old woman with a 10-year history HIV presents to the pain clinic for initial evaluation of bilateral pain in her feet and hands for the past 3–4 years. She was untreated for HIV for her first 6 years with the disease, but she has been on antiretroviral treatment for the past 4 years, now with excellent control of her disease. She started experiencing minimal pain symptoms about 8 years ago; however, her pain has become more severe over the past 3–4 years. She states that the pain is most intense on the bottom of her feet, but she also feels numbness and a tingling sensation up to the mid-calf in both lower extremities. The bottom of her feet have an intense burning and are in constant pain. She feels similar pain in her fingertips and notes numbness at the wrist bilaterally. She is awakened multiple times a night from the pain. Examination reveals decreased sensation to light touch over the dorsal and palmar aspects of both hands and all 10 toes with mild hypersensitivity to light touch over the plantar aspect of both feet. There is no edema, and no lesions or changes are noted in skin color. She has 5/5 strength in all extremities.

INTRODUCTION

HIV-associated sensory neuropathy has become the most common neurological disorder associated with AIDS. It is associated with use of effective antiretroviral medications along with a decline in central nervous system (CNS) opportunistic infection and HIV-related dementia. The prevalence of HIV-related neuropathy is also thought to rise in the United States as highly active antiretroviral therapy (HAART) usage and HIV survival rates increase. This will likely lead to more of these patients being referred to and treated by pain practitioners nationally.[1,2]

DEFINITION

HIV polyneuropathy can cause the patient to experience unusual sensations, parasthesias, dysesthesias, numbness, and pain in the body, most often in their hands and feet. Even nonpainful stimuli can elicit painful sensations. In later stages of HIV polyneuropathy, patients may experience muscle weakness. HIV-related polyneuropathy is typically related to axonal degeneration as well as reduced density of mostly unmyelinated nerve fibers.

EPIDEMIOLOGY

A review of 37 cohort and cross-sectional studies reported variation in the prevalence of HIV polyneuropathy ranging from 1.2% to 69%, and annual development of neuropathy in HIV-positive patients ranging from 0.7 to 39.7 per 100 persons per year. Greater risk of peripheral neuropathy was reported among patients with more severe HIV disease and in older populations.[3,4]

Peripheral neuropathies have been documented since very early reports of patients infected with the HIV virus, in the 1980s.[5-7] However, large variability exists in epidemiology literature. There is minimal to no uniformity in the diagnostic criteria used for HIV peripheral neuropathy in many series published. Clinical, electrophysiological, and pathological evaluations vary greatly among studies.[5] Even the most common form of HIV peripheral neuropathy does not have uniform diagnostic criteria. Autopsy studies have shown the percentage of peripheral neuropathies encountered in HIV-infected patients is close to 30%.[5,8]

PATHOPHYSIOLOGY

HIV-associated painful neuropathy may arise from two different sources: direct neurotoxicity via infection of neurons by the virus itself, and indirect neurological damage via release of viral proteins and inflammatory response.[9,10] It is unclear whether the virus can invade neurons, given that there has been a lack of evidence revealing CD4 receptor expression on the surface of neurons.[11] Several HIV-related proteins have been found to play a role in HIV-related nervous system disease, such as trans-activator of transcription (Tat), negative regulatory factor (Nef), stromal cell–derived factor 1-alpha (SDF-1α), and regulated on activation, normal T cell expressed and secreted (RANTES).[10]

Glycoprotein (Gp) 120 has been studied extensively with the strongest evidence for indirect neurotoxic effects of HIV on the peripheral nervous system. Gp120 is exposed on the surface of the HIV envelope, and its involvement in the pathogenesis of HIV-related distal symmetrical polyneuropathy has been shown in vitro and in vivo. Gp120 can induce neuronal cell lysis in cultured dorsal root ganglion (DRG) cells[10,12] and can activate macrophages which lead to the release of neurotoxic inflammatory mediators such as tumor necrosis factor-alpha (TNF-α) and interleukin-1 (IL-1).[10,13] Gp120 also can induce Schwann cells to release RANTES, which in turn causes DRG glial cells to produce TNF-α, leading to neuronal cell death through TNF receptor 1–mediated neurotoxicity.[10,14,15] Application of Gp120 to the sciatic nerve in rats leads to neuronal swelling and macrophage infiltration, similar to the inflammatory process observed in patients with HIV.[10,14-16] Clinically speaking, polyneuropathies arising from either HIV or antiviral medications are difficult to distinguish from one another. However, the pathophysiology of nucleoside analog reverse-transcriptase inhibitors (NRTIs) leading to neuropathy is different. NRTIs may produce mitochondrial dysfunction by inhibiting mitochondrial DNA polymerase gamma, axonal cell loss, dying back of epidermal nerve fiber (EDNFs), and macrophage infiltration into the DRG.[10,17]

Mitochondrial DNA damage is more significant in patients suffering from distal symmetrical polyneuropathy than in HIV-negative patients and HIV patients without distal peripheral neuropathy. Mitochondrial DNA damage is also higher in the distal sural nerve than in the DRG, which suggests that mitochondrial dysfunction may contribute to the clinical phenotype of length-dependent neuropathy.[10,18,19]

There are a number of different types of HIV polyneuropathies, classified according to the time of onset during HIV disease stage and by clinical course and major symptoms. In the next sections, we discuss the six main types.

DISTAL SYMMETRICAL NEUROPATHY

Distal symmetrical polyneuropathy (DSP) is the most common type of HIV-related neuropathy. Distal symmetrical neuropathy is a typical length-dependent neuropathy in that symptoms typically start at the most distal peripheral part, the toes, and progressively migrate higher up the lower extremities. Symptoms may then start at the fingertips and progressively move up the hands and mid-arms. DSP can present with numbness, pain, dysesthesias, burning sensation, pins-and-needles type sensation, and allodynia.[5] This form of neuropathy typically occurs in the intermediate and late stages of AIDS. Subclinical and neuropathological signs and symptoms may be noted earlier in the disease stage.[5] The most characteristic pathological feature is axonal degeneration of long axons in distal regions. In DSP, the density of both small and large myelinated fibers is affected; however, the density of the unmyelinated fibers is reduced most.[5,20] An average of 27% reduction in myelinated fibers has been shown in DSP, which resembles the magnitude of fiber reduction in diseases such as diabetic neuropathy that also predominantly affects small sensory fibers. Prominent macrophage activation has been seen in immunopathological studies with areas of axonal degeneration and release of proinflammatory cytokines. Cases of subtle to prominent infiltration of lymphocytes of the epineurium have also been seen in patients with distal symmetrical neuropathy.[5]

On neurological exam, the most common signs of DSP are depressed or absent ankle reflexes.[11,21] Vibratory thresholds are increased in the feet while joint position remains relatively normal. Pain and temperature sensations are reduced in a stocking-and-glove distribution. Examination of the feet may reveal some muscle atrophy and weakness, typically restricted to the intrinsic foot muscles.[4,11]

The diagnosis of DSP consists of a comprehensive neurological history and examination. Appropriate blood studies help to exclude other potential causes of neuropathy, such as diabetes mellitus, vitamin deficiencies, hereditary factors, alcoholism, and infectious causes such as cytomegalovirus (CMV) and/or Lyme disease. In complex patients, cerebrospinal fluid (CSF) analysis, electrodiagnostic studies, and sural nerve biopsies may be helpful.

Antiretroviral toxic neuropathies can be indistinguishable from distal symmetrical neuropathy and has been classified as such in much research.[2,22,23] The difference is mainly the fact that exposure to nucleoside antiretroviral medications is the cause of this neuropathy. Studies of the neuropathology of both distal symmetrical neuropathy and antiretroviral toxic neuropathies share similar features, including axonal degeneration and loss of unmyelinated fibers prominently.[2,24] Another major contributing factor is the prominent mitochondrial disruption and cristae abnormalities that have been described with use of antiretroviral agents. Specifically, these medications have shown to interfere with mitochondrial DNA synthesis. Changes in myelin, including myelin splitting and edema, have been noted in animal models of peripheral neurotoxicity caused by antiretroviral agents.[2,25–27] The most-studied antiretroviral agents that have been shown to be neurotoxic and play a role in DSP associated with HIV are zalcitabine, didanosine, and stavudine.[10,28] The neurotoxic effect is dose dependent for these agents. It has been estimated to occur in 15%–30% HIV patients receiving each of these drugs.[24,29] Symptoms of neuropathy are usually reversible after discontinuation of these drugs. A number of patients are able to tolerate reintroduction of these medications after resolution of the neuropathy.[29] In antiretroviral toxic neuropathies, once the neurotoxic antiretroviral agent is discontinued, resolution of neuropathic symptoms typically occurs in 4 to 8 weeks. However, resolution can take up to 16 weeks in certain patients. Patients have reported experiencing a "coasting period" of 4 to 8 weeks after withdrawal of the antiretroviral agent, during which time the neuropathic symptoms may intensify.[11]

INFLAMMATORY DEMYELINATING POLYNEUROPATHIES

The prevalence of inflammatory demyelinating polyneuropathies, both acute and chronic, is relatively less common than distal sensory polyneuropathy. There are two main clinical forms of inflammatory demyelinating polyneuropathies: acute inflammatory demyelinating polyneuropathy and chronic inflammatory demyelinating polyneuropathy. Acute inflammatory demyelinating polyneuropathy is a monophasic illness with spontaneous recovery usually occurring after 3–4 weeks. Chronic inflammatory demyelinating polyneuropathy has been described as having a relapsing and remitting course that typically lasts more than 8 weeks. Chronic inflammatory demyelinating polyneuropathy is thought to occur more frequently in the HIV population.[4] Acute inflammatory demyelinating polyneuropathy is clinically characterized by rapidly progressive ascending weakness as well as generalized areflexia and a relative sparing of sensory symptoms.[4,11] Chronic inflammatory demyelinating polyneuropathy can also present with ascending muscle weakness and loss of reflexes with sensory sparing; however, the chronic form is distinguished by its slower progression and can be either monophasic or relapsing.[4]

The pathogenesis of both inflammatory types of demyelinating polyneuropathies is thought to be autoimmune. Early in the process of chronic inflammatory demyelinating polyneuropathy, lymphocytic and macrophage infiltration and demyelination are the notable pathological causes. Later stages show signs of remyelination, decrease of lymphocytic infiltration, and reduction in the density of small myelinated and unmyelinated fibers as the main pathological features. Conversely, acute inflammatory demyelinating polyneuropathy has two different types of presenting forms: a demyelinating form, which is more common, and an axonal form.[2,21] The demyelinating form associated with HIV, an immune attack which appears to be mediated by macrophages, occurs on the Schwann cell or myelin structure. In this case, the inflammatory infiltration is mostly made up of CD8 lymphocytes. In only a few cases has the pathology of the HIV acute inflammatory demyelinating polyneuropathy axonal subtype been studied. In a nerve biopsy performed at Johns Hopkins Hospital, one patient showed Wallerian degeneration changes, mild inflammation, and no evidence of demyelination.[2]

CSF studies cannot be reliably used to confirm the diagnosis of inflammatory demyelinating polyneuropathy, especially in patients with high CD 4 counts. CSF lymphocytic pleocytosis (10–50 cell/mm^3) can help distinguish HIV patients with inflammatory demyelinating neuropathies from those without the HIV infection. However, HIV-positive patients who are asymptomatic with high CD4 counts may have high protein levels in their CSF sample with minimal lymphocytic pleocytosis. Therefore, HIV infection must still be considered in all patients with inflammatory demyelinating polyneuropathy.[2,4,30] The extension of CMV cytopathic effects has been shown to involve endothelial cells. These effects of CMV have also been seen in nerves, roots, DRG, and the spinal cord.[2,30]

PROGRESSIVE POLYRADICULOPATHY

Progressive polyradiculopathy most commonly presents in advanced immunosuppression in HIV patients, when CD4 counts are less than 50 cells/mm^3 and with the presence of other AIDS-defining opportunistic infections. A number of patients also suffer from coexistent systemic CMV infections, for example, CMV retinitis. The most common cause of progressive polyradiculopathy in patients with HIV/AIDS is CMV, less commonly followed by neurosyphilis and lymphomatous meningitis.[11,31]

Progressive polyradiculopathy can present as a rapidly progressive flaccid paraparesis. It may also present with numbness and mild sensory loss, radiating pain and parasthesias in the cauda equina distribution, loss of reflexes in the lower extremities, and frequently with sphincter dysfunction. Some patients may present with a thoracic sensory level of symptoms. Upper extremities can also be involved later in the course of progressive polyradiculopathy.[11,31,32]

CSF analysis in CMV-related progressive polyneuropathy reveals a discernible polymorphonuclear pleocytosis, increased protein levels (above 50 mg), and low glucose levels. Radiological studies of the spinal cord are recommended to eliminate any concern regarding focal compressive lesions of the cauda equina. Additionally, a polymerase chain reaction (PCR) test for CMV in the CSF is recommended.[11]

MONONEUROPATHY MULTIPLEX

Mononeuropathy multiplex is manifested by multifocal sensory or motor abnormalities involving individual peripheral cutaneous and mixed nerves, nerve roots, or cranial nerves.[11,33] Mononeuropathy multiplex can occur in both early and late stages of HIV infection. Signs and symptoms of mononeuropathy multiplex may have common characteristics with distal sensory polyneuropathy and inflammatory demyelinating polyneuropathy. In patients infected with HIV with CD4 counts of greater than 200 cells/mm^3, mononeuropathy multiplex presents with the acute onset of sensory deficits, with numbness and tingling, limited to one or two peripheral or cranial nerves. In patients with early HIV infection, mononeuropathy multiplex is thought to be immune mediated and is typically self-limited neuropathy or vasculitis.[8,11] The initial multifocal and random neurological features may progress. In the late stages of HIV infection, or in patients with CD4 counts less than 50, mononeuropathy multiplex is most commonly associated with CMV; it has also been associated with varicella zoster[32] and hepatitis C infections.[34] A more extensive and rapidly progressive form of mononeuropathy multiplex may occur in this late stage of the disease and as the immune system continues to weaken. The initial multifocal random neurological features may progress to symmetrical neuropathy. In this case, mononeuropathy multiplex can involve multiple nerves in two or more extremities. It can also result from direct CMV infection of peripheral nerves. CMV-associated mononeuropathy multiplex is characterized by CMV inclusions in endothelial cells, Wallerian degeneration, and focal demyelination.[11,35]

CSF analysis reveals nonspecific abnormalities, such as elevated protein and mild mononuclear pleocytosis. PCR for CMV DNA and nerve biopsy can provide more specific diagnosis.[11] Electrophysiological examination may reveal a multifocal pattern of reduction in evoked sensory and motor compound muscle action potential amplitudes and aid in making the diagnosis of mononeuropathy multiplex.[8]

AUTONOMIC NEUROPATHY

Autonomic neuropathy has been reported as case series mainly in the HIV-infected population. The exact prevalence is unknown. It has been noted to be more severe in patients with advanced disease.[5] Patients with HIV who are otherwise neurologically asymptomatic have been reported to have subclinical autonomic nervous system involvement, whereas patients with advanced HIV disease have more frequent and severe autonomic involvement. Failure of the parasympathetic autonomic system is manifested clinically by resting tachycardia, impotence, and urinary dysfunction. Sympathetic system abnormalities include orthostatic hypotension, syncope, diarrhea, and anhidrosis. There are many contributing factors to autonomic dysfunction, including central and peripheral nervous system abnormalities, dehydration, malnutrition, and certain medications such as vincristine, tricyclic antidepressants, and pentamidine.[5,11]

DIFFUSE INFILTRATIVE LYMPHOCYTOSIS SYNDROME

Diffuse infiltrative lymphocytosis syndrome (DILS) is found almost exclusively in HIV-infected patients[5] and typically in patients with higher CD4 counts and fewer opportunistic infections.[8] DILS is characterized by a persistent CD 8 hyperlymphocytosis and is associated with multivisceral CD8 T-cell infiltration,[5,36] including salivary glands, lungs, kidneys, gastrointestinal tract, and peripheral nerves, which causes it to closely resemble Sjogren's syndrome.

Clinically, DILS may present as acute or subacute painful multifocal, and usually symmetrical, neuropathy. Electrophysiological studies show axonal neuropathy. Nerve biopsy specimens show marked angiocentric CD8 cell infiltration without mural necrosis and abundant expression of HIV p24 in macrophages.[5,8]

TREATMENT

Treatments for the HIV-related neuropathies have been studied mostly in patients with DSP. Symptomatic treatments and regenerative treatments have been studied clinically.

Numerous successful trials have been conducted of pharmacological therapies for chronic neuropathic pain; however, there have been fewer trials with patients with HIV-related DSP. Moreover, many of the agents that have been successful in treating pain in chronic neuropathic pain have not been proven to be effective in HIV-DSP. A meta-analysis of 14 randomized controlled trials of pharmacological agents used to treat HIV-DSP[37] found that only a few agents, including smoked cannabis, recombinant human nerve growth factor, and high-dose capsaicin 8% transdermal patch, have been shown efficacy in this population.[4,37] The difference in treatment efficacy is thought to be due to the difference in underlying pathophysiology of HIV-DSP compared to other types of neuropathic pain, such as that due to vitamin deficiencies and diabetes.

Among topical agents, capsaicin has produced promising results for reducing HIV-DSP pain. Capsaicin 8% transdermal patch showed significant improvement of pain scores in HIV patients with DSP in an initial randomized control trial in 2008.[38] Since then, multiple other studies have confirmed these results.[39–41] In contrast, a randomized control trial of topical 5% lidocaine

gel and other topical agents did not show these agents to be effective in significantly reducing patients' pain associated with HIV-DSP.[42]

First-line oral analgesic agents, such as nonopioid analgesics, acetaminophen, and NSAIDs, have shown limited efficacy in the treatment of HIV-DSP.[43] Trials of antidepressant and anticonvulsants have typically been unsuccessful in producing significant benefit over placebo in randomized clinical trials. Amitriptyline and duloxetine have not shown any significant pain relief over placebo in randomized control trials.[44–46] A small trial of gabapentin did show promising results by significantly relieving pain in patients with HIV-DSP compared to placebo.[47] However, a large randomized controlled trial studying 302 patients, comparing pregabalin to placebo, did not show significant pain reduction for HIV DSP.[48] Both peptide T and mexilitine also did not show significant benefit.[37,49] In different controlled trials, lamotrigine was found to be effective and well tolerated, particularly among patients receiving HAART therapy.[50,51] Typically, a multimodal approach to controlling DSP-related pain in HIV patients, combining different agents on an individual basis, is what may be the best treatment. Trials of smoked cannabis have shown improvement in pain symptoms when compared to placebo.[52,53] These trials reported significant and up to 30% pain relief with cannabis compared to that with placebo.

Nonpharmacological therapies have been studied in this population as well. A trial randomized HIV-DSP patients to receive acupuncture complimented by burning of mugwort root moxibustion or receive fake acupuncture.[54] A significant effect was found on their first follow-up, and afterward the treatment group retained only a nonsignificant trend toward improvement. A similar trial with a larger randomized, placebo-controlled trial of acupuncture alone, amitriptyline alone, and the combination of the two in patients with HIV-DSP failed to show superiority of any of the interventions compared to placebo.[45] Hypnosis has also been tested in this patient population with some promising results.[55] This study trained 36 HIV patients with DSP in self-hypnosis for pain management. Patients improved their pain scores regardless of the current analgesic regimen at that time. Another trial looked at lower extremity splinting, which reduces sleep disturbances and discomfort from external stimuli. This trial showed a trend toward improvement in pain but no significant difference in pain reduction.[56]

Regenerative treatments are disease-modifying therapies that may improve symptoms by repairing nerve damage and thus promoting nerve regrowth. A number of agents have been tested, but only recombinant human nerve growth factor (rhNGF), a neurotrophin that regulates small sensory nerve fiber activity, showed significant benefit over placebo. However, clinical trials with rhNGF did not show significant disease modifying in neuropathy, thus further trials were halted. Other disease-modifying therapies, such as prosaptide, peptide T, and acetyl-L-carnitine, were unsuccessful in demonstrating significant pain relief from HIV neuropathy. Some of these therapies were successful in other neuropathy trials. For example, acetyl-L-carnitine was shown to be important in mitochondrial function and thought to have neurotrophic/supportive effects on peripheral nerves, including activating nerve growth factor receptors.[57] When given intramuscularly, acetyl L-carnitine reduced pain ratings.[57] Subsequent treatment with oral acetyl L-carnitine reduced pain ratings as well.

There have been case reports of successful use of spinal cord stimulation (SCS) in patients with severe, unrelenting HIV-related polyneuropathy. Two patients obtained over 90% pain relief with both the SCS trial and post-implantation. One of the patients was able to be weaned off all narcotic medications after undergoing SCS, while the other was opioid naïve and able to titrate down multiple analgesic medications.[58]

Both acute and chronic inflammatory demyelinating polyneuropathy are treated with intravenous immunoglobulin or plasmapheresis (4–5 exchanges).[4,11,59] There may be a role for corticosteroids; however, these should be used with caution in the HIV population. Patients with severe immunosuppression may respond to treatment of CMV infection.[11,60]

Progressive polyradiculopathy can have a good response to early therapy, which requires early diagnosis and treatment to avoid any irreversible damage to nerve roots that may lead to necrosis.[11] Progressive polyradiculopathy has been shown to respond to treatment for CMV infection as well, if the patient is infected with CMV.

Mononeuropathy multiplex may affect the peripheral nerves. The peripheral nerves of the early form of HIV-related mononeuropathy multiplex may spontaneously improve without treatment within several months.[11] Immunomodulation therapy should be considered in patients with incomplete recovery, including corticosteroids, plasmapheresis, or high-dose intravenous immunoglobulin therapy.

Autonomic neuropathy should be first treated by discontinuing all agents that may be leading to autonomic neuropathy, including tricyclic antidepressants. If patients are orthostatic, volume depletion should be treated, if present. Supportive management includes supportive stockings, abdominal binders, increased intake of caffeine, fluids, and salt, and multiple small meals. Sitting, standing, and reconditioning exercises may be helpful. Starting medications such as fludrocortisones and oral midodrine may be useful.[11]

Treatment of DILS consists primarily of standard antiretroviral therapy and/or corticosteroids. In a study of HIV patients affected with DILS, zidovudine therapy was associated with improvement of DILS in six out of six patients, and steroid therapy provided relief of symptoms in four out of five patients.

CONCLUSION

HIV-related neurological complications are frequent and due to improved HAART treatment. HIV-related polyneuropathy is the most common neurological complication. HIV-related distal symmetrical sensory polyneuropathy is the most common and most studied neuropathy in this population. However, multiple forms of polyneuropathy may occur, including both acute and chronic inflammatory demyelinating polyneuropathies, progressive polyradiculopathy, mononeuropathy multiplex, autonomic neuropathy, and diffuse infiltrative lymphocytosis syndrome. Prompt diagnosis and treatment is important; typically a multimodal form of therapy is required to control symptoms in these patients. With more patients surviving longer with the use of HAART therapy, there is likely to be an increase in patients suffering from HIV-related polyneuropathies.

GUIDING QUESTIONS

- Can you describe the pathophysiology of HIV polyneuropathy due to the virus itself versus from antiretroviral treatment therapy?
- Can you distinguish between the six main HIV-associated polyneuropathies?

- What are the treatment options for each of the different HIV-associated polyneuropathies?

KEY POINTS

- HIV polyneuropathy may leads to painful or unusual sensations, parasthesias, dysesthesias, numbness, and pain, most commonly in the hands and feet.
- The prevalence of HIV-related polyneuropathy is thought to increase because of the effectiveness of antiretroviral medications leading to increased HIV survival rates and use of antiretroviral therapy itself.
- The most common cause of HIV polyneuropathy is likely indirect neurological damage via release of viral proteins and the inflammatory response; however, the HIV virus itself may lead to direct damage.
- Use of antiretrovirals may contribute to mitochondrial damage, macrophage infiltration, and axonal cell loss, leading to HIV-related polyneuropathy.
- Diagnosis of HIV-related polyneuropathy can be made clinically on the basis of signs, symptoms, history of HIV, and possible HAART therapy exposure. Differential diagnosis includes diabetic neuropathy, alcohol abuse, and vitamin B12 deficiency.
- Treatment of HIV-related polyneuropathy includes removal of the offending agent and pharmacological and nonpharmacological treatments.
- Pharmacological treatments include anticonvulsants, antidepressants, topical agents such as capsaicin, regenerative treatments, and analgesics.
- Nonpharmacological therapies include acupuncture and spinal cord stimulation.

REFERENCES

1. Pillay P, Wadley AL, Cherry CL, Karstaedt AS, Kamerman PR. Pharmacological treatment of painful HIV-associated sensory neuropathy. *S Afr Med J*. 2015;105(9):769–772. doi:10.7196/SAMJnew.7908
2. Pardo CA, McArthur JC, Griffin JW. HIV neuropathy: insights in the pathology of HIV peripheral nerve disease. *J Peripher Nerv Syst*. 2001:6:1–27. doi:10.1046/j.1529-8027.2001.006001021.x
3. Ghosh S, Chandran A, Jansen JP. Epidemiology of HIV-related neuropathy: a systematic literature review. *AIDS Res Hum Retroviruses*. 2012;28(1):36–48. doi:10.1089/aid.2011.0116
4. Kaku M, Simpson DM. HIV neuropathy. *Curr Opin HIV AIDS*. 2014;9(6):521–526. doi:10.1097/COH.0000000000000103
5. Gabbai AA, Castelo A, Oliveira ASB. HIV peripheral neuropathy. *Handb Clin Neurol*. 2013;115:515–529. doi:10.1016/B978-0-444-52902-2.00029-1
6. Snider WD, Simpson DM, Nielsen S, Gold JW, Metroka CE, Posner JB. Neurological complications of acquired immune deficiency syndrome: analysis of 50 patients. *Ann Neurol*. 1983;14:403–418. doi:10.1002/ana.410140404
7. Levy J, Hollander H, Shimabukuro J, Mills J, Kaminsky L. Isolation of AIDS-associated retroviruses from cerebrospinal fluid and brain of patients with neurological symptoms. *Lancet*. 1985;326(8455):585–588. doi:10.1016/S0140-6736(85)90587-2
8. Ferrari S, Vento S, Monaco S, et al. Human immunodeficiency virus-associated peripheral neuropathies. *Mayo Clin Proc*. 2006;81(2):213–219. doi:10.4065/81.2.213
9. Flatters SJL. The contribution of mitochondria to sensory processing and pain. *Prog Mol Biol Transl Sci*. 2015;131:119–146. doi:10.1016/bs.pmbts.2014.12.004
10. Schütz SG, Robinson-Papp J. HIV-related neuropathy: current perspectives. *HIV/AIDS Res Palliat Care*. 2013;5:243–251. doi:10.2147/HIV.S36674
11. Wulff EA, Wang AK, Simpson DM. HIV-associated peripheral neuropathy: epidemiology, pathophysiology and treatment. *Drugs*. 2000;59(6):1251–1260. doi:10.2165/00003495-200059060-00005
12. Apostolski S, McAlarney T, Hays AP, Latov N. Complement dependent cytotoxicity of sensory ganglion neurons mediated by the gp120 glycoprotein of HIV-1. *Immunol Invest*. 1994;23(1):47–52. doi:10.3109/08820139409063432
13. Jones G, Zhu Y, Silva C, et al. Peripheral nerve-derived HIV-1 is predominantly CCR5-dependent and causes neuronal degeneration and neuroinflammation. *Virology*. 2005;334(2):178–193. doi:10.1016/j.virol.2005.01.027
14. Keswani SC, Polley M, Pardo CA, Griffin JW, McArthur JC, Hoke A. Schwann cell chemokine receptors mediate HIV-1 gp120 toxicity to sensory neurons. *Ann Neurol*. 2003;54(3):287–296. doi:10.1002/ana.10645
15. Wallace VCJ, Blackbeard J, Segerdahl AR, et al. Characterization of rodent models of HIV-gp120 and anti-retroviral-associated neuropathic pain. *Brain*. 2007;130(Pt 10):2688–2702. doi:10.1093/brain/awm195

16. Wallace VCJ, Blackbeard J, Pheby T, et al. Pharmacological, behavioural and mechanistic analysis of HIV-1 gp120 induced painful neuropathy. *Pain*. 2007;133(1–3):47–63. doi:10.1016/j.pain.2007.02.015

17. Estanislao L, Thomas D, Simpson D. HIV neuromuscular disease and mitochondrial function. *Mitochondrion*. 2004;4(2–3):131–139. doi:10.1016/j.mito.2004.06.007

18. Burdo TH, Miller AD. Animal models of HIV peripheral neuropathy. *Future Virol*. 2014;9(5):465–474. doi:10.2217/fvl.14.28

19. Lehmann HC, Chen W, Borzan J, Mankowski JL, Höke A. Mitochondrial dysfunction in distal axons contributes to human immunodeficiency virus sensory neuropathy. *Ann Neurol*. 2011;69(1):100–110. doi:10.1002/ana.22150

20. McCarthy BG, Hsieh ST, Stocks A, et al. Cutaneous innervation in sensory neuropathies: evaluation by skin biopsy. *Neurology*. 1995;45(10):1848–1855. doi:10.1212/WNL.45.10.1848

21. Cornblath DR, McArthur JC. Predominantly sensory neuropathy in patients with AIDS and AIDS-related complex. *Neurology*. 1988;38(5):794–796. doi:10.1212/WNL.38.5.794

22. Moyle G. Clinical manifestations and management of antiretroviral nucleoside analog-related mitochondrial toxicity. *Clin Ther*. 2000;22(8):911–936. doi:10.1016/S0149-2918(00)80064-8

23. Moyle GJ, Sadler M. Peripheral neuropathy with nucleoside antiretrovirals: risk factors, incidence and management. *Drug Saf*. 1998;19(6):481–494.

24. Simpson DM, Tagliati M. Nucleoside analogue-associated peripheral neuropathy in human immunodeficiency virus infection. *J Acquir Immune Defic Syndr Hum Retrovirol*. 1995;9(2):153–161.

25. Chen C, Vazquez-Padua M, Cheng Y. Effect of anti-human immunodeficiency virus nucleoside analogs on mitochondrial DNA and its implication for delayed toxicity. *Mol Pharmacol*. 1991;39(5):625–628.

26. Lewis W, Day BJ, Copeland WC. Mitochondrial toxicity of NRTI antiviral drugs: an integrated cellular perspective. *Nat Rev Drug Discov*. 2003;2(10):812–822. doi:10.1038/nrd1201

27. Hao S. The molecular and pharmacological mechanisms of HIV-related neuropathic pain. *Curr Neuropharmacol*. 2013;11(5):499–512. doi:10.2174/1570159X11311050005

28. Morgello S, Estanislao L, Simpson D, et al. HIV-associated distal sensory polyneuropathy in the era of highly active antiretroviral therapy: the Manhattan HIV Brain Bank. *Arch Neurol*. 2004;61(4):546–551. doi:10.1001/archneur.61.4.546

29. Moore RD, Wong WEM, Keruly JC, Mcarthur JC. Incidence of neuropathy in HIV-infected patients on monotherapy versus those on combination therapy with didanosine, stavudine and hydroxyurea. *AIDS*. 2000;14(3):273–278. doi:10.1097/00002030-200002180-00009

30. Cornblath DR, McArthur JC, Kennedy PG, Witte AS, Griffin JW. Inflammatory demyelinating peripheral neuropathies associated with human T-cell lymphotropic virus type III infection. *Ann Neurol*. 1987;21(1):32–40. doi:10.1002/ana.410210107

31. Eidelberg D, Sotrel A, Vogel H, Walker P, Kleefield J, Crumpacker 3rd CS. Progressive polyradiculopathy in acquired immune deficiency syndrome. *Neurology*. 1986;36(7):912–916.

32. Said G, Lacroix C, Chemouilli P, et al. Cytomegalovirus neuropathy in acquired immunodeficiency syndrome: a clinical and pathological study. *Ann Neurol*. 1991;29(2):139–146.

33. Miller RG, Parry GJ, Pfaeffl W, Lang W, Lippert R, Kiprov D. The spectrum of peripheral neuropathy associated with ARC and AIDS. *Muscle Nerve*. 1988;11(8):857–863. doi:10.1002/mus.880110810

34. Caniatti LM, Tugnoli V, Eleopra R, Tralli G, Bassi R, De Grandis D. Cryoglobulinemic neuropathy related to hepatitis C virus infection. Clinical, laboratory and neurophysiological study. *J Peripher Nerv Syst*. 1999;1(2):131–138.

35. Anders HJ, Goebel FD. Cytomegalovirus polyradiculopathy in patients with AIDS. *Clin Infect Dis*. 1998;27(2):345–352.

36. Chahin N, Temesgen Z, Kurtin PJ, Spinner RJ, Dyck PJB. HIV lumbosacral radiculoplexus neuropathy mimicking lymphoma: diffuse infiltrative lymphocytosis syndrome (DILS) restricted to nerve? *Muscle and Nerve*. 2010;41(2):276–282. doi:10.1002/mus.21507

37. Phillips TJC, Cherry CL, Cox S, Marshall SJ, Rice ASC. Pharmacological treatment of painful HIV-associated sensory neuropathy: a systematic review and meta-analysis of randomised controlled trials. *PLoS One*. 2010;5(12). doi:10.1371/journal.pone.0014433

38. Simpson DM, Brown S, Tobias J. Controlled trial of high-concentration capsaicin patch for treatment of painful HIV neuropathy. *Neurology*. 2008;70(24):2305–2313. doi:10.1212/01.wnl.0000314647.35825.9c

39. Noto C, Pappagallo M, Szallasi A. NGX-4010, a high-concentration capsaicin dermal patch for lasting relief of peripheral neuropathic pain. *Curr Opin Investig Drugs*. 2009;10(7):702–710.

40. Backonja MM, Malan TP, Vanhove GF, Tobias JK. NGX-4010, a high-concentration capsaicin patch, for the treatment of postherpetic

neuralgia: a randomized, double-blind, controlled study with an open-label extension. *Pain Med*. 2010;11(4):600–608. doi:10.1111/j.1526-4637.2009.00793.x

41. Clifford DB, Simpson DM, Brown S, et al. A randomized, double-blind, controlled study of NGX-4010, a capsaicin 8% dermal patch, for the treatment of painful HIV-associated distal sensory polyneuropathy. *J Acquir Immune Defic Syndr*. 2012;59(2):126–133. doi:10.1097/QAI.0b013e31823e31f7

42. Estanislao L, Carter K, McArthur J, Olney R, Simpson D, Group L-HN. A randomized controlled trial of 5% lidocaine gel for HIV-associated distal symmetric polyneuropathy. *J Acquir Immune Defic Syndr*. 2004;37(5):1584–1586. doi:10.1097/00126334-200412150-00010

43. Stavros K, Simpson DM. Understanding the etiology and management of HIV-associated peripheral neuropathy. *Curr HIV/AIDS Rep*. 2014;11(3):195–201. doi:10.1007/s11904-014-0211-2

44. Kieburtz K, Simpson D, Yiannoutsos C, et al. A randomized trial of amitriptyline and mexiletine for painful neuropathy in HIV infection. AIDS Clinical Trial Group 242 Protocol Team. *Neurology*. 1998;51(6):1682–1688. doi:10.1212/WNL.51.6.1682

45. Shlay JC, Chaloner K, Max MB, et al. Acupuncture and amitriptyline for pain due to HIV-related peripheral neuropathy: a randomized controlled trial. Terry Beirn Community Programs for Clinical Research on AIDS. *JAMA*. 1998;280(18):1590–1595. doi:10.1016/S0965-2299(99)80027-2

46. Harrison T, Miyahara S, Lee A, et al. Experience and challenges presented by a multicenter crossover study of combination analgesic therapy for the treatment of painful hiv-associated polyneuropathies. *Pain Med (United States)*. 2013;14(7):1039–1047. doi:10.1111/pme.12084

47. Hahn K, Arendt G, Braun JS, et al. A placebo-controlled trial of gabapentin for painful HIV-associated sensory neuropathies. *J Neurol*. 2004;251(10):1260–1266. doi:10.1007/s00415-004-0529-6

48. Simpson DM, Schifitto G, Clifford DB, et al. Pregabalin for painful HIV neuropathy: a randomized, double-blind, placebo-controlled trial. *Neurology*. 2010;74(5):413–420. doi:10.1212/WNL.0b013e3181ccc6ef

49. Simpson DM, Dorfman D, Olney RK, et al. Peptide T in the treatment of painful distal neuropathy associated with AIDS: results of a placebo-controlled trial. The Peptide T Neuropathy Study Group. *Neurology*. 1996;47(5):1254–1259.

50. Simpson DM, Olney R, McArthur JC, Khan A, Godbold J, Ebel-Frommer K. A placebo-controlled trial of lamotrigine for painful HIV-associated neuropathy. *Neurology*. 2000;54(11):2115–2119.

51. Simpson DM, McArthur JC, Olney R, et al. Lamotrigine for HIV-associated painful sensory neuropathies: a placebo-controlled trial. *Neurology*. 2003;60(9):1508–1514. doi:10.1212/01.WNL.0000063304.88470.D9

52. Ellis RJ, Toperoff W, Vaida F, et al. Smoked medicinal cannabis for neuropathic pain in HIV: a randomized, crossover clinical trial. *Neuropsychopharmacology*. 2009;34(3):672–680. doi:10.1038/npp.2008.120

53. Abrams DI, Jay CA, Shade SB, et al. Cannabis in painful HIV-associated sensory neuropathy: a randomized placebo-controlled trial. *Neurology*. 2007;68(7):515–521. doi:10.1212/01.wnl.0000253187.66183.9c

54. Anastasi JK, Capili B, McMahon DJ, Scully C. Acu/moxa for distal sensory peripheral neuropathy in HIV: a randomized control pilot study. *J Assoc Nurses AIDS Care*. 2013;24(3):268–275. doi:10.1016/j.jana.2012.09.006

55. Dorfman D, George MC, Schnur J, Simpson DM, Davidson G, Montgomery G. Hypnosis for treatment of HIV neuropathic pain: a preliminary report. *Pain Med (United States)*. 2013;14(7):1048–1056. doi:10.1111/pme.12074

56. Sandoval R, Roddey T, Giordano TP, Mitchell K, Kelley C. Randomized trial of lower extremity splinting to manage neuropathic pain and sleep disturbances in people living with HIV/AIDS. *J Int Assoc Provid AIDS Care*. 2013. doi:10.1177/2325957413511112

57. Youle M, Osio M, Cassetti I, et al. A double-blind, parallel-group, placebo-controlled, multicentre study of acetyl l-carnitine in the symptomatic treatment of antiretroviral toxic neuropathy in patients with HIV-1 infection. *HIV Med*. 2007;8(4):241–250. doi:10.1111/j.1468-1293.2007.00467.x

58. Knezevic NN, Candido KD, Rana S, Knezevic I. The use of spinal cord neuromodulation in the management of HIV-related polyneuropathy. *Pain Physician*. 18(4):E643–E650.

59. Exchange P, Syndrome SG, Group T. Randomised trial of plasma exchange, intravenous immunoglobulin, and combined treatments in Guillain-Barré syndrome. Plasma Exchange/Sandoglobulin Guillain-Barré Syndrome Trial Group. *Lancet*. 1997;349(9047):225–230. doi:10.1016/S0140-6736(96)09095-2

60. Roullet E, Assuerus V, Gozlan J, et al. Cytomegalovirus multifocal neuropathy in AIDS: analysis of 15 consecutive cases. *Neurology*. 1994;44(11):2174–2182.

18

Immune-Related Neuropathy

WHIT BRADDY

More and more we are learning that the immune system plays an important role in the development and maintenance of chronic pain. However, there are instances where we have determined the immune system to be the predominant source of pain. Here we will examine the most common causes of immune-related peripheral neuropathy. There are numerous reports, but in keeping with our objective, we will delve into those that often present with painful peripheral neuropathy. These sources of immune-related pain fall into four broad categories: viral, vasculitis, autoimmune disease, and paraneoplastic syndromes.

Internists, neurologists, and oncologists normally treat these diseases. However, as these diseases often present with pain, the skilled pain management physician should be able to recognize these conditions, make appropriate referrals, and understand how to treat the associated pain. Therefore, let us delve into some topics less familiar to us and see how we might broaden our understanding and our ability to treat immune-related pain.

VIRAL

Case 1: You are seeing one of your long-time patients today. He is doing well and continues to see improvement from the recent epidural he received. Near the end of the visit he asks for your opinion on his wife's symptoms. She is a little embarrassed, but divulges that her hands and feet hurt. On further questioning she notes that they feel like they are on fire. It started a week ago with just the tips of her fingers, but now involves the whole hand and foot and she is having trouble tying her shoes and walking. A quick exam reveals profound loss of strength in her hands and feet and absent Achilles reflexes.

Acute inflammatory demyelinating polyneuropathy (AIDP) in its most common form, Guillain-Barré syndrome (GBS), was first described in 1916[1] and remains a well-recognized autoimmune disease. After 100 years of research it continues to occur at a rate of 1–2 cases per 100,000 individuals. Like many autoimmune conditions, it occurs more frequently in females and more frequently as we grow older.

GBS is an autoimmune disease that is usually triggered by a mild respiratory or gastrointestinal illness. It is most frequently attributed to a previous *Campylobacter jejuni*[2] or cytomegalovirus infection,[3] but has also been associated with the Epstein-Barr virus, varicella zoster, *Mycoplasma pneumoniaie*, and, most recently, the Zika virus. These infections seem to initiate the development of autoantibodies directed at Schwann cells. Antibodies and activated complement bind and initiate demyelination, which disrupts nerve conduction, causing the symptoms associated with Guillain-Barré.

Now, here's where it gets interesting. The initial presentation of Guillain-Barré is pain, paresthesia, or weakness in the hands or feet. Symptoms progress proximally for 1 to 3 weeks after diagnosis, causing weakness and areflexic paralysis in the effected areas.[4] However, pain remains throughout treatment. A recent study found that pain was the presenting symptom in one-third of cases. Two-thirds of patients experience pain during the treatment phase of GBS, and this pain becomes chronic in one-third of patients. The patterns of pain at presentation were muscle pain, painful peripheral paresthesias, and radicular pain.[5]

Diagnosis is based primarily on clinical presentation. However, lumbar puncture and cerebrospinal fluid (CSF) examination are usually performed to rule out other causes and to evaluate for supporting evidence. CSF samples in GBS usually exhibit an elevation in protein with a normal white blood cell count. Particular antibodies that tend to cause the demyelination have been isolated, but such specific testing is not commonly available.

Treatment is supportive care and immunomodulation. Since 25% of patients[6] develop respiratory insufficiency, this often involves intubation and mechanical ventilation. Plasmaphoresis removes the offending autoantibodies from the patient's circulation. This is usually performed five times over the course of 2 weeks. The other approach growing in popularity is intravenous immunoglobulin (IVIG), a treatment whose function is not well understood. It appears that IVIG interrupts the immune system at multiple points. Different studies have determined that it inhibits T-cell signaling that stimulates antibody production,[7] inhibits the binding of these antibodies,[8] interrupts the complement pathway,[9] and contains antibodies against the offending autoantibodies.[10]

Despite these treatments, GBS remains a disabling and deadly disease. Up to 20% of patients become severely disabled and 5% of cases are fatal.[11] Our dilemma, however, is how to treat the large percentage of patients that experience pain, both in the acute setting and after discharge. Traditionally, NSAIDs and opioids have been utilized. There is little research on the subject; however, gabapentin has been specifically evaluated for acute GBS pain and found to be highly effective with fewer side effects than placebo with breakthrough opioids.[12]

Case 2: A new patient presents to your clinic. She is happy to finally meet you and notes that it took forever to get in to see you so you must be good. Her primary care provider (PCP) sent her to you because she was having burning pain running down the side of her leg and he thought she might need an epidural. However, over the past 2 months, she has noticed that she now has pain throughout both lower legs and her hands and feels clumsy. She appears normal on exam, but has altered sensation in these areas and absent Achilles reflex.

Chronic inflammatory demyelinating polyneuropathy (CIDP) includes a spectrum of acquired neuropathies. CIDP is differentiated from AIDP by symptom severity and the time to maximal effect. AIDP symptoms peak within 4 weeks, whereas CIDP develops more slowly and peaks after 8 weeks. CIDP occurs most frequently between the ages of 40 and 60, has a slight predilection for men,[13] and occurs at a rate of 5–9 cases per 100,000 people.[14]

Symptoms, therefore, are similar to those of GBS but more insidious in their development. The classic presentation is slowly developing symmetrical proximal and distal weakness with loss of sensation. These symptoms usually begin in the lower extremities. Patients indicate difficulties associated with the developing weakness. They may have new onset of difficulty walking, rising from a chair, or climbing stairs. Upper extremity weakness often presents as a loss in fine motor skills of the hands, such as difficulty tying shoelaces or using utensils. Sensory changes cause a loss of balance and even a history of falls.[13] Physical exam usually reveals impaired proprioception, decreased or absent reflexes, but no apparent atrophy. This is an important differentiation. Demyelination causes sensory and motor deficiencies, whereas axonal loss usually presents with atrophy.

Just as pain is a common presenting complaint with GBS, so, too, can it present with CIDP. Several studies have found that a significant number of these patients experience pain to be a prominent symptom.[15,16] In each study all patients presented with pain in the lower extremities that was often radicular in nature. It is unclear if the authors based this on physical exam or only a description of the pain. However, CIDP-induced nerve root inflammation has been documented[17] and could cause a straight-leg raise test to indicate radicular signs. These symptoms were present in addition to the traditional findings of distal paresthesias and decreased lower extremity reflexes.

CIDP is commonly accepted to be an autoimmune disorder, and it is effectively treated by immune-modulating techniques. However, its exact mechanisms remain elusive. Autopsy studies have revealed that pathological changes are evident in nerve roots, plexuses, and nerve trunks, which are thought to cause these symptoms.[18,19] On histological examination it is the nodes of Ranvier and paranodal regions that are disrupted. While exact antibodies have yet to be identified, it is assumed that they are directed toward molecules in this region.

Diagnosis of CIDP depends on an appropriate clinical presentation and an electromyogram (EMG) that indicates demyelination. However, a diagnosis of CIDP is only the beginning of the workup. CIDP is often the result of a wide array of other autoimmune, infectious, and neoplastic disorders[13] (see Box 18.1). We will investigate several of these individually, but you can see how

BOX 18.1
CIDP-ASSOCIATED DISORDERS

PARAPROTEIN-ASSOCIATED DISORDERS
Monoclonal gammopathy of undetermined significance (MGUS)
Osteosclerotic myeloma (POEMS syndrome)
Multiple myeloma
Waldenstrom macroglobulinemia
Amyloidosis
Castleman disease

CHRONIC INFECTIONS
HIV infection
Huan T-lymphotropic virus type 1
Lyme disease
Hepatitis C
Cat-scratch disease
Epstein-Barr infection

CONNECTIVE TISSUE AND AUTOIMMUNE DISORDERS
Systemic lupus erythematosus
Sjogren syndrome
Rheumatoid disease
Giant-cell arteritis
Sarcoidosis
Inflammatory bowel disease
Myasthenia gravis
Chronic active hepatitis
Multiple sclerosis

SYSTEMIC MEDICAL DISORDERS
Diabetes mellitus
Thyrotoxicosis
Chronic renal failure requiring dialysis
Membranous glomerulonephropathy

MALIGNANCY
Hepatocellular carcinoma
Melanoma
Pancreatic carcinoma
Colon adenocarcinoma
Lymphoma
Paraneoplastic demyelinating neuropathy

MEDICATIONS
Interferon alpha
Procainamide
Tacrolimus
Tumor necrosis factor antagonists

OTHER POSSIBLE ASSOCIATIONS
Vaccinations
Solid organ transplantation
Hereditary neuropathy

Reprinted with permission. Gorson KC, Katz J. Chronic inflammatory demyelinating polyneuropathy. Neurol Clin. 2013;2:511–532.

arriving at a diagnosis of CIDP implies an obligation for further investigation and appropriate referral. To that end, obtaining a lumbar puncture and CSF protein and cell count is a reasonable step. Most patients will exhibit an elevated CSF protein level. Further testing can be guided by symptoms and history to rule out other potential causes.

Treatment, much like for AICP, is immunomodulation. Again, the debate centers on plasma exchange, IVIG, or immunosuppressing medications such as steroids. If we accept that CIDP is caused by circulating antibodies, then removing these antibodies with plasma exchange is logical. The evidence, including a Cochrane review, suggests that plasma exchange is highly effective, however the benefits disappear when treatment is discontinued and the body continues to produce autoantibodies. The IVIG in the CIDP Efficacy (ICE) Trial established the dosing and exhibited a 54% efficacy of IVIG in treating CIDP. The second phase of the trial also showed that half of responders remained in remission after 6 months of discontinuing IVIG.[20] Steroids remain the easiest and least expensive form of treatment but side effects are always a concern. One comparison between IVIG and pulsed-dose methylprednisolone found the steroid to be equally as effective as IVIG. The benefit of steroids took longer to develop but appeared to be more enduring after discontinuation.[21]

VASCULITIS
Case 3: A new patient presents to your clinic. She is a very nice retired nurse. She comes in today

because she thinks she needs an epidural. She describes a burning pain from the knee down the side of the leg and across the top of the foot. On exam she looks exhausted, has bleary eyes, and a rash on her ankles.

The vasculitides are a diverse collection of diseases characterized by an autoimmune-inflicted vascular necrosis. They may be primary autoimmune diseases or they may develop secondarily as a result of drugs, infection, connective tissue disease, or neoplasm. The vasculitides are categorized by the size of the vessel affected in accordance with the Chapel Hill Consensus Conference.[22] Since blood supply is basic to the functionality of all tissues, vasculitis can manifest as dysfunction of any tissue or organ. Therefore, it should not be surprising that it can and does frequently affect the peripheral nervous system.

The peripheral nervous system effects of vasculitis are predominantly indirect. As the autoimmune assault on blood vessels progresses, the vasa nervorum, which supplies blood to peripheral nerves, can be affected. Breakdown of blood supply results in ischemia to peripheral nerves, and it is this ischemia that results in the peripheral neuropathy and pain associated with vasculitis. However, this ischemia upsets the natural blood–nerve barrier that normally protects nervous tissue from the immune system. Cellular immune infiltration of peripheral nerves may be enhanced by dysfunction of this barrier.[23] While these are believed to be the mechanism, the trigger remains to be determined.

Fortunately, the vasculitides are relatively rare. A Norwegian study found the rates of these particular vasculitides to be at least 10 in 100,000.[24] However, within individual subtypes, peripheral neuropathic pain is common. Previous studies indicate that it occurs in up to 75% of patients with polyarteritis nodosa,[25] 67% of those with granulomatosis with polyangiitis (formerly Wegeners),[26] 78% of those with Churg-Strauss,[27] and 58% of those with microscopic polyangiitis.[28] Furthermore, these are the presenting symptom in up to 55% of patients.[29] The symptoms generally have an acute onset in the lower extremity, affecting one particular nerve distribution before spreading to involve other nerves. These symptoms most often affect the peroneal nerve, but also commonly affect the tibial, ulnar, median, or radial nerves.[30] This type of presentation is known as mononeuritis multiplex.

The diagnosis of a vasculitis-induced peripheral neuropathy rests primarily on diagnosing vasculitis. If and when appropriate testing for the suspected vasculitis has been exhausted, then tissue biopsy should be considered. However, in the setting of mononeuritis multiplex, biopsy should be performed immediately. It is recommended that a combined nerve/muscle biopsy be performed of the sural or superficial peroneal nerve.[31] A positive biopsy would reveal vasculitic skip lesions requiring the examination of several adjacent samples. Unfortunately, biopsy has only proven a 60%–70% sensitivity.[32]

Much like diagnosis, the treatment of vasculitis peripheral neuropathy depends largely on treating the underlying condition. Systemic remission is generally induced with oral prednisolone 1 mg/kg/day with cyclophosphamide 2 mg/kg/day for severe systemic cases or with oral prednisolone and methotrexate for milder cases. This is followed by low-dose maintenance therapy. Systemic vasculitis and progression of nerve injury can be arrested with proper treatment. However, the sensorimotor deficits and pain may remain, requiring continuing treatment. There is little research into the management of post-vasculitis pain syndromes, simply owing to the rarity of this condition. But, the injury is not unique. Vasculitis causes neuropathic pain secondary to ischemia, which has been well studied. For instance, diabetic peripheral neuropathy is largely attributed to ischemia, and we are adept at treating this pain with common neuropathic agents.

AUTOIMMUNE DISEASE

Case 4: A 50-year-old woman comes to see you with face and hand pain. On discussion, she's not really sure how long it has been going on, it's just been getting worse. She appears exhausted, with red eyes. On exam, her hands and face have altered sensation, but you can't seem to relate the distribution to one particular structure or nerve. Review of symptoms (ROS) reveals frequent use of eye drops and frequent urination, but she thinks that's because she drinks lots of fluids.

Sjogren syndrome (SS) is now considered to be one of the most common autoimmune disorders. Approximately 0.6% to 1% of adults may be affected.[33] The predominant symptoms of SS are due to glandular dysfunction. However, 65% of patients experience extraglandular symptoms, predominantly of the peripheral nervous system. Therefore, odds are, if you are not treating patients with Sjogren peripheral neuropathy, you are missing the diagnosis.

Sjogren syndrome is caused by lymphocytic invasion and eventual destruction of exocrine glands, specifically the lacrimal and salivary glands.[34] As with many autoimmune diseases, there has been much investigation into viral triggers. Epstein-Barr virus and Coxsackie virus have been implicated, but no single agent has been established. Autoantibodies, however, have been isolated. Anti-SSA/Ro and Anti-SSB/La are commonly associated with SS in more than 50% of patients and are used in diagnosis.

Patients with SS are almost always females approximately 50 years of age. The predominant symptom is dry eyes, or keratoconjunctivitis sicca. Patients will recount intolerance to contact lenses, a constant foreign body sensation, decreased visual acuity, or frequent use of eye drops. The second most common symptom is dry mouth, xerostomia. Patients will often note increased fluid intake or difficulty in chewing or swallowing. There is also a high degree of association with other autoimmune conditions, especially rheumatoid arthritis and thyroid disease. Neurological symptoms involve debilitating fatigue and neuropathic pain. Neuropathic pain is estimated to occur in approximately 10% of patients,[35] usually presenting as a painful small-fiber neuropathy affecting the face, torso, proximal extremities, or a stocking-and-glove distribution.

Sjogren syndrome is diagnosed with the revised European-American criteria and requires four of six criteria. These include ocular symptoms and confirmatory tests, oral symptoms and confirmatory tests, as well as antibody testing for anti-SSA or ant-SSB, and a salivary gland biopsy showing lymphocytic invasion.[36] The painful small-fiber neuropathy is also diagnosed with a punch biopsy and comparison of intraepidermal nerve fiber density against standardized norms.[37]

Unfortunately, there are no good data for systemic treatment of SS. A recent review found little benefit from available immunosuppressants, including corticosteroids and biologics. Standard recommendations continue to center around eye drops and oral hygiene.[38] Furthermore, there is no direct evidence for the treatment of small-fiber neuropathy. The treatment guidelines are based on research into neuropathic pain. Therefore, the usual neuropathic medications can be employed. Expert opinion recommends against tricyclic antidepressant (TCA) medications, which may exacerbate dry eyes and dry mouth, and to titrate medications slowly due to chronic fatigue associated with this disease.

Case 5: A 30-year-old woman is referred to you by her PCP. She has multiple sclerosis and is having trouble controlling her "MS pain." Her PCP has been prescribing oxycodone but because of new opioid guidelines, he has referred her to you. She also notes pain shooting down her back, with pain and numbness in her leg. She asks you if an epidural would help her.

Multiple sclerosis (MS) is second only to trauma as a cause of neurological disability in young adults.[39] MS occurs mainly in Europe and the societies who originated there, such as the United States, Canada, Australia, and New Zealand, and is rare in Asia. The disease afflicts women more than men, at approximately a 2:1 ratio. Interestingly, the rates of MS increase with latitude, moving away from the equator both north and south. In the United States the incidence is estimated to be 90 per 100,000 people.

Like many of the diseases discussed in this chapter, MS causes demyelination. However, MS is unique in that its demyelination occurs within the central nervous system (CNS). The etiology of MS, like many causes of pain, is not completely elucidated. However, most experts agree that this is an autoimmune disease. Plaque biopsy studies have revealed complement deposition, immunoglobulins, T cells, and large numbers of macrophages containing myelin debris.[40] What causes this autoimmune reaction continues to be debated. Like many diseases, MS likely occurs at the intersection of genetic susceptibility and an environmental trigger. Genetic studies have repeatedly identified gene variants associated with developing MS[41] and a significant volume of data implicates the Epstein-Barr virus as a trigger.

Multiple sclerosis generally presents between the ages of 20 and 40 years. The presenting event is an acute neurological deficit. This is often optic neuritis (transient loss of vision) or transverse myelitis (transient sensory or motor loss). These symptoms are caused by the development of CNS plaques and are confirmed by MRI. The McDonald criteria are used for definitive diagnosis. There are currently 13 FDA-approved disease-modifying treatments (DMT). These treatments have been shown to reduce the frequency and severity of attacks and slow the progression of disability, though there is conflicting evidence for each.

Despite treatment, however, patients with MS experience significant symptoms. Commonly reported symptoms include fatigue, spasticity, ataxia, vision problems, pain, and depression.[42] A recent meta-analysis of pain experienced in MS indicated the prevalence of headache to be 43%, peripheral neuropathy 26%, back pain 20%, spasms 15%, Lhermitte sign 16%, and trigeminal neuralgia 3.8%.[43] Despite the prevalence of pain in these patients, there are limited data on its treatment. Small studies on gabapentin[44] and pregabalin[45] showed significant benefit to peripheral neuropathic pain. Again, only small studies have evaluated treatments of trigeminal neuralgia in MS, however, they do indicate benefit from carbamazepine, lamotrigine, and topiramate.

PARANEOPLASTIC SYNDROME

Case 6: One of your longtime patients comes to see you. He is a 70-year-old man with spinal stenosis who doesn't want surgery. He comes in for caudal epidurals three to four times each year. You've tried to get him to exercise, and talked to him about how smoking reduces blood flow to his spine, but he just keeps coming back for epidurals. Today, however, he presents with burning pain in his arm that has been worsening over the past month. He wants to know if he has stenosis up top, too.

Paraneoplastic syndrome (PS) is a remote symptom caused by the body's reaction to a malignancy. These are not effects caused directly by the neoplasm, local invasion, or distant metastasis. Traditionally, these syndromes are an immune response to malignancy that leads to neurological symptoms. These syndromes can occur for a variety of different neoplasms. For our purposes, the most important condition to consider is small-cell lung cancer (SCLC). Lung cancer is the second most common cause of cancer in both men and women, and approximately 10% to 15% of lung cancer is SCLC. This results in approximately 70 cases per 100,000 people. Nine percent of these patients will develop a paraneoplastic syndrome.[46]

Like most things too small to see, our understanding of the exact mechanisms continue to evolve. At this point, it is generally accepted that paraneoplastic syndromes are due to the body mounting an immunological defense against the invading neoplasm. However, unlike an immune response to bacteria, responding to a neoplasm involves reacting to a mutation of one's own tissue. In doing so, the body can develop a sensitivity to self-antigens. When these antibodies react with native tissue, paraneoplastic syndromes develop.

These antigens can be expressed on the cell surface or intracellularly. Surface antigens become the targets of autoantibodies anti-Hu and anti-CV2[47] and intracellular antigens appear to be targeted by T cells. Interestingly, patients found to have a PS have also been found to have a lower tumor burden and decreased metastasis.[48]

Perhaps the most important thing to remember from this discussion is that paraneoplastic syndromes often present months before the diagnosis of cancer.[49] Obviously, the time to diagnosis and treatment can have profound effects on outcome. Unfortunately, paraneoplastic neuropathy presents much like the other causes of neuropathy we have discussed. It can present as a sensory, motor, demyelinating, autonomic, or vasculitic neuropathy. Fortunately, there are some clues that a painful neuropathy may be secondary to cancer. These neuropathies tend to have a subacute, yet progressive course with early involvement of the upper extremities. Paraneoplastic neuropathies also tend to be painful and asymmetrical.

Guidelines for the diagnosis of paraneoplastic peripheral neuropathy have been published and they recommend monitoring for the presentation just discussed. They note specifically that the diagnosis should be considered in cases with a subacute onset of numbness or pain in an asymmetrical pattern involving the arms with loss of proprioception.[50] These guidelines are more useful when used in the context of the whole patient. As we have discussed, most paraneoplastic peripheral neuropathies develop as a result of SCLC. Rates of SCLC parallel population smoking rates. Therefore, these symptoms in a smoker should lower our threshold for testing. If there is no previously diagnosed tumor, guidelines recommend testing for the most common autoantibodies: anti-Hu, Yo, CV2, Ri, Ma2, and amphiphysin.[50] If initial thoracic CT is normal then a full-body PET scan is indicated and repeated every 3 to 6 months until neoplasm can be diagnosed or ruled out.[51]

The outcome for SCLC is notoriously poor. The 5-year mortality predicted for this disease in 2015 was 90%.[52] This is due to its rapid growth, early metastasis, and tendency to relapse after treatment. However, there is significant variability, based on progression at the time of diagnosis. Those who present with localized disease have a 2-year survival of approximately 30%,[53] whereas those with advanced disease have an average survival of 10 months. Clearly, then, the focus is treating the underlying malignancy.[54] Fortunately, it has been shown that treatment of the tumor is associated with improvement in paraneoplastic syndromes.[47] Many additional treatments have been attempted, but there are no large randomized trials to guide us in treating the accompanying neuropathic pain. However, as we have seen, progressing through this chapter, autoimmune assault on the peripheral nervous system is a common mechanism of pain. Based on other diseases with this mechanism, it is reasonable to consider the treatments that have proven effective in those conditions.

CONCLUSION

The immune system is quite capable of causing pain, and the nervous system is a vulnerable target. It is interesting how frequently viruses are suspected to be the initiating event. Just as we are now finding viruses to be the cause of many neoplasms, we may one day reveal them to be common sources of pain. Unfortunately, we live in a time when the immune system remains poorly understood and our treatments inelegant.

The diseases we have discussed fall outside the standard training of pain physicians, but their symptoms will present in our practices. Were we to look only at the low stated incidence of each of these conditions, we might be tempted to dismiss their importance and simply treat what we know. However, using the estimated incidences of each, in addition to the estimated incidence of cervical radiculopathy[55] and lumbar radiculopathy,[56] we can see that the numbers are significant (see Figure 18.1). Overall, these conditions represent 12% of the common causes of peripheral neuropathy. Misdiagnosis and incorrect treatment

of such conditions likely contribute to the difficulty in helping all of our patients and in definitively documenting the benefit of many of our therapies and procedures.

Despite the differing causes of these conditions, they impact the peripheral nervous system in common ways. From what we understand, they cause demyelination, small-fiber neuropathy, or ischemia—each of which we are familiar with treating. Given the difficulty of collecting large numbers of patients with uncommon conditions, there are only small studies to guide us. However, in this chapter we have reviewed the available data for treating these conditions with common agents. The most commonly studied is gabapentin, but there are small studies that support the usage of pregabalin, tricyclics, carbamazepine, lamotrigine, and topiramate as well. In the end, each of these conditions causes neuropathic pain that yields to well-known neuropathic agents.

A PRACTICAL APPROACH

As with all new information, we must ask how we can incorporate this knowledge into our practice. In the end, we need a practical approach to remain efficient practitioners while increasing our ability to diagnose less common causes of peripheral neuropathy.

The case-based approach is useful, as each condition we discussed has a common presentation. Simply knowing the presentation and having these diagnoses in our differential will greatly increase our ability to recognize them when they present. Above all, remember that a significant percentage of your patients will have peripheral neuropathy that is not due to the anatomy of their spine. Many of these conditions require an astute pain physician and timely referral to improve survival and care of these patients.

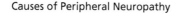

Causes of Peripheral Neuropathy

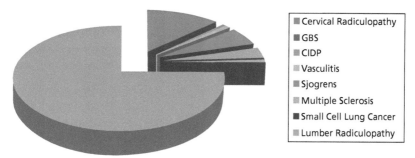

FIGURE 18.1. Distribution of causes of peripheral neuropathy. CIDP, chronic inflammatory demyelinating polyneuropathy; GBS, Guillain-Barré syndrome.

REFERENCES

1. Guillain G, Barré JA, Strohl A. Sur un syndrome de radiculonévrite avec hyperalbuminose du liquide céphalo-rachidien sans réaction cellulaire: remarques sur les caractères cliniques et graphiques des reflexes tendineux. *Bulletins et mémoires de la Société des Médecins des Hôpitaux de Paris.* 1916;40:1462–1470.

2. Poropatich KO, Walker CL, Black RE. Quantifying the association between *Campylobacter* infection and Guillain-Barré syndrome: a systematic review. *J Health Popul Nutr.* 2010;28:545–552.

3. Hadden RDM, Karch H, Hartung HP, et al. Preceding infections, immune factors, and outcome in Guillain-Barre syndrome. *Neurology.* 2001;56:758–765.

4. Hiraga A, Mori M, Ogawara K, Hattori T, Kuwabara S. Differences in patterns of progression in demyelinating and axonal Guillain-Barré syndromes. *Neurology.* 2003;61:471–474.

5. Ruts L, Drenthen J, Jongen JL, Hop WC, Visser GH, Jacobs BC, et al.; Dutch GBS Study Group. Pain in Guillain-Barré syndrome: a long-term follow-up study. *Neurology.* 2010 Oct;75(16):1439–1447. doi: 10.1212/WNL.0b013e3181f88345.

6. Hughes RAC, Wijdicks EF, Benson E, et al. Supportive care for patients with Guillain-Barré syndrome. *Arch Neurol.* 2005;62:1194–1198.

7. Pashov, A., Kaveri, A., Kazatchkine, M.D., Bellon, B. Suppression of experimental autoimmune encephalomyelitis by intravenous immunoglobulin. Kazatchkine MD, Morell A, eds. *Intravenous Immunoglobulin: Research and Therapy.* New York: Parthenon Publishing; 1996:317–318.

8. Kondo N, Kasahara K, Kameyama T, et al. (Intravenous immunoglobulins suppress immunoglobulin productions by suppressing Ca(2+)-dependent signal transduction through Fc gamma receptors in B lymphocytes. *Scand J Immunol.* 1994;40:37–42.

9. Malik U, Oleksowicz L, Latov N, Cardo LJ. Intravenous gamma-globulin inhibits binding of anti-GM1 to its target antigen. *Ann Neurol.* 1996;39:136–139.

10. Jacob S, Rajabally Y. (Current proposed mechanisms of action of intravenous immunoglobulin in inflammatory neuropathies. *Curr Neuropharmacol.* 2009;7:337–342.

11. Yuki N, Hartung H-P. Guillain-Barré syndrome. *N Engl J Med.* 2012;366:2294–2304.

12. Pandey CK, Bose N, Garg G, Singh N, Baronia A, Agarwal A, et al. Gabapentin for the treatment of pain in Guillain-Barre syndrome: a double-blinded, placebo-controlled, crossover study. *Anesth Analg.* 2002;95(6):1719–1723.

13. Gorson KC, Katz J. Chronic inflammatory demyelinating polyneuropathy. *Neurol Clin.* 2013; 2: 511–532.

14. Laughlin RS, Dyck PJ, Melton LJ, et al. Incidence and prevalence of CIDP and the association of diabetes mellitus. *Neurology.* 2009;73:39–45.

15. Boukhris S, Magy L, Khalil M, Sindou P, Vallat JM. Pain as the presenting symptom of chronic inflammatory demyelinating polyradiculoneuropathy (CIDP). *J Neurol Sci.* 2007;254:33–38.

16. Goebel A, Lecky B, Smith LJ, Lunn MP. Pain intensity and distribution in chronic inflammatory demyelinating polyneuropathy. *Muscle Nerve.* 2012;46:294–295.

17. Schady W, Goulding PJ, Lecky BR, King RH, Smith CM. Massive nerve root enlargement in chronic inflammatory demyelinating polyneuropathy. *J Neurol Neurosurg Psychiatry.* 1996;61(6):636–640.

18. Hyland HH, Russell WR. Chronic progressive polyneuritis, with report of a fatal case. *Brain.* 1930;53(3):278–289.

19. Dyck PJ, Lais AC, Ohta M, Bastron JA, Okazaki H, Groover RV. Chronic inflammatory polyradiculoneuropathy. *Mayo Clin Proc.* 1975;50(11):621–637.

20. Hughes RA, Donofrio P, Bril V, et al, ICE Study Group. Intravenous immune globulin (10% caprylate-chromatography purified) for the treatment of chronic inflammatory demyelinating polyradiculoneuropathy (ICE study): a randomized placebo-controlled trial. *Lancet Neurol.* 2008;7:136–144.

21. Nobile-Orazio E, Cocito D, Jann S, et al. Intravenous immunoglobulin versus intravenous methylprednisolone for chronic inflammatory demyelinating polyradiculoneuropathy: a randomised controlled trial. *Lancet Neurol.* 2012;11:493–502.

22. Jennette JC, Falk RJ, Andrassy K, et al. Nomenclature of systemic vasculitides. Proposal of an international consensus conference. *Arthritis Rheum.* 1994;37:187–192.

23. Pagnoux C, Guillevin L. Peripheral neuropathy in systemic vasculitides. *Curr Opin Rheumatol.* 2005;17:41–48.

24. Haugeberg G, Bie R, Bendvold A, Larsen AS, Johnsen V. Primary vasculitis in a Norwegian community hospital: A retrospective study. *Clin Rheumatol.* 1998;17:364–368.

25. Moore PM, Cupps TR: Neurological complications of vasculitis. *Ann Neurol.* 1983, 14:155–167.

26. Fauci AS, Haynes BF, Katz P, et al. Wegener's granulomatosis: prospective clinical and therapeutic experience with 85 patients for 21 years. *Ann Intern Med.* 1983;98:76–85.

27. Sehgal M, Swanson JW, DeRemee RA, et al. Neurologic manifestations of Churg-Strauss syndrome. *Mayo Clin Proc.* 1995;70:337–341.

28. Guillevin L, Durand-Gasselin B, Cevallos R, et al. Microscopic polyangiitis: clinical and laboratory findings in eighty-five patients. *Arthritis Rheum.* 1999;42:421–430.

29. Bouche P, Leger JM, Travers MA, et al. Peripheral neuropathy in systemic vasculitis: clinical and electrophysiologic study of 22 patients. *Neurology.* 1986, 36:1598–1602.

30. Said G. [Neurological manifestations of systemic necrotizing vasculitis] (in French). *Rev Neurol (Paris).* 2002;158:915–918.

31. Vrancken AFJE, Gathier CS, Cats EA, et al. The additional yield of combined nerve/muscle biopsy in vasculitic neuropathy. *Eur J Neurol.* 2010;18:49–58.

32. Zwinderman AH, Voskuyl AE, Schelhaas DD, et al. Diagnostic strategies for the histological examination of muscle biopsy specimens for the assessment of vasculitis in rheumatoid arthritis. *Stat Med.* 2000;19:3433–3447.

33. Fox RI. Sjogren's syndrome. *Lancet.* 2005;366:321–331.

34. Gutta R, McLain L, McGuff SH. Sjögren syndrome: a review for the maxillofacial surgeon. *Oral Maxillofacial Surg Clin N Am.* 2008;20:567–575.

35. Birnbaum J. Peripheral nervous system manifestations of Sjogren syndrome: clinical patterns, diagnostic paradigms, etiopathogenesis, and therapeutic strategies. *Neurologist.* 2010;16:287–297.

36. Vitali C, Bombardier S, Jonsson R, et al. Classification criteria for Sjogren's syndrome: a revised version of the European criteria proposed by the American European group. *Ann Rheum Dis.* 2002;61:554–558.

37. Kennedy WR, Wendelschafer-Crabb G, Walk D. Use of skin biopsy and skin blister in neurologic practice. *J Clin Neuromuscul Dis.* 2000;1:196–204.

38. Ramos-Casals M, Tzioufas AG, Stone JH, Sisó A, Bosch X. Treatment of primary Sjögren syndrome: a systematic review. *JAMA.* 2010;304(4):452–460.

39. Hauser SL, Oksenberg JR. The neurobiology of multiple sclerosis: genes, inflammation, and neurodegeneration. *Neuron.* 2006;52:61–76.

40. Prineas JW, Graham JS. Multiple sclerosis: capping of surface immunoglobulin G on macrophages engaged in myelin breakdown. *Ann Neurol.* 1981; 10(2):149–158.

41. Nylander A, Hafler DA. Multiple sclerosis. *J Clin Invest.* 2012;122(4):1180–1188.

42. Nicholas R, Rashid W. Multiple sclerosis. *Am Fam Physician.* 2013;87:712–714.

43. Foley PL, Vesterinen HM, Laird BJ, et al. Prevalence and natural history of pain in adults with multiple sclerosis: systematic review and meta-analysis. *Pain.* 2013;154(5):632–642. doi: 10.1016/j.pain.2012.12.002

44. Houtchens MK, Richert JR, Sami A, Rose JW. Open label gabapentin treatment for pain in multiple sclerosis. *Mult Scler.* 1997;3:250–253.

45. Solaro C, Boemker M, Tanganelli P. Pregabalin for treating paroxysmal symptoms in multiple sclerosis: a pilot study. *J Neurol.* 2009;256:1773–1774.

46. Gozzard P, Woodhall M, Chapman C, et al. Paraneoplastic neurologic disorders in small cell lung carcinoma: a prospective study. *Neurology.* 2015; 85:235.

47. Rudnicki SA, Dalmau J. Paraneoplastic syndromes of the peripheral nerves. *Curr Opin Neurol.* 2005;18:598–603.

48. Rauer S, Andreou I. Tumor progression and serum anti-HuD antibody concentration in patients with paraneoplastic neurological syndromes. *Eur Neurol.* 2002;47(4):189Y195.

49. Graus F, Keime-Guibert F, Rene R, et al. Anti-Hu-associated paraneoplastic encephalomyelitis: analysis of 200 patients. *Brain.* 2001; 124:1138–1148.

50. Graus F, Delattre JY, Antoine JC et al. Recommended diagnostic criteria for paraneoplastic neurological syndromes. *J Neurol Neurosurg Psychiatry.* 2004;75:1135–1140.

51. Koike H., Tanaka F., Sobue G. Paraneoplastic neuropathy: wide-ranging clinicopathological manifestations. *Curr Opin Neurol.* 2011;24(5):504–510.

52. Luna, GA, Espinosa, DM. Treatment for small cell lung cancer, where are we now—a review? *Transl Lung Cancer Res.* 2016;5(1):26–38.

53. van Meerbeeck JP, Fennell DA, De Ruysscher DK. Small cell lung cancer. *Lancet.* 2011;378:1741–1755.

54. Foster NR, Qi Y, Shi Q, et al. Tumor response and progression-free survival as potential surrogate endpoints for overall survival in extensive stage small-cell lung cancer: findings on the basis of North Central Cancer Treatment Group trials. *Cancer.* 2011;117:1262–1271.

55. Radhakrishnan K, Litchy W, O'Fallon W, et al. Epidemiology of cervical radiculopathy. A population-based study from Rochester, Minnesota, 1976 through 1990. *Brain.* 1994;117(Pt 2):325–335.

56. Schoenfeld AJ, Laughlin M, Bader JO, Bono CM. Characterization of the incidence and risk factors for the development of lumbar radiculopathy. *J Spinal Disord Tech.* 2012;25: 163–167.

19

Metabolic, Endocrine, and Other Toxic Neuropathies

MARTIN J. CARNEY, MARK R. JONES, PREYA K. JHITA, HAROLD J. CAMPBELL, MICHELLE ST. ROMAIN, MARK MOTEJUNAS, AND ALAN D. KAYE

In this chapter, we focus on peripheral neuropathy related to hypothyroidism, alcoholism, and vitamin and copper deficiency. Diabetic neuropathy and chemotherapy-related neuropathy are covered in Chapters 16 and 18, respectively.

CASE

A 42 year old cachectic male with a three decade history of heavy ethanol abuse presents with pins and needles, bilateral from his soles to his knees. This symptoms have worsened over the past 12 months. The patient has reduced sensation to pinprick with reduced lower extremity reflexes. Abnormal liver enzymes were identified on a liver function panel. Abnormal tibial H-reflext and nerve conduction studies are identified in both lower extremities. Positive sharp waves and fibrillation potentials are seen on needle electromyography. Multivitamins, including benfotiamine, alpha-lipoic acid, N-acetylcystine, gabapentin, opportunities to discontinue drinking including the use of disulfiram, topical capsaicin, and physical therapy are employed. The patient also agrees to see a psychologist.

ALCOHOLIC NEUROPATHY

Definition

Alcohol is one of the most commonly used substances, and the effects of alcohol abuse are seen daily in healthcare settings around the world. *Alcohol abuse* is defined as a pattern of drinking that may cause harm to one's health, personal relationships, or ability to work. Excessive alcohol commonly affects the peripheral nervous system and can lead to peripheral neuropathy. *Alcoholic neuropathy* refers to the axonal degeneration of both the sensory and motor nerves, typically starting at the most distal end of the nerve in the body, or the feet and hands, and extending proximally.[1] The sensory disturbances caused by this nerve degeneration can lead to pain, the focus of this section.

Epidemiology

Worldwide, the incidence of alcoholic neuropathy ranges from 10% to 50%, while in the United States, the prevalence is 25%–66% of chronic drinkers.[2]

There is a higher incidence in females than in males, as studies have shown females' peripheral nerves are more sensitive to the toxic effects of alcohol.[3] As alcoholic neuropathy is more common among chronic drinkers, rather than episodic drinkers, the chance of developing nerve degeneration increases with age.[4]

Clinical Features and Diagnosis

Alcoholic peripheral neuropathy has a gradual onset, which progresses over months to years. Degeneration of nerve fibers affects both sensory and motor function and can eventually lead to gait abnormalities. Initially, sensory dysfunction causes painful paresthesias with or without a burning sensation, most often first occurring in the toes and feet. The paresthesias cause diminished vibratory and pinprick sensation as well as thermal and proprioceptive sensation. If axonal degeneration continues, weakness of the distal extremities can occur. Both the sensory and motor deficits eventually extend proximally and symmetrically into the extremities and ultimately can cause gait abnormalities.[5] Patients commonly present with difficulty walking or increased falls.

There is no specific laboratory test to diagnose alcoholic neuropathy; it is primarily a clinical diagnosis. Neuropathy can be confirmed with nerve conduction studies showing abnormal conduction velocity and action potentials. Alcoholic neuropathy predominately has small-fiber axonal loss. Needle electromyography studies may also demonstrate signs of denervation in the extremities.[5]

Pathophysiology

The pathophysiology behind alcoholic neuropathy is multifactorial. The exact mechanisms are not yet fully understood, but there are various theories. Thiamine deficiency, which is commonly seen in chronic alcohol use, can induce neuropathy. Thiamine, or vitamin B1, plays an important role in many cellular processes, including those involving the peripheral nervous system. Ethanol's effect on thiamine includes diminishing absorption of thiamine in the intestines, reducing stores of thiamine in the liver, and affecting the phosphorylation of thiamine into its active form. Chronic alcoholics also have deficiencies from not consuming the necessary amount of important vitamins and nutrients, thereby further depleting thiamine stores.

Ethanol also has a direct toxic effect on neurons. It has been shown that the total lifetime amount of ethanol consumed is directly related to the severity of neuropathy. Acetaldehyde, a toxic metabolite of ethanol, can form acetaldehyde advanced glycation end products, leading to increased neuronal cell death.[2]

Furthermore, ethanol induces oxidative stress, leading to free radical damage of the nerves. Reactive oxygen species have been shown to activate secondary messengers involved in central sensitization of the cells in the dorsal horn of the spinal cord. They also activate spinal glial cells involved in chronic neuropathic pain expression. Chronic alcohol use leads to a disturbance in the balance of pro-oxidants and antioxidants, resulting in oxidative damage of fats, proteins, and DNA. Ultimately, this causes neuronal injury manifested as alcoholic neuropathy. Figure 19.1 demonstrates the complex pathophysiology of this disease process.

Treatment

In a clinical setting, gabapentin, amitriptyline, aspirin, and acetaminophen are often used for the management of painful parasthesias from alcoholic neuropathy. However, these only manage acute pain and do not halt the progression of nerve damage. Furthermore, the potential side effects and limited efficacy of these drugs make them not ideal for long-term use. Other treatment options are being explored but require clinical trials before regular usage.

Benfotiamine, a synthetic derivative of thiamine (vitamin B1), has been shown to be

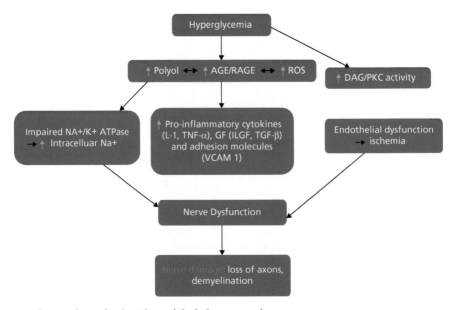

FIGURE 19.1. The complex pathophysiology of alcoholic neuropathy.

Modified from Chopra K, Tiwari V. Alcoholic neuropathy: possible mechanisms and future treatment possibilities. *Br J Clin Pharmacol.* 2012;73(3):348–362.

beneficial in patients with alcoholic neuropathy by increasing concentrations of the active coenzyme form of thiamine, thiamine diphosphate, as well as total thiamine overall. Thiamine is usually deficient in chronic alcoholics because of lack of nutritional intake and reduced hepatic storage, subsequently inducing neuropathy. Taking benfotiamine is generally believe to improve motor function and paralysis while decreasing neuropathic symptoms.

Alpha-lipoic acid is a nutrient that has been successfully used in other countries for peripheral neuropathy. It is believed to increase overall nerve health and is therefore likely a viable option for use in alcohol-induced neuropathy.

Vitamin E and its isoforms have been show to decrease pain associated with neuropathy, including hyperalgesia and allodynia. However, these effects have only been seen in rats so there is a need for clinical trials in patients.[2]

A common manifestation of vitamin B12 deficiency is peripheral neuropathy. Administration of vitamin B12 provides overall symptomatic relief of neuropathic pain.

Myo-inositol is a component of the phospholipids that form the nerve cell membrane.

Its role has been explored in the setting of diabetic neuropathy, as low nerve myo-inositol concentrations have been seen in diabetics with neuropathy (Figure 19.2). Supplementation of this constituent in rats was shown to prevent a reduction in nerve conduction velocity. Furthermore, higher levels of myo-inositol are associated with nerve regeneration, which could play an important role in preventing the progression of alcoholic neuropathy.[2]

N-acetylcysteine also shows potential in alleviating neuropathy. In animal studies, this amino acid corrected nerve conduction velocity reductions, as well as endoneurial blood flow reductions. N-acetylcystine also acts as an antioxidant and helps block apoptosis of neurons.[2]

Topical capsaicin cream has been shown to provide symptomatic relief from neuropathic pain. Capsaicin stimulates afferent group C nerve fibers, which initially causes burning and irritation. Repeated stimulation results in a decrease of the initial burning and irritation, thereby providing an analgesic effect. Long-term use of topical capsaicin potentially can decrease pain intensity in neuropathy.

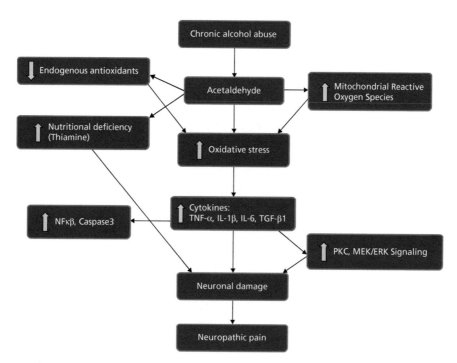

FIGURE 19.2. The complex pathophysiology of diabetic neuropathy.

Modified from Yagihashi S, Mizukami H, Sugimoto K. Mechanism of diabetic neuropathy: where are we now and where to go? *J Diabetes Investig.* 2011;2(1).

Lastly, anticonvulsants, such as gabapentinoid agents, are also first-line drugs in the symptomatic treatment of neuropathic pain. They alleviate pain through anticholinergic effects, sedative effects, and blocking reuptake of norepinephrine and serotonin. These drugs have various side effects that should be monitored for carefully if prescribed.

To rebuild strength lost due to neuropathic changes, physical therapy should be prescribed, as it plays an important role in recovery. Stretching and strengthening the lower extremities helps to prevent permanent gait abnormalities.

Prevention

Once alcoholic neuropathy is diagnosed, the goal is to prevent further damage to the nerves. Ultimately, alcohol abstinence, along with a healthy diet, is the best way to halt the disease process. Those that suffer from alcoholism would also benefit from rehabilitation including psychotherapy, nutritional consults, and substance abuse support groups, to lead to a more sustainable recovery overall.

VITAMIN DEFICIENCY NEUROPATHY

Definition

Vitamin deficiency neuropathy is caused by nutritional deficiencies in certain vitamins and trace minerals. Depending on the particular deficiency, neuropathy may present as acute, subacute, or chronic; demyelinating, axonal, or myeloneuropathy; and upper motor neuron deficit, lower motor neuron deficit, or both. Malnutrition is a major cause of vitamin deficiency, which affects patients with alcohol abuse or eating disorders or who are of older age, are pregnant, homeless, or of lower socioeconomic status.[6] Medical conditions that affect the gastrointestinal (GI) system, especially following bariatric surgery, can impair absorption of essential vitamins. Similarly, patients receiving total parental nutrition (TPN) may also be at risk for developing vitamin and trace mineral deficiencies. A deficiency in thiamine, vitamin B12, vitamin E, vitamin B6, or copper may cause neuropathy.

Vitamin B1 (Thiamine)

Thiamine is a water-soluble B complex vitamin in which a deficiency can cause beriberi, Wernicke's encephalopathy, or Korsakoff's syndrome. Thiamine, after being absorbed in the GI system and converted to thiamine diphosphate (TDP), becomes an essential cofactor in cellular respiration, ATP production, synthesis of glutamate and GABA, and myelin sheath maintenance. Since only enough thiamine for about 20 days is stored in the body, symptoms can present within a few weeks.[6] Initial symptoms of deficiency present as fatigue, irritability, and muscle cramps. Clinical features of beriberi may include distal sensory loss, pain of a burning quality, and paresthesia and cramping of lower distal extremities. Neuropathy may progress, causing ascending weakness in the lower extremities and sensory motor neuropathy in the distal upper extremities. Neuropathy may also involve the recurrent laryngeal nerve and cranial nerves, causing hoarseness and facial weakness. If the ocular motor nerve is involved, ocular motor muscle weakness and the nystagmus may present if not otherwise attributed to Wernicke's encephalopathy, which manifests as ophthalmoplegia, ataxia, nystagmus, and encephalopathy. Since blood and urine assays of thiamin deficiency are not reliable, the measurement of thiamine pyrophosphate (TPP) or erythrocyte transketolase activation is preferred to assess thiamine deficiency. These assays must be taken before thiamin supplementation is administered, for an accurate measurement. Axonal sensorimotor polyneuropathy can be seen on electrodiagnostic testing, and nerve biopsies show axonal degeneration. Thiamine supplementation should be administered if thiamin deficiency is suspected, at an initial dose of 100 mg intravenously or intramuscularly, followed by 100 mg per day thereafter. Neurological improvement may take up to 6 months; motor symptoms usually improve before sensory symptoms. Patients can expect a slow recovery; however, patients with severe neuropathy may have permanent neurological impairment.

Vitamin B12 (Cobalamin)

Vitamin B12 is a water-soluble B-complex vitamin in which a deficiency causes neurological symptoms. B12 is an important component in the formation of tetrahydrofolate, a precursor of nucleotide synthesis, and succinyl coenzyme A, essential in myelin sheath formation. After ingestion, B12 binds to R proteins in the GI system and is then released in the small intestine to bind to intrinsic factor. Bound to intrinsic factor, B12 is absorbed in the terminal ileum. Deficiency may be caused by pernicious anemia, malnutrition,

GI surgery, medications such as proton pump inhibitors and metformin, or chronic exposure to nitrous oxide. Vitamin B12 deficiency has been observed in 5%–20% of older adults. Unlike thiamine, symptoms of B12 deficiency may not appear for years, because enough B12 for several years is stored in the liver.[7]

Clinical features of neurological involvement may include subacute combined degeneration, neuropsychiatric symptoms, peripheral neuropathy, and optic neuropathy. Myeloneuropathy often presents with proprioception and vibration deficiencies, increased tone, brisk knee and arm reflexes, Hoffman's signs in the fingers, and extensor plantar responses in the toes.

Diagnosis of B12 deficiency is made in the presence of specific neurological symptoms, hematological abnormalities, and serum B12 levels less than 200 pg/mL. Since a significant number of patients with vitamin B12 deficiency have normal serum vitamin B12 levels, serum methylmalonic acid (MMA) and homocysteine measurement may improve sensitivity of testing. Elevated MMA and homocysteine suggest vitamin B12 deficiency; however, one must rule out renal insufficiency and hypovolemia, which may similarly elevate MMA and homocysteine.

Pernicious anemia may be diagnosed via anti-intrinsic factor and anti-parietal cell antibody testing. In MRI studies, an increased T2 signal intensity can be seen in the posterior column of the spinal cord. If deficiency is suspected, an initial dosage of 1000 mcg intramuscularly is delivered daily for 5–7 days, then 1000 mcg intramuscularly monthly thereafter. Neurological response usually takes place during the first 6 months of treatment. Treatment may prevent further impairment; however, patients may also suffer some permanent neurological impairment despite treatment.

Vitamin E

Vitamin E (alpha-tocopherol) is a fat-soluble vitamin. After ingestion, vitamin E is incorporated into chylomicrons and absorbed in the intestines, requiring bile acids, fatty acids, and monoglycerides to be absorbed. Vitamin E deficiency usually stems from malabsorption problems. Patients with cystic fibrosis may also develop vitamin E deficiency secondary to fat malabsorption. Neurological involvement of vitamin E deficiency has been hypothesized to be caused by the loss of antioxidant and free radical scavenger properties that vitamin E has, which protects the nervous system.

Abetalipoproteinemia is a rare autosomal dominant disorder that also leads to vitamin E deficiency. Abetalipoproteinemia results from mutations in the microsomal triglyceride transfer protein, which results in fat malabsorption and, therefore, deficiencies in fat-soluble vitamins such as vitamins A, D, E, and K. Vitamin E deficiency may result in pigmented retinopathy, loss of vibration and proprioception, loss of deep tendon reflexes, ataxia, cerebellar degeneration, and generalized muscle weakness. Symptoms of vitamin E deficiency may take 5–10 years to present, because its active form, alpha-tocopherol, is stored in adipose tissues. Clinical features of deficiency may mimic Friedreich's ataxia with symptoms including ataxia, hyporeflexia, and loss of proprioception and vibration.

Diagnosis of vitamin E deficiency is made by serum alpha-tocopherol levels. As alpha-tocopherol levels may be normal in patients with deficiency, serum vitamin E–to–total serum lipid concentration ratio may increase the sensitivity of the test. Sensory predominant axonal neuropathy may be seen on nerve conduction studies, whereas electromyography may be normal or show mild denervation. If vitamin E deficiency is suspected, an initial dose of 400 international units of vitamin E is given orally twice daily, gradually increasing the dose until serum vitamin E levels normalized. Patients with abetalipoproteinemia may require large doses to normalize serum vitamin E levels. Patients with malabsorption syndromes may require water-miscible or intramuscular doses of vitamin E.

Copper

Copper is a trace mineral that is important in many oxidative reactions in the body in which a deficiency may cause myelopathy or myeloneuropathy. Copper is both passively and actively absorbed in the GI system after it is solubilized by gastric acid. It is then bound to plasma proteins and transported to the liver. The bound copper is incorporated into ceruloplasmin for distribution and delivery to cells. Cells tightly regulate absorption and excretion of copper because of free radical generation by reactions in which it is involved.

Copper deficiency can be seen prior to gastric surgery, excessive zinc or iron supplementation, and malabsorption syndromes. Patients with copper deficiency may present similarly to those with B12 deficiency. Clinical features of copper deficiency include gait difficulty, paresthesias in the lower extremities, loss of proprioception and vibration, upper motor neuron signs such as bladder dysfunction, brisk knee jerks, and extensor plantar reflexes. Motor neuron deficits may also present.

A diagnosis of copper deficiency is made with low serum copper, low ceruloplasmin, and low urinary excretion of copper. Since ceruloplasmin is an acute-phase reactant, it is often not an adequate marker for copper deficiency. Zinc may also be high. Anemia or myelodysplastic syndrome may be seen on blood studies. MRI can show increased T2 signal in the posterior columns of the spinal cord. Mixed motor and sensory axonal polyneuropathy will be seen on nerve conduction studies.

Treatment of copper deficiency depends on the cause. Excessive zinc intake should be discontinued if it is a factor. Oral supplementation of 2 mg of elemental copper three times daily is preferred, although intravenous infusion is also available. Copper supplementation will stop progression of neurological symptoms; however, some permanent damage may be expected.

CHEMOTHERAPEUTIC NEUROPATHY

Definition

Chemotherapy-induced peripheral neuropathy (CIPN) is a concerning and, at times, dose-limiting side effect of many chemotherapeutic agents. The clinical presentation of a patient suffering from symmetrical stocking-glove peripheral neuralgias postoncological treatment is characteristic for CIPN. However, in more severe cases, patients can suffer permanent and quite debilitating neuropathic pain in combination with possible motor and autonomic involvement. The severity of symptoms is positively correlated with the cumulative dose administered and can be compounded if a patient has a preexisting neuropathy such as diabetes, alcoholism, or age-related axonal loss. The drugs most commonly associated with CIPN are the taxanes, vinca-alkaloids, platinum compounds, bortezomib, and thalidomide. In the setting of improved patient survival and increasingly effective treatments of many of the other side effects of these drugs, the symptomatic treatment and prevention of CIPN is an important aspect of maximizing patients' quality of life.

Pathophysiology

The pathogenesis of chemotherapy-induced peripheral neuropathy is drug specific, but the two core mechanisms of action proposed are axonopathy and neuronopathy. *Axonopathy* is the destruction of a nerve fiber, beginning at the most vulnerable peripheral tip of the axon with progressive retrograde involvement. *Neuronopathy* is the destruction of the nerve body itself, specifically the cells of the dorsal root ganglion. These mechanisms of action can operate synergistically and are not mutually exclusive.

Taxanes

Taxanes act by disrupting microtubule structure, which in turn impairs the cell's ability to perform axoplasmic transportation. Without the ability to transport anterograde, the cells undergo progressive axonopathy. In addition to its peripheral effects, paclitaxel has been shown to act centrally on the mitochondrial permeability transition pore. Opening this pore leads to a calcium release from the mitochondria and, in turn, neurotoxicity.[8]

Symptoms of taxanes-induced neuropathy are classically strictly sensory, consisting of bilateral, distal symmetrical numbness, tingling, and burning. Both small (pinprick and temperature) and large (proprioception and vibration) nerve fibers are affected equally. Achilles reflexes may be absent or subdued. The onset of symptoms can range from within the first 24 to 72 hours after initial treatment but more classically only result after multiple drug administrations. The neurotoxic threshold is estimated at 1000 mg/m² for paclitaxel and 400 mg/m² for docetaxel.[9]

Vinca-Alkaloids

Similar to taxanes, vinca-alkaloids act to interrupt microtubule formation by inhibiting the polymerization of dimer bodies into the elongating microtubule. With the disruption, once again, of the cell's major transport system, the cell is thought to undergo progressive axonopathy.

Classically, several weeks after the first treatment, sensory symptoms such as numbness and tingling of the hands and feet develop. However, rarely patients may suffer from muscle pain in their jaw and legs immediately after the first infusion. Unlike the taxanes, vinca-alkaloids often involve a patient's motor and autonomic nerves. More than a third of patients develop autonomic neuropathy characterized by orthostatic hypotension, constipation, ileus, and impotence.[8]

Patients' symptoms have the potential to worsen months after discontinuation of the drug; this is a phenomenon referred to as "coasting."

Platinum Derivatives

These compounds act to inappropriately cross-link DNA molecules, thereby inhibiting DNA synthesis. This mechanism of action has been found to be neurotoxic primarily to the cells of the dorsal root ganglion. Oxaliplatin uniquely contributes to the chelation of calcium within a cell and, in turn, transient activation of the voltage-gated sodium channels, which creates a state of hyperexcitability.

The CIPN clinical presentation is largely sensory. Patients may experience pain and numbness in their distal extremities which can spread proximally. These symptoms may continue to worsen 3–6 months after therapy (coasting) and have the potential to become chronic. Lhermitte's sign may also occur, which is characterized by the sensation on a nonpainful electric shock traveling down one's spine in response to neck flexion. A cumulative dose of 240–300 mg/m^2 of cisplatin has the potential to lead to CIPN.[9] Lipoplatin and carboplatin have been found to be less toxic than cisplatin.

Bortezomib

Bortezomib is a proteasome inhibitor. Experimental studies predict that accumulation of various cytoplasmic aggregates is the cause of early neurotoxicity seen in the cells of the dorsal root ganglion. Neuropathic pain is the predominant feature; vibratory sense and Achilles reflexes are often preserved. An estimated 10% of patients may develop a form of autonomic dysfunction. The peripheral neuropathy usually does not present until the fifth cycle of bortezomib at a cumulative dose of roughly 26 mg/m^2.[8]

Thalidomide

Thalidomide is a glutamic acid derivative and acts to induce the production of interferon-gamma and interleukin-2 while inhibiting tumor necrosis factor-alpha and angiogenesis. The mechanism of action of the neurotoxic effect of thalidomide is unknown. Patients may present with numbness in their hands and feet with diminished or absent Achilles reflexes. Between 80% and 90% of patients suffer from autonomic neuropathy in the form of constipation.[8]

Clinical Features and Diagnosis

The diagnosis of CIPN is largely clinical; however, nerve conduction velocity (NCV), sensory nerve action potential (SNAP), and compound muscle action potential (CMAP) in combination with electromyography (EMG) are the standard neurophysiological tests used to confirm the diagnosis. Axonopathy can be illustrated by decreased SNAP and NCV amplitude measurements. The utility of skin biopsies is being explored in the evaluation of CIPN; nerve biopsies are rarely indicated. Genetic studies have been found to positively correlate certain genes with the development of CIPN but have not become a standard method of diagnosis.

Treatment

The treatment for CIPN is largely symptomatic. Drugs directed against neuropathic pain, such as anticonvulsants, tricyclic antidepressants, opioids, and topical anesthetics, are all options depending on the severity of the symptoms. If there is autonomic, motor, or debilitative proprioceptive involvement, patients can benefit from both occupational and physical rehabilitation.

Prevention

Multiple drugs have been used in an attempt to prevent CIPN and have been found to have differing levels of success, depending on the dose and type of chemotherapeutic agent they are used with. Vitamin E, amifostine, and glutamine have all been found to decrease the neuropathic symptoms of paclitaxel. Pyridoxine with pyridostigmine has helped counteract the effects of vincristine. Calcium and magnesium infusions are routinely used to prophylactically treat oxaliplatin neuropathy. Likewise, evidence suggests that delivering the same cumulative dose of a chemotherapeutic agent but in smaller, spaced intervals has been shown to decrease the incidence CIPN while having no effect on tumor suppression. Lastly, changing the treatment regimen to a less toxic option can also help mitigate a patient's CIPN symptoms.

KEY POINTS

- As alcohol is one of the most commonly used substances, the effects of alcohol abuse are seen daily in medical clinics and hospitals around the world. The incidence of alcoholic neuropathy ranges from 10% to 50%, while in the United States, the prevalence is 25%–66% of chronic drinkers.

- Alcoholic peripheral neuropathy is a gradual process, progressing over months to years. Degeneration of nerves affects both sensory and motor function and can eventually lead to gait abnormalities.
- Malnutrition is a foremost contributor to vitamin deficiencies. Patients with medical conditions that affect the gastrointestinal system, most notably following bariatric surgery, are also at risk for developing these neuropathies.
- Deficiencies in thiamine, vitamin B12, vitamin E, vitamin B6, and copper may all cause varying degrees of neuropathies. The symptoms may present as acute, subacute, or chronic demyelinating, axonal, or myeloneuropathy and can affect upper as well as lower motor neurons.
- Chemotherapy-induced peripheral neuropathy (CIPN) is a concerning and, at times, dose-limiting side effect of many chemotherapeutic agents. The severity of symptoms is positively correlated with the cumulative dose administered and can be compounded if a patient has a preexisting neuropathy.
- Various preventive strategies and treatments exist to mitigate the severity of CIPN. These treatments are largely based on the specific oncological agent used.

SUGGESTED READING

Chopra K, Tiwari V. Alcoholic neuropathy: possible mechanisms and future treatment possibilities. *Br J Clin Pharmacol.* 2012; 73(3):348–362.

Hammond N, Yunxia W, Mazen D, Barohn R. Nutritional neuropathies. *Neurol Clin.* 2013; 31(2): 477–489.

Tesfaye S, Vileikyte L, Rayman G, et al. Painful diabetic peripheral neuropathy: consensus recommendations on diagnosis, assessment and management. *Diabetes Metab Res Rev.* 2011;27:629–638.

REFERENCES

1. Koike H and Sobue G. Alcoholic neuropathy. *Curr Opin Neurol.* 2006;19(5):481–486.
2. Chopra K and Tiwari V. Alcoholic neuropathy: possible mechanisms and future treatment possibilities. *Br J Clin Pharmacol.* 2012;73(3):348–362.
3. Ammendola A, Gemini D, Iannaccone S, et al. Gender and peripheral neuropathy in chronic alcoholism: a clinical-electroneurographic study. *Alcohol Alcohol.* 2000;35(4):368–371.
4. Zambelis T, Karandreas N, Tzavellas E, Kokotis P, Liappas J. Large and small fiber neuropathy in chronic alcohol-dependent subjects. *J Peripher Nerv Syst.* 2005;10(4):375–381.
5. Azhary H, Farooq M, Bhanushali M, Majid A, Kassab M. Peripheral Neruopathy: Differential Diagnosis and Management. *Am Fam Physician.* 2010;81(7):887–892.
6. Hammond N, Wang Y, Dimachkie M, Barohn RJ. Nutritional neuropathies. *Neurol Clin.* 2013;31(2):477–489.
7. Becker D, Balcer L, Galetta S. The neurological complications of nutritional deficiency following bariatric surgery. *J Obes.* 2012; 1–8.
8. Miltenburg N, Boogerd W. Chemotherapy-induced neuropathy: a comprehensive survey. *Cancer Treat Rev.* 2014; 40(7); 872–882.
9. Grisold W, Cavaletti G, Windebank A. Peripheral neuropathies from chemotherapeutics and targeted agents: diagnosis, treatment, and prevention. *Neuro-Oncology.* 2012; 14(4): Iv45–v54.

PART IV

Lesions of the Central Nervous System

20

Spinal Cord Injury

JUSTIN F. AVERNA, ALEXANDER BAUTISTA, GEORGE C. CHANG CHIEN,
AND MICHAEL SAULINO

CASE

A 29-year-old man with L1 paraplegia, sustained from a gunshot wound injury to the spinal cord at the age of 26, reports having constant burning, stabbing, crushing pain in his bilateral legs and feet; a tight, band-like pain at the level of his injury; warmth and cramping from his right low back and hip; and right shoulder pain. His right shoulder pain is exacerbated by prolonged wheelchair propulsion and overhead activities. On examination, he has reduced range of motion in his right shoulder, especially with abduction and external rotation. There is warmth to palpation at the right inguinal region. Complete paraplegia with significant spasticity in his bilateral legs was noted. There are no signs of allodynia or hyperalgesia in his legs. For his right shoulder pain, diagnostic ultrasound demonstrates a partial-thickness tear of his supraspinatus tendon. For his right low back and hip pain, radiographic imaging demonstrates signs of early heterotrophic ossification in the femoral-acetabular joint.

DEFINITION

Spinal cord injury (SCI) causes multiple areas of dysfunction in the nervous systems, such as neuronal hyperexcitability in the spinal cord, brainstem, thalamus, and cortex.[1] Pain from SCI has been regarded as one of the most difficult problems to manage, its greatest impact being on physical, psychological, and social functioning.

Over the years, the terminology regarding SCI pain has evolved. In order for clinicians to communicate clearly, the International Association of the Study of Pain (IASP) established a Spinal Cord Injury Task Force to put forward classification and taxonomy of SCI pain. The current taxonomy describes at least four major types of pain associated with SCI. This classification includes musculoskeletal, visceral, and neuropathic pain. Neuropathic pain includes the at-level pain that occurs in a dermatomal or segmental distribution at the level of injury, and below-level pain, which is a more diffuse type of pain below the neurological insult.[2] The nociceptive component of pain may arise from extensive damage to deep somatic tissue such as bones, joints, discs, ligaments, and muscles.

PATHOPHYSIOLOGY

The underlying mechanisms of SCI-associated pain is complex. The multidimensional nature of SCI pain affects the neural system, including autonomic nervous system dysregulation, and alters metabolic and biochemical processes throughout the body. There is growing evidence to suggest involvement of supraspinal structures and damaged nerve roots in the periphery.[3] In incomplete injuries, the damaged nerve roots may give rise to pain at the level of the injury. In complete transection of the spinal cord, there may be a residual transmission of nociceptive impulses, a phenomenon called "sensory incomplete" lesion, that may not evident on physical examination.[4] In the spinal cord, the trauma itself may lead to structural remodeling of the terminal primary afferents within the dorsal horn. The presence of these pathologies often results in abnormal spontaneous neuronal activities, which are associated with increased background activity, increased responsiveness to peripheral stimulation, and prolonged firing following a stimulus.[4,5] There may also be a reduction in GABAergic inhibitory tone and amplification of ascending input. In addition, glial activation, cytokine and prostaglandin release, and structural reorganization have been linked to the development of SCI pain.[6]

Supraspinal mechanisms have long been suspected in the development of neuropathic pain. Patients had continued neuropathic pain despite peripheral sympathetic spinal blockade and surgical removal of cord segments above the level of injury.[7] In animal models, lesions of the spinothalamic tract resulted in an increase in spontaneous and evoked thalamic neuronal activities linked with changes in thalamic NMDA receptor function, sodium channel expression, and microglial activation.[6] Electroencephalography (EEG) has demonstrated changes in the rhythmicity of thalamic neurons that may underlie pain. Chemical changes on magnetic resonance spectroscopy (correlation of pain intensity and concentration of N-acetylaspartate and myoinositol in the thalamus) suggest neuronal loss or dysfunction.

Pain following SCI is also associated with structural and functional changes at a cortical level. In people with complete thoracic injuries and below-level neuropathic pain, reorganization of the somatosensory cortex has been shown to occur and correlates with pain intensity. The extent to which supraspinal changes and pain are dependent on preserved ascending fiber tracts remains unclear. Clinical electrophysiological studies suggest that 50% of patients with clinically complete injuries still have preserved transmission in spinal pathways. Therefore, preserved spinal cord pathways that transverse the injury site have been proposed as an important factor underlying the development of below-level neuropathic pain following SCI.

EPIDEMIOLOGY

The occurrence of pain following SCI is very common. The prevalence of pain is about 65%–85% in patients with SCI and around 30% of these patients will have severe pain.[8] About 40% of patients at 6 months after injury[9] and 59% after 5 years[8,10] will complain of musculoskeletal pain. There is also an increased prevalence of at-level and below-level neuropathic pain more than 5 years after SCI.[8] In a most recent meta-analysis, no demonstrable difference in SCI pain prevalence related to gender, injury completeness, and paraplegia and tetraplegia was found. However, it has been shown that the time of injury and the presence of depression are factors that increase pain prevalence. The severity of pain is associated with the presence of disturbed mood and acceptance of disability. A definitive statement with regard to SCI-related pain prevalence has not been achieved owing to heterogeneity of the study population.[11]

CLINICAL FEATURES AND DIAGNOSIS OF SPINAL CORD INJURY

Clinical Features

The factors that contribute to development of pain after SCI remain an enigma. These patients may present with varying degrees of musculoskeletal pain and neuropathic pain depending on the level of injury.

Musculoskeletal Pain

Musculoskeletal pain is evident in paraplegic patients with SCI and is secondary to overuse syndromes of the upper limbs.[12] This type of pain maybe secondary to disruption of ligaments, joints, and fractures of bone, resulting in instability of the spine. The upper limb and shoulder joints are particularly susceptible because they bear the weight of the body for mobility and assist in transfers and wheelchair propulsion. Patients also frequently present with muscle spasm that may exacerbate musculoskeletal pain. The mechanism of spasticity is the imbalance of excitatory and inhibitory modulatory synaptic influences on the alpha motor neurons resulting in hyperactivity of the stretch reflex arc.[13] Spasticity usually occurs late in the disease process and is often seen in patient with incomplete SCI.

At-Level Neuropathic Pain

Segmental deafferentation/girdle (border or transitional) pain is a variation of neuropathic pain that occurs within a band of two to four segments above or below the level of SCI. It often occurs in anesthetized skin or at the border of normal skin sensation. This may present with cramp-like pain in the neck, shoulder, or both, with or without allodynia to light touch or hyperalgesia of the affected region. This typical type of pain may resolve over time.[2]

Below-Level Neuropathic Pain

Patients with this pain usually complain of constant, throbbing, stabbing pain that is diffusely located below the SCI. The pain is typically associated with hyperalgesia and may gradually worsen over time. The pain may occur with spontaneous or evoked episodes and usually worsens in the presence of infection, sudden noise, or jarring movement. These presentations are part of the central dysesthesia syndrome and/or de-afferentation pain.[2] There may be a syrinx or an abnormal cyst in the spinal cord with this type of pain. The onset is often delayed by a mean of 6 years. Damage to the central part of the spinal cord with cervical injuries results in the central cord syndrome, which is characterized by pain and weakness of the arms and relatively strong but spastic leg function.[13]

DIAGNOSIS

Like any chronic pain syndrome, evaluation of SCI pain requires a multidisciplinary assessment. The initial information based on the history should include an inventory of pain characteristics, its onset, quality, distribution, and aggravating and alleviating factors for pain and spasms; interventions and treatments received; problems encountered that include but are not limited to spasms, infections, and pressure sores; and the patient's level of functioning. Of paramount importance, a detailed account regarding the patient's initial SCI should be obtained that includes date and mechanism of injury, associated injuries, a description of vertebral column stabilization procedures, and comorbidities.

Pain assessment always includes some component of self-report. This can supplement information obtained during the clinical interview and provides a means of evaluating the success or failure of treatment strategies. The most commonly used measure of pain, both for SCI-related pain and pain general, is the numerical rating scale (NRS). A number of studies have established the NRS as a reliable measure of pain intensity.[14] Another typical measure of pain intensity is the visual analog scale (VAS). Typically, a clinically meaningful change in pain intensity is approximately 33% decrement in a visual analog score.[15] There are scales that have been used to assess the multidimensional component of SCI pain and may assist in the rehabilitation part of managing SCI pain. This will aid in appropriate planning of the treatment program. Examples of such scales are Graded Chronic Pain Disability Scale, the Brief Pain Inventory, and the Multidimensional Pain Inventory.

It is essential to conduct a thorough physical examination with a focus on identifying the potential etiology of the pain and the presence of abnormal sensation and movement. Neurological evaluation is based on the guidelines established by the International Standard for Neurological Classification of SCI.[16] To assess spasticity, the modified Ashworth Spasticity Scale can be used both for initial assessment and response to treatment. Wheelchair propulsion, the patient's posture and gait, including determination of appropriate comfort and fit of assistive devices and orthosis, should be observed to assess plausible contributors to pain.

The use of ancillary tests may help determine the cause of pain, level and extent of injury, and presence of specific pain syndromes. Conditions associated with at-level and below-level lesions may pose a challenge to the diagnosis. Imaging modalities such as magnetic resonance imaging (MRI) may be of utility for diagnosing syringomyelia and may provide useful information to assess segmental instability or compression about the site of injury, spinal nerve impingement, orthopedic hardware loosening, and fluid collection. Electrodiagnostic studies such as quantitative sensory testing, somatosensory evoked potentials, and motor evoked potentials may be warranted to document the extent of injury and delineate the varying degrees of dissociated sensory loss.[13] Reversible abnormalities should also be ruled out; hence, determination of hypovitaminosis, particularly of B12 and D, complete blood count, erythrocyte sedimentation rate, C-reactive protein, and hormonal assessment should be undertaken.

TREATMENT

The heterogeneous nature of SCI pain warrants a multidisciplinary approach to treatment, which should be tailored individually to enhance motivation and participation in the treatment plan. Expectations should be realistic, rational, and relevant in the formulation of the management plan. The goals should be catered to addressing pain and spasms, as well as improvement of function for the patient in order to achieve independent living and possibly return to work. The treatment plan should encompass four domains: pain management, spinal rehabilitation, psychological treatment, and social and environmental modification.[13]

Nonpharmacological Treatments

Many nonpharmacological treatments have been studied in patients post–SCI pain. The effectiveness of exercise programs on SCI-related shoulder pain has been demonstrated in several studies with small sample size. The efficacy of environmental modifications and adaptive equipment was shown in nonrandomized, noncontrolled studies. Long-term exercise diminishes pain over time. Synergy between osteopathic manipulative treatment and pharmacological interventions was suggested in a small, randomized study. A positive effect of using healing touch and progressive relaxation for chronic neuropathic pain was demonstrated in a small, nonrandomized, noncontrolled study. Efficacy of acupuncture and transcutaneous electrical nerve stimulation (TENS) appears to be better for at-level pain syndromes, as shown in quasi-randomized studies. Physical therapy has been shown to improve musculoskeletal pain, including shoulder pain, overuse syndromes, and pressure-related pain.[17] However, there is minimal evidence for the utility of massage therapy, which is the most common nonpharmacological intervention used in this population.

Pharmacological Therapy

Pharmacological interventions have more compelling evidence regarding their effectiveness, although generalized definitive recommendations are difficult to formulate. Guidelines are available to provide a general approach that may be tailored to each individual patient. Patients with SCI-related chronic pain use NSAIDs most commonly, although no formal studies have evaluated their efficacy. Spasmolytics are appropriate for pain associated with muscle imbalances from involuntary co-contraction. Oral baclofen, a $GABA_B$ receptor agonist that works at spinal and supraspinal sites, is considered first line, despite not being extensively studied in a formal way. Tizanidine, a central alpha-2-adrenergic receptor agonist, has proven efficacy for spasticity and possibly for pain but has not formally been studied either.

Anticonvulsants like pregabalin, which binds the alpha-2-delta subunit of the voltage-dependent calcium channel, have demonstrated positive results in two randomized controlled trials (RCTs)—approximately 30% decrement in pain scores after 3–4 months with average dosing between 350 and 450 mg/day. Pregabalin is the only pharmaceutical that has FDA indication for SCI-associated pain. The most common adverse effect was development or worsening of edema (10%–20%); other adverse effects include somnolence, dizziness, dry mouth, fatigue, and blurred vision. The best evidence after pregabalin is that for gabapentin: a handful of studies support its use and it appears to be better tolerated, with average dosing 1800 mg/day.

Antidepressants, in particular tricyclic antidepressants (TCAs), are considered second line for SCI-associated neuropathic pain. Amitriptyline is the best studied, with limited support for nortriptyline. There is evidence to suggest increased efficacy when used in combination with anticonvulsants. TCAs' side effects have been well established and include sedation, dry mouth, blurred vision, constipation, urinary retention, orthostatic hypotension, weight gain, and cardiac dysrhythmias, and overdose can lead to death. There are good data to support TCA use when pain and depression are both present. Dual serotonin-norepinephrine reuptake inhibitors (SRNIs), such as duloxetine, appear to modulate pain independent of their antidepressant properties. A small RCT of duloxetine for central neuropathic pain (in stroke or SCI) failed to show a reduction in pain intensity but did demonstrate changes in other aspects of these chronic pain syndromes, including allodynia. Traditional selective serotonin reuptake inhibitors (SSRIs) have no proven benefit and can exacerbate spasticity.

Cannabinoids have anecdotal evidence for treatment of SCI-related neuropathic pain, but trials with synthetic cannabinoids have not been promising. Cannabis contains 60 or more cannabinoids, the most abundant of which are delta-9-tetrahydrocannabinol (THC) and cannabidiol (CBD). Dronabinol is a pure isomer of THC with conflicting data, more negative than positive, with most common side effects being sedation and weight gain. A small RCT of dronabinol showed no relief in below-level neuropathic pain. Nabilone is an enriched THC preparation with minimal data to support its use, although it has been indicated for used with chemotherapy-related nausea and vomiting. Sativex is a fixed ratio of THC/CBD in an oral mucosal spray that is approved in Spain, the United Kingdom, Canada, and New Zealand for multiple sclerosis–related spasticity. Effects on pain are somewhat variable, and the most common side effects are fatigue and dizziness.

Some patients with SCI-related neuropathic pain respond to parenteral opioids. However, sustained relief with oral opioids is often difficult to obtain and long-term benefit is commonly reduced by constipation, drowsiness, tolerance, and dependence. An RCT of tramadol found significant improvement in pain in comparison to placebo but was associated with a high rate of adverse events, including tiredness, dry mouth, and dizziness.[17]

Neuromodulation

Neuromodulation options include spinal cord stimulation (SCS), deep brain stimulation, and use of an intrathecal pump to treat pain and spasticity. SCS may be effective in some patients with neuropathic SCI pain, although it depends on the type of injury and type of pain. At least partial preservation of sensation in the area of pain is normally required to obtain success. SCS may be more useful if the spinal cord lesion is incomplete, and it appears to be more effective for at-level neuropathic SCI pain. While both SCS and deep brain stimulation may be of benefit, there is little evidence showing its efficacy over a long period of time.[18]

Intrathecal therapies have demonstrated promising pain relief, but the intrathecal route is also associated with long-term side effects and tolerance, which can reduce its benefit. Intrathecal baclofen has been effective in the treatment of spasm-related pain, and intrathecal morphine bolus had positive effects in an RCT for central pain. Combination therapy shows promise with varying degrees of success; morphine and clonidine have demonstrated synergistic benefit and reduction in pain. Intrathecal gabapentin failed to have a therapeutic effect in a generalized pain population.[17]

Surgical Treatment

Orthopedic and neurosurgical procedures that stabilize the spine immediately after trauma and decompress impinged nerve roots can be very effective at eliminating pain caused by instability or nerve root compression. Syrinx procedures have better outcomes for neurosurgical symptoms than for pain. The pain associated with the syrinx may persist even when the syrinx has decompressed.

Other surgical options include cordotomy, myelotomy, and dorsal root entry zone lesioning (DREZ). DREZ lesions that involve two to three spinal segments have been proposed to be effective in management of SCI pain. Its effectiveness is thought to be due to elimination of abnormal activity in dorsal horn neurons close to the level of injury, interruption of ascending pain pathways, or rebalancing of inhibitory and excitatory input within a damaged sensory network. Most studies indicate that 50%–85% of patients will obtain good (>50%) relief of their pain.[19] Those with unilateral, radicular, cauda equina pain or intermittent, at-level neuropathic pain are more likely to have a favorable outcome, whereas those who have sacral, continuous, below-level neuropathic pain or a syrinx are less likely to do well. Cordotomy, cordectomy, and myelotomy are associated with severe adverse effects with either poor or no relief of below-level neuropathic pain.[20]

Spinal Rehabilitation

The goal of rehabilitation therapy is to restore functional independence and improve quality of life. Treatment includes exercise, hydrotherapy, postural training, pressure relief, utilization of physical aids (i.e., crutches, orthotics, wheelchairs), and other physical modalities (TENS and ultrasound). While these interventions have some utility in the management of biomechanical pain, these modalities do not help reduce neuropathic pain.[21]

Psychological Therapy

Reduction of psychological distress, improvement of quality of life, and enhancement of social integration are the main focus of psychological therapy. Interventions include pain-coping skills, cognitive-behavioral therapy, exposure to social, sexual, and communication skill training, and family dynamics.[13] A recent study performed of patients with SCI suggests that although cognitive-behavioral approaches may not produce significant reductions in pain, they can provide improvements in other aspects of function, such as mood.[22] Cognitive impairment due to concomitant brain injury may limit the utility of psychological interventions.

Social or Environmental Modification

The chronic nature of SCI pain often results in patients' inability to adapt to their present condition and they usually struggle to go back to normalcy and return to work. Environmental factors need to be addressed that include need for homecare, adaptive equipment, family education, availability of appropriate employment opportunities, and workplace adjustment.[23]

FUTURE DIRECTIONS

Electrical stimulation of the various brain regions, including the thalamus, periventricular gray matter, internal capsule, and motor cortex, has been used for the treatment of neuropathic SCI pain and may be beneficial in a limited number of intractable cases.[24] Transcranial direct current stimulation (tDCS) was superior to a sham intervention when the estimates of two studies were combined. However, overall evidence for the effectiveness of tDCS in reducing chronic pain in SCI is scarce and inconclusive. Brain stimulation and motor cortex stimulation are both invasive and have associated serious adverse events and questionable long-term efficacy.

GUIDING QUESTIONS

- What is the mechanism for developing pain from spinal cord injury (SCI)?
- How do you properly assess SCI pain?
- What are the treatment goals and options for SCI pain?

KEY POINTS

- SCI pain is one of the pain syndromes that is recalcitrant to treatment. SCI pain is associated with substantial impact on the patient's life, interfering with activities of daily living, effective rehabilitation, and quality of life.
- SCI pain is a result of injury associated with mechanical trauma and vascular compromise of the spinal cord parenchyma. The underlying mechanism for the development of SCI pain includes neuronal hyperexcitability, reduced inhibition, and neuronal reorganization and plasticity.
- The diverse factors associated with SCI pain warrant the need for an interdisciplinary approach tailored to individual patients. The goals of treatment should encompass four domains: pain management, spinal rehabilitation, psychological treatment, and social and environmental modification.

REFERENCES

1. Gwak YS, Kim HY, Lee BH, Yang CH. Combined approaches for the relief of spinal cord injury-induced neuropathic pain. *Complement Ther Med.* 2016;25:27–33.
2. Siddall PJ, Yezierski RP, Loeser JD. Taxonomy and epidemiology of spinal cord injury pain. In: *Spinal Cord Injury Pain: Assessment, Mechanisms, Management Progress in Pain Research and Management*, Vol. 23. Seattle: IASP Press; 2002:9–24.
3. Siddall PJ. Management of neuropathic pain following spinal cord injury: now and in the future. *Spinal Cord.* 2009;47(5):352–359.
4. Sherwood AM, Dimitrijevic MR, McKay WB. Evidence of subclinical brain influence in clinically complete spinal cord injury: discomplete SCI. *J Neurol Sci.* 1992;110(1–2):90–98.
5. Hao JX, Xu XJ, Yu YX, Seiger A, Wiesenfeld-Hallin Z. Transient spinal cord ischemia induces temporary hypersensitivity of dorsal horn wide dynamic range neurons to myelinated, but not unmyelinated, fiber input. *J Neurophysiol.* 1992;68(2):384–391.
6. McMahon S, Koltzenburg M, Tracey I, Turk DC. *Wall and Melzack's Textbook of Pain.* 6th ed. Philadelphia: Elsevier/Saunders, 2013.
7. Melzack R, Loeser JD. Phantom body pain in paraplegics: evidence for a central "pattern generating mechanism" for pain. *Pain.* 1978;4(3):195–210.
8. Siddall PJ, McClelland JM, Rutkowski SB, Cousins MJ. A longitudinal study of the prevalence and characteristics of pain in the first 5 years following spinal cord injury. *Pain.* 2003;103(3):249–257.
9. Siddall PJ, Taylor DA, McClelland JM, Rutkowski SB, Cousins MJ. Pain report and the relationship of pain to physical factors in the first 6 months following spinal cord injury. *Pain.* 1999;81(1–2):187–197.
10. Gerhart KA, Johnson RL, Whiteneck GG. Health and psychosocial issues of individuals with incomplete and resolving spinal cord injuries. *Paraplegia.* 1992;30(4):282–287.
11. Mehta S, McIntyre A, Dijkers M, Loh E, Teasell RW. Gabapentinoids are effective in decreasing neuropathic pain and other secondary outcomes after spinal cord injury: a meta-analysis. *Arch Phys Med Rehabil.* 2014;95(11):2180–2186.
12. Dalyan M, Cardenas DD, Gerard B. Upper extremity pain after spinal cord injury. *Spinal Cord.* 1999;37(3):191–195.
13. Que JC, Siddall PJ, Cousins MJ. Pain management in a patient with intractable spinal cord injury pain: a case report and literature review. *Anesth Analg.* 2007;105(5):1462–1473.
14. Jensen MP, Turner JA, Romano JM, Fisher LD. Comparative reliability and validity of chronic pain intensity measures. *Pain.* 1999;83(2):157–162.
15. Hanley MA, Jensen MP, Ehde DM, et al. Clinically significant change in pain intensity ratings in persons with spinal cord injury or amputation. *Clin J Pain.* 2006;22(1):25–31.
16. Kirshblum SC, Waring W, Biering-Sorensen F, et al. Reference for the 2011 revision of the International Standards for Neurological Classification of Spinal Cord Injury. *J Spinal Cord Med.* 2011;34(6):547–554.
17. Saulino M. Spinal cord injury pain. *Phys Med Rehabil Clin N Am.* 2014;25(2):397–410.
18. Finnerup NB, Sang CN, Burchiel KJ, Jensen TS. Treatment of spinal cord injury pain. *Pain Clin Updates.* 2001;IX:1–6.
19. Denkers MR, Biagi HL, Ann O'Brien M, Jadad AR, Gauld ME. Dorsal root entry zone

lesioning used to treat central neuropathic pain in patients with traumatic spinal cord injury: a systematic review. *Spine (Phila Pa 1976)*. 2002;27(7):E177–E184.

20. Finnerup NB, Johannesen IL, Sindrup SH, Bach FW, Jensen TS. Pain and dysesthesia in patients with spinal cord injury: a postal survey. *Spinal Cord*. 2001;39(5):256–262.

21. Turk DC, Rudy TE. Toward an empirically derived taxonomy of chronic pain patients: integration of psychological assessment data. *J Consult Clin Psychol*. 1988;56(2):233–238.

22. Turk DC. Customizing treatment for chronic pain patients: who, what, and why. *Clin J Pain*. 1990;6(4):255–270.

23. Summers JD, Rapoff MA, Varghese G, Porter K, Palmer RE. Psychosocial factors in chronic spinal cord injury pain. *Pain*. 1991;47(2):183–189.

24. Mehta S, McIntyre A, Guy S, Teasell RW, Loh E. Effectiveness of transcranial direct current stimulation for the management of neuropathic pain after spinal cord injury: a meta-analysis. *Spinal Cord*. 2015;53(11):780–785.

21

Brain Infarction (Thalamus and Brainstem)

THEODORE G. ECKMAN AND JIANGUO CHENG

CASE

A 75-year-old man presents to the pain clinic with severe right-sided facial and upper extremity pain. He suffered a cerebrovascular accident (CVA) 5 months ago that resulted in right-sided (predominantly upper extremity) numbness. However, the numbness evolved to include tingling and then to outright pain that is now described as "burning" and "severe." He has a history of hypertension and diabetes mellitus. A thorough neurological exam reveals right-sided motor weakness (upper extremity more than lower extremity). Light touch elicits painful response and light pinprick induces an exaggerated amount of pain. These responses are limited to the right side of the face and upper extremity. A review of prior MRI imaging reveals an old lacunar infarct in the left medial thalamus.

DEFINITION

Central post-stroke pain (CPSP) is a type of central pain syndrome that occurs following a CVA. There are no universally accepted diagnostic criteria for CPSP. At the very minimum, CPSP represents the onset of neuropathic pain within areas of sensory disturbances from a prior CVA. The lesion can affect anywhere in the central nervous system's (CNS) sensory processing pathways, but usually the lesion includes the spinothalamocortical tract and its associated projections (see Figure 21.1). The first clinical condition of CPSP was reported in 1906 by Dejerine and Roussy, in which they described severe hemibody pain contralateral to prior thalamic CVAs.[1] This led to the development of terms such as "thalamic syndrome" and "Dejerine-Roussy syndrome," which is misleading because any part of the spinothalamocortical tract, not just the thalamus, can be involved. In fact, later studies have suggested that approximately only one-fourth to one-third of CPSP cases are attributed

to intrathalamic lesions.[2] Because of the varied locations for the CVA lesions, it is not unexpected that patient presentations and complaints can vary, and different pain descriptors are often used, such as burning, lacerating, numbness, coldness, and stabbing. Allodynia, hyperalgesia, and stimulus-evoked dysesthesia are frequently observed in CPSP, and these clinical findings are considered hallmarks of CPSP as they are representative of central neuropathic pain.

In a broader context, CPSP is a form of post-stroke pain. There are other pain conditions commonly encountered in post-stroke patients including headaches, hemiplegic shoulder pain, contractures, spasticity, and other musculoskeletal pain conditions. Post-stroke patients often suffer from cognitive and expressive difficulties secondary to their stroke. Therefore, the combination of multiple and possibly coexisting causes of pain, cognitive dysfunction, and a latency of onset for CPSP symptoms following the initial stroke confounds the overall clinical picture. It is therefore not surprising that CPSP is most likely underreported and underdiagnosed. CPSP should be considered in any post-stroke patients when their affected side (corresponding to a lesion seen on MRI or CT scan) demonstrates allodynia, hyperalgesia, or stimulus-evoked dysesthesia, when other neuropathic pain syndromes or pain conditions have been excluded.

PATHOPHYSIOLOGY

As previously mentioned, the development of pain following a CVA has been documented for over a century, with Dejerne and Roussy's first description occurring in 1906. Shortly thereafter, Head and Holmes, in 1911, postulated the disinhibition theory to explain the condition.[3] In this theory, injury to the lateral thalamus frees the medial thalamus from its inhibition, thus providing a "disinhibited" state. This was believed

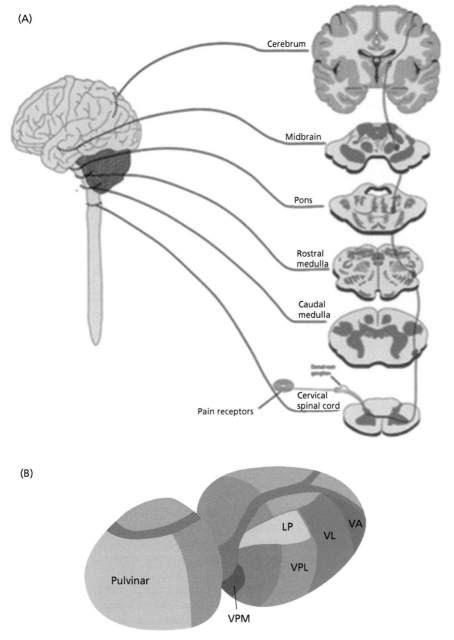

FIGURE 21.1. A. The spinothalamocortical tract. **B.** The nuclei of the thalamus. LP, lateral posterior nucleus; VA, ventral anterior nucleus; VL, ventral lateral nucleus; VPL, ventral posterolateral nucleus; VPM, ventral posteromedial nucleus.

Reprinted with permission from Treister AK, Hatch MN, Cramer SC, et al. Demystifying poststroke pain: from etiology to treatment. *Phys Med Rehab*. 2017;9:63–75, Fig. 1, p. 65.

to provide an explanation for the development of allodynia and spontaneous pain. However, this cannot be the entire story, as sensory deficit alone is insufficient to predict CPSP, by the simple acknowledgment that more than half of patients with thermal sensory deficits do not develop CPSP. Further, it has since been shown that any injury to the spinothalamocortical tract leads to increased activity of the lateral thalamus. In addition to this theory of central disinhibition, both central sensitization and an imbalance of stimuli are thought to also contribute to the onset and maintenance of CPSP; these will be described next.

Central sensitization is both an incompletely understood and complex phenomenon. While lesions can occur anywhere in the spinothalamocortical tract to produce CPSP, the thalamus is profoundly responsible for pain processing and is an important relay center for this tract. There are at least two types of neurons found in the thalamus: relay cells that project to the cerebral cortex, and GABAergic interneurons that produce inhibition.[4] These neurons are collectively responsible for two firing patterns: bursting when the cell membranes are hyperpolarized, and single-spike activity when the cell membranes are depolarized.[5] There is also additional GABAergic inhibition from the dorsal and lateral aspects surrounding the thalamus in the reticular formation. Therefore, a lesion to one of these sensitive areas produces altered metabolic activity that leads to a deviation from the normal nociceptive and sensory processing in this network. The deafferented cells are then capable of generating intrinsic activity, and this provides an explanation and a possible mechanism for spontaneous neuronal activity and, therefore, the onset of central sensitization following a lesion in this area.

As just described, the proposed mechanisms for central disinhibition and central sensitization explain how different components of the spinothalamocortical tract can become hypo- or hyperfunctioning following a lesion that disrupts this delicate pain processing network. It is important to recognize that this altered neuronal activity is accompanied by an alteration in the neurotransmitters that play a fundamental role in neuronal functioning. This is of critical importance, because this provides a rationale for the use of medications to address these neurotransmitters and their interactions with receptors. Thalamic neuronal activity, for example, is under the influence of noradrenergic, serotonergic, and cholinergic input.[4] Norepinephrine from the locus ceruleus and serotonin from the dorsal raphe nuclei have been shown to mediate thalamic burst firing via their reticular and relay nuclei.[6] This provides a rationale for the use of tricyclic antidepressants (TCAs) and selective serotonin and/or norepinephrine reuptake inhibitors (SSRIs/SNRIs). Furthermore, glutamate, an excitatory amino acid neurotransmitter, is thought to mediate both nociceptive and non-nociceptive inputs to the thalamic nuclei,[4] and this likewise provides a rationale for the use of ketamine, an NMDA-receptor antagonist.

In summary, the spinothalamocortical tract and its projections are integral for pain processing, and there are complex interactions (feedback, inhibition, relay, etc.) that govern normal nociceptive and other sensory processing. A CNS lesion in this area disrupts this normal processing and, through the proposed mechanisms (central disinhibition, central sensitization, imbalance of stimuli, etc.), there is the potential onset of CPSP with its hallmark neuropathic features of allodynia, hyperalgesia, and stimulus-evoked dysesthesia. It is important to recognize that this is an incomplete understanding and potentially inaccurate explanation based on the current available information that exists for the onset and the pathophysiology of CPSP. The last pivotal piece of information that explains the clinical aspects that appear for each patient, as well as the diversity of symptoms seen across different patients, is the location of the lesion within the spinothalamocortical tract, discussed further later in the chapter.

EPIDEMIOLOGY

Approximately 795,000 people in the United States suffer a CVA annually. Among these patients, it is unclear how many develop either post-stroke pain or CPSP. The estimates range from as low as 2.8% for the development of CPSP[7] to as high as 74% for the development of post-stroke pain in general.[8] The complicating factors for determining an accurate incidence and prevalence for CPSP in post-stroke patients include the latency of onset of symptoms, comorbid expressive and cognitive dysfunction, comorbid pain conditions, and the lack of universal diagnostic criteria. Nonetheless, most authorities believe the incidence to be 8%–14% for the onset of CPSP following a stroke.[4] Conservatively, this would account for approximately 50,000 new cases of CPSP annually. As there are 7 million stroke survivors in the United States, CPSP is clinically relevant now and expected to be more so in the future with a continuously aging population. Important risk factors associated with the development of CPSP following a CVA include increased stroke severity, previous depression, diabetes mellitus, female gender, alcohol intake, statin use, antithrombotic regimen, and peripheral vascular disease.[7]

CLINICAL FEATURES AND DIAGNOSIS

CPSP is defined as the presence of neuropathic pain within the distribution of somatosensory dysfunction following a CVA with concordant imaging findings, as previously described. It is an important distinction that motor dysfunction does not correlate with pain in CPSP.[2] Some authors suggest that the presence of somatosensory dysfunction is a prerequisite for the diagnosis of CPSP[9]; however, there are no universally agreed upon diagnostic criteria for CPSP. There is often a latency of the pain symptoms following the CVA such that 80% of patients have pain within 2 months and nearly all cases of CPSP have symptoms within 6 months.[4] The contralateral arm and leg, trunk, and face are commonly affected, and the most common pattern is contralateral hemibody (see Figure 21.2). The most common descriptors include burning (more common in younger patients[10]), lacerating, aching, shooting, squeezing, and stabbing. The pain may be spontaneous (continuous or paroxysmal) or evoked (by nociceptive and non-nociceptive stimuli) and variable in both intensity and quality. There is often sparing of joint position and vibration sensations. Allodynia, stimulus-evoked dysesthesia, and hyperalgesia are usually noted on exam. Clinical examination will also demonstrate impaired pinprick, temperature, and touch sensation in most patients that reflects somatosensory involvement.

The location of the lesion along the spinothalamocortical pathway has been shown to be important for the specific characteristics of the pain pattern observed with CPSP. Admittedly, CPSP patients often have multiple lesions that may or may not be the pain generators, thus the following generalizations should be cautiously employed. The first distinction is that thalamic lesions, most notably those involving the ventroposterolateral (VPL) portion of the thalamus, are the most likely to produce pain in a hemibody distribution than any other lesion.[4] The second distinction is between lesions that are supratentorial and those that are infratentorial. Supratentorial lesions are more likely to affect an extremity and have an observed sensory deficit to sharpness or coldness.[4] This is likely because of the predominant involvement of A-delta fibers. Conversely, infratentorial lesions are more likely to affect the face and involve a deficit of temperature sensation and heat pain.[4] This is likely because of the predominant involvement of C fibers.

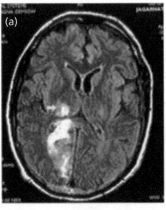

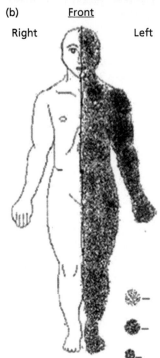

FIGURE 21.2. **A.** Cranial MRI with FLAIR sequence demonstrating right thalamic and occipital region infarct. **B.** Schematic diagram of same patient showing areas of central post-stroke pain (CPSP) with differing severities based on density of black dots.

Reprinted with permission from Kumar B, Kalita J, Kumar G, et al. Central poststroke pain: a review of pathophysiology and treatment. *Anesth Analg.* 2009;108(5):1645–1657, Fig. 3, p. 1648.

Additional distinctions with location concern whether the lateral or medial medulla is involved. Wallenberg syndrome, also known as lateral medullary syndrome, is a classically described lateral medullary wedge infarction that results in a syndrome that can include a combination of dysphagia, slurred speech, ataxia, vertigo, nystagmus, Horner's syndrome, diplopia, and palatal myoclonus, as well as severe facial pain.[4] In fact, 25% of these patients develop severe ipsilateral periorbital pain with or without contralateral limb pain that is described as constant and severe.[11] These lateral medullary lesions often produce pain that is more often described as numbness, burning, and cold.[11] They likely represent dysfunction of both the spinothalamic and trigeminothalamic pathways.[11] In contrast, medial medullary syndrome often spares the spinothalamic pathways (which traverse in the more lateral position in the medulla) and predominantly involves the lemniscal pathways.[12] The pain is often contralateral to the lesion in an extremity; however, there can be ipsilateral features, such as tongue deviation, observed as well. This pain is rarely described as burning whereas other terms, such as numbness, squeezing, and coldness, are often used.[12]

TREATMENT

There are no consensus guidelines for the treatment of CPSP. Often, clinicians resort to using medications that have a history for treating peripheral neuropathic pain conditions that have not been studied in CPSP. Therefore, these treatments are anecdotal and not evidence based. Some practical suggestions for treating CPSP include the following. Address and treat other comorbid pain conditions (hemiplegic shoulder, headaches, etc.) as these conditions, if left untreated, will heighten central pain conditions like CPSP. Start with medications that have the best evidence with the least amount of side effects; progress to using other neuropathic pain medications as necessary. Optimize treatment to address comorbid conditions, such as depression, seizures, or both. Maximize a multidisciplinary care model and seek out additional opinions regarding invasive options when the prior interventions have failed to provide an adequate result. The following few paragraphs will highlight the different pharmacological options for the treatment of CPSP with an emphasis on best available evidence in the literature for this specific condition. This will be followed by a discussion of nonpharmacological therapies available for the treatment of CPSP.

One of the most studied drug classes for the treatment of CPSP is antidepressants. Amitriptyline, a TCA, has evidence

(double-blinded, placebo-controlled, crossover study) for its use in CPSP dating back to 1989.[13] This was a small study ($n = 15$) but demonstrated statistically significant pain reduction with a dose of 75 mg/day. Amitriptyline has also been shown to be helpful with the treatment of other central pain states such as pain seen in spinal cord injury.[14] There have been attempts to delineate whether amitriptyline even has a role for prophylaxis to prevent the onset of CPSP, but the studies have been underpowered and haven't yielded significant results.[15] TCAs are often associated with numerous side effects secondary to a high anticholinergic load (dry mouth, urinary retention, somnolence, confusion, etc.) that may not be tolerated in this elderly population. In addition, TCAs can lower the seizure threshold, which would be undesirable for a CPSP patient who may have post-stroke seizure disorders. However, numerous authors and clinicians suggest amitriptyline as the first-line agent for the treatment of CPSP.[16]

The success and long-standing history of amitriptyline for the treatment of CPSP and other central pain states has contributed to an enthusiasm and willingness to try other antidepressants for treatment. However, data range from being scarce to nonexistent in support of efficacy for most other antidepressants. Certainly, if amitriptyline is not well tolerated, other antidepressants with adrenergic properties (nortriptyline, desipramine, imipramine, doxepin, and venlafaxine) can be used for treatment, but current available data are insufficient to support their efficacy. SSRIs and SNRIs have a pivotal role in the treatment of neuropathic pain in general as they are considered first-line treatment as per the International Association for the Study of Pain's (IASP) neuropathic pain special interest group (NeuPSIG) guidelines.[17] That notwithstanding, the only SSRI with evidence to support its use for the treatment of CPSP is fluvoxamine,[18] but this study only demonstrates mild relief, and only if started within 1 year. However, as is often the case when data are insufficient to provide guidance for which medications to use, most clinicians feel comfortable extrapolating the use of antidepressants for the treatment of CPSP, based on their success with the treatment of peripheral neuropathic pain conditions. This is especially true if comorbid depression is present.

Another medication class that is often employed to treat CPSP is anticonvulsants (antiepileptic medications). Within this class, lamotrigine has the best evidence to support its use for the treatment of CPSP. Lamotrigine is a novel antiepileptic medication that works through presynaptic inhibition of sodium channels and suppression of glutamate release. Two case series and one randomized, double-blinded, placebo-controlled study have demonstrated that lamotrigine can achieve statistically significant pain reduction in CPSP.[19] This was shown with a modest dose of 200 mg/day, and it is believed that higher doses might further result in a dose-dependent pain reduction. Lamotrigine, as is true of some of the other antiepileptic medications, is associated with potentially serious side effects, such as Stevens-Johnson syndrome and agranulocytosis. Therefore, surveillance for these conditions is warranted. While there are some other antiepileptic medications that have shown modest effect with the treatment of CPSP, such as zonisamide, topiramate, and phenytoin, other medications, including carbamazepine, valproic acid, and levetiracetam, have not been consistently shown to provide pain reduction.[16,20]

Two other antiepileptic medications deserve attention because of their association with the treatment of neuropathic pain conditions: gabapentin and pregabalin. The current NeuPSIG guidelines recommend these two medications as first-line therapy for the treatment of neuropathic pain, but studies are limited to suggest their use for the treatment of central neuropathic pain and, specifically, CPSP. Gabapentin has not been studied in the treatment of CPSP. There are, however, numerous other studies to suggest it is a useful adjunct for the treatment of peripheral nerve injury, neuropathic pain syndromes, and central pain from spinal cord injury.[14] On the other hand, pregabalin has been studied in CPSP and the results are mixed. In one randomized, double-blind, controlled trial, pregabalin failed to demonstrate statistically significant pain reduction, but secondary outcome measures (sleep disturbance, anxiety, and global impression of change) were all improved.[21] In a different open-label, 52-week study evaluating pregabalin's effectiveness for treating central pain conditions in which 60% of patients had CPSP, there was a 30% pain reduction observed in 50% of this patient population.[22] Taken together, these studies suggest that pregabalin can potentially decrease pain and improve other metrics seen in patients with CPSP, although the data are modest and comparatively weak compared to data for amitriptyline and lamotrigine.

There are additional medications from a variety of classes that have been used and studied for the treatment of CPSP, with varying degrees of success. Opioid receptor agonists and opioid receptor antagonists have not been shown to improve pain scores, and there is currently an emphasis against the use of opioid receptor agonists for the treatment of neuropathic pain because of the myriad number of undesirable side effects.[14,17] Infusions of lidocaine and ketamine have been shown to be efficacious, especially if patients have comorbid features of complex regional pain syndrome and/or spinal cord injury,[23,24] but optimal dosing, frequency, and length of infusion are still unknown. Intrathecal baclofen also has evidence to support its efficacy for the treatment of CPSP,[25] and this medication should be strongly considered if comorbid spasticity is present. Unfortunately, oral baclofen has not been shown to improve CPSP.[25] There is insufficient evidence to suggest if intrathecal delivery of ziconotide may play a role in the treatment of CPSP; however, this medication is FDA approved for the treatment of neuropathic pain and there is potential for it to be used for this condition. While there is little evidence to suggest benefit for topical medication such as lidocaine and capsaicin, they are low-risk interventions and therefore represent second-line treatment options.[17]

As discussed earlier, there are numerous noninvasive and invasive therapies that can be considered for the treatment of CPSP. There are several surgical procedures such as cordotomy, sympathectomy, and thalamotomy that have been attempted, but none of them have been studied in a controlled fashion, and the pain often returns. These surgical options are not currently recommended.[16] There are other, less invasive therapies such as electrical motor cortex stimulation and repetitive transcranial magnetic stimulation that are gaining more attention. While there is insufficient evidence to suggest they are efficacious, these therapies appear to be mostly benign and with a low-risk profile. Lastly, deep brain stimulation (DBS) has emerged as a potentially viable treatment option. While some authors have declared that DBS is not effective for CPSP, there are new data to support its use. In one study, there was a 53% responder rate for the trial and 58% had long-term pain reduction following implantation.[26] Some of the targets include the periventricular gray matter and the VPL of the thalamus. While the invasiveness of DBS precludes its use early in the treatment of CPSP, there is optimism that this therapy can offer significant pain reduction for CPSP patients.

GUIDING QUESTIONS

- How common is central post-stroke pain (CPSP) following a cerebrovascular accident (CVA)?
- What are important features found in CPSP?
- How would you diagnose CPSP?
- What are the best treatment options for CPSP?

KEY POINTS

- Any lesion caused by a CVA affecting the spinothalamocortical system or its projections has the potential to lead to CPSP.
- There are no universally accepted diagnostic criteria for CPSP, but the condition represents the onset of central neuropathic pain as evidenced by allodynia, hyperalgesia, and stimulus-evoked dysesthesia in an area of sensory disturbance from a prior CVA.
- The pathophysiology and mechanism for CPSP remain unclear, but central disinhibition, central sensitization, and an imbalance of stimuli all appear to be involved in the development and maintenance of pain.
- The highest level of evidence for the treatment of CPSP exists for the use of amitriptyline and lamotrigine.
- Deep brain stimulation, motor cortex stimulation, and repetitive transcranial magnetic stimulation are promising areas of research for potential new treatment modalities.

SUGGESTED READING

Hansson P, Boivie J. Chapter 20: Central neuropathic pain. In: Simpson DM, McArthur JC, Dworkin RH eds. *Neuropathic Pain* .1st ed. New York: Oxford University Press; 2012:339–349.

Kim JS. Pharmacological management of central post-stroke pain: a practical guide. *CNS Drugs.* 2014;28:787–797.

Kumar B, Kalita J, Kumar G, et al. Central poststroke pain: a review of pathophysiology and treatment. *Anesth Analg.* 2009;108(5):1645–1657.

Treister AK, Hatch MN, Cramer SC, et al. Demystifying poststroke pain: from etiology to treatment. *Phys Med Rehab.* 2017;9:63–75.

REFERENCES

1. Dejerine J, Roussy G. Le syndrome thalamique. *Rev Neurol.* 1906;12:521–32.
2. Leijon G, Boivie J, Johansson I. Central post-stroke pain: neurological symptoms and pain characteristics. *Pain.* 1989;6:13–25.
3. Head H, Holmes G. Sensory disturbances from cerebral lesions. *Brain.* 1911;34:102–254.
4. Kumar B, Kalita J, Kumar G, et al. Central poststroke pain: a review of pathophysiology and treatment. *Anesth Analg.* 2009;108(5):1645–1657.
5. Steriade M, Timofeev I, Grenier F, et al. Role of thalamic and cortical neurons in augmenting responses and self-sustained activity: dual intracellular recordings in vivo. *J Neurosci.* 1998;18:6425–6443.
6. McCormick DA, Wang Z. Serotonin and noradrenaline excite GABAergic neurons of the guinea-pig and cate nucleus reticularis thalami. *J Physiol.* 1991;442:235–255.
7. O'Donnell MJ, Diener HC, Sacco RL, et al. Chronic pain syndromes after ischemic stroke: PRoFESS trial. *Stroke.* 2013;44:1238–1243.
8. Murinova N, Creutzfesldt C, Krashin D, Kaye AD. Chapter 3: Patient with poststroke pain. In: Kaye AD, Shah RV. eds. *Case Studies in Pain Management.* 1st ed. Cambridge, UK: Cambridge University Press; 2015:22–29.
9. Hansson P, Boivie J. Chapter 20: Central neuropathic pain. In: Simpson DM, McArthur JC, Dworkin RH eds. *Neuropathic Pain.* 1st ed. New York: Oxford University Press; 2012;339–349.
10. Bowsher D, Leigon G, Thuomas K. Central poststroke pain: correlation of MRI with clinical pain characteristics and sensory abnormalities. *Neurology.* 1998;51:1352–1358.
11. MacGowan DJ, Janal MN, Clark WC, et al. Central poststroke pain in and Wallenger's lateral medullary infarction: frequency, character, and determinants in 63 patients. *Neurology.* 1997;49:120–125.
12. Kim JS, Choi-Kwon S. Sensory sequelae of medullary infarction, differences between lateral and medial medullary syndrome. *Stroke.* 1999;30:2697–2703.
13. Leijon G, Boivie J. Central post-stroke pain: a controlled trial of amitriptyline and carbamazepine. *Pain.* 1989;36:27–36.
14. Rintala DH, Holmes SA, Courtade D, et al. Comparison of the effectiveness of amitriptyline and gabapentin on chronic neuropathic pain in

persons with spinal cord injury. *Arch Phys Med Rehabil.* 2007;88:1547–1560.

15. Lampl C, Yazdi K, Roper C. Amitriptyline in the prophylaxis of central post-stroke pain: preliminary results of 39 patients in a placebo-controlled, long-term study. *Stroke.* 2002;33:3030–3032.

16. Kim JS. Pharmacological management of central post-stroke pain: a practical guide. *CNS Drugs.* 2014;28:787–797.

17. Finnerup NB, Attal N, Haroutounian S, et al. Pharmacotherapy for neuropathic pain in adults: a systematic review and meta-analysis. *Lancet Neurol.* 2015;14:162–173.

18. Shimadozono M, Kawahira K, Kamishita T, et al. Reduction of central poststroke pain with the selective serotonin reuptake inhibitor fluvoxamine. *Int J Neurosci.* 2002;112:1173–1181.

19. Vestergaard K, Anderson G, Gottrup H, et al. Lamotrigine for central poststroke pain: a randomized controlled trial. *Neurology.* 2001;56:184–190.

20. Treister AK, Hatch MN, Cramer SC, et al. Demystifying poststroke pain: from etiology to treatment. *Phys Med Rehabil.* 2017;9:63–75.

21. Kim JS, Bashford G, Murphy TK, et al. Safety and efficacy of pregabalin in patients with poststroke pain. *Pain.* 2011;152:1018–1023.

22. Onouchi K, Koga H, Yokoyama K, et al. An open-label, long-term study examining the safety and tolerability of pregabalin in Japanese patients with central neuropathic pain. *J Pain Res.* 2014;7:439–447.

23. Attal N, Gaude V, Brasseur L, et al. Intravenous lidocaine in central pain: a double-blind, placebo-controlled, psychophysical study. *Neurology.* 2000;54:564–574.

24. Eide PK, Stubhaug A, Stenehjem AE. Central dysesthesia pain after traumatic spinal cord injury is dependent on N-methyl-D-aspartate receptor activation. *Neurosurgery.* 1995;37:1080–1087.

25. Taira T, Tanikawa T, Kawaumura H, et al. Spinal intrathecal baclofen suppresses central pain after a stroke. *J Neurol Neurosurg Psychiatry.* 1994;57:381–382.

26. Bittar RG, Kar-Purkayastha I, Owen SL, et al. Deep brain stimulation for pain relief: a meta-analysis. *J Clin Neurosci.* 2005;12:515–519.

22

Spinal Cord Infarction

RANDALL P. BREWER, SAI MUNJAMPALLI, AND ALIZA KUMPINSKY

CASE

A 59-year-old men presents to the emergency department, complaining of severe mid-thoracic pain after lifting a heavy object. Neurological examination reveals paraplegia without deep tendon reflexes, loss of pain and temperature sensation, and paresthesias to light touch below approximately T10. Proprioception and vibratory sensation are intact. He cannot feel the urge to void and rectal tone and has no cremasteric reflex. MRI scans of the thoracic and lumbar spine show signal hyperintensities on T2-weighted images at T10–12 spinal cord, and anterior spinal artery syndrome from compression by a herniated intervertebral disc is diagnosed. The patient was treated with corticosteroid for spinal cord infarction. After 2 months of physical therapy, he was able to flex both legs without assistance. However, neurological deficit has remained unchanged 1 year after the presumptive diagnosis was made and the patient has developed burning pain in both of his legs.

EPIDEMIOLOGY AND ETIOLOGY

Spinal cord infarctions are rare, comprising approximately 1% of all strokes,[1] but its consequences are devastating. Most patients have at least one vascular risk factor for arteriosclerosis.[2] The incidence of spinal cord infarction has increased with improved surgical advances in the repair of aortic aneurysms. Anterior spinal artery syndrome is the most common neurological complication following repair of the abdominal aorta below the renal arteries.[3] The highest risk relates to the extent of aortic repair, particularly type II aneurysm repair of the entire descending thoracic aorta.[3] During open procedures, clamping of the aorta for greater than 20 to 30 minutes carries the highest risk, although the risk is not eliminated with less invasive approaches.[2] It has been reported that the incidence of spinal cord infarction is 5%–21% after open surgery and 3%–12% after endovascular repair.[4]

Other procedures associated with spinal cord infarction, though less commonly, include spinal surgery, femoral-arterial bypass, and coronary bypass surgery.[4,5] Case reports of transforaminal steroid injections (cervical, thoracic, and lumbar) causing spinal cord infarctions indicate that the infarctions are likely due to injury of the vertebral artery or the radiculomedullary arteries.[6] The embolization of particulate corticosteroids has been implicated in the etiology of vascular occlusion. Surgical procedures that increase thoracic venous pressure, such as ligation of esophageal varices, have been recognized as causes of spinal venous infarction. Measures such as cerebrospinal fluid (CSF) drainage and use of intraoperative monitoring of somatosensory-evoked potentials are purported to reduce spinal ischemic complication rates of aortic surgery.[2,5]

Systemic hypotension is another major precipitant of spinal cord ischemia. Unfortunately, since anoxic encephalopathy overshadows the clinical presentation, the myelopathy can be missed initially. The lumbosacral segment was most commonly at risk in this scenario.[7]

Aortic atherosclerosis can present with intermittent spinal ischemic symptoms, similar to cerebral transient ischemic attacks (TIAs). The symptoms tend to manifest as activity-induced, transient symptoms of myelopathy, and these spinal TIAs may precede spinal cord infarction similar to cerebral TIAs heralding a stroke.[8] Atherosclerotic lesions tend to respond well to aortofemoral bypass procedures.

Thrombosis can cause both acute and stepwise spinal cord dysfunction, and can be embolic or in situ. Known embolic sources include cardiac valves affected by either rheumatic heart disease or bacterial endocarditis; atrial myxoma; nitrogen bubbles from decompression sickness; and iatrogenic emboli from surgical procedures to thrombose renal, bronchial, or dural arteries.[9] Primary thrombosis can stem from a variety of conditions. Culprits include systemic inflammatory conditions such as Crohn's disease, polyarteritis nodosa, and giant cell arteritis. Local inflammation, for example from meningovascular syphilis or bacterial meningitis, can also lead to spinal cord ischemia. Sickle cell disease, intrathecal chemical irritants, vasospastic agents such as cocaine, angiographic contrast material, the postpartum state, and intravascular neoplastic invasion all predispose to thrombosis and spinal cord infarction.[9] Venous infarction without hemorrhage can be seen in association with systemic thrombophlebitis.

Fibrocartilaginous emboli caused by traumatic rupture of intervertebral disks can cause an ischemic syndrome. The elasticity of the nucleus pulposus is reduced with aging and accompanies degenerative changes in the disks.[10] Arterial events are seen in about half of these cases, whereas the remaining cases have mixed arterial and venous involvement. Local fracture from trauma can force the fragments of disk material into the bone marrow sinusoids, thereby increasing pressure into the spinal vertebral plexus and arterial channels and leading to cord infarction.[11]

Radiation therapy can produce myelopathy from occlusive changes in the arterioles of the spinal cord parenchyma. The degree of myelopathy depends on the length of the irradiated segment, total radiation dose, and dose per fraction. Two syndromes have been described: transient (acute) radiation myelopathy and delayed (chronic) radiation myelopathy. The course can be progressive or marked by remissions.[12]

Spinal cord dysfunction can also be caused by hemorrhage into the subarachnoid, subdural, or epidural spaces.[13] The onset is usually sudden and painful. Spinal subarachnoid hemorrhage (SAH) presents with sudden, severe back pain that initially localizes near the level of the bleed. The most common identifiable cause is spinal angioma; others include coarctation of the aorta, rupture of a spinal artery, mycotic and other aneurysms of the spinal artery, vascular malformations, polyarteritis nodosa, spinal tumors, lumbar puncture, blood dyscrasias, and therapeutic thrombolytic and anticoagulant usage.[13] Spinal epidural hemorrhage and spinal subdural hemorrhage are very rare, and the clinical presentation is often similar in both of these

TABLE 22.1. ETIOLOGIES OF SPINAL CORD INFARCTION ACCORDING TO ANATOMICAL LEVEL

Spinal Cord Anatomical Region	Etiologies
Cervical	Steroid injections, vertebral artery dissection, postradiation vasculopathy, fibrocartilaginous emboli, cocaine use, venous thrombosis, coagulopathy, vasculitis
Thoracic	Perioperative, global hypoperfusion, aortic rupture or thrombosis, atherosclerosis, coagulopathy, vasculitis, dural arteriovenous fistula
Lumbar	Perioperative, global hypoperfusion, aortic rupture or thrombosis, atherosclerosis, coagulopathy, vasculitis

conditions. Table 22.1 summarizes the most common etiologies of spinal cord infarction according to anatomical segment.

VASCULAR ANATOMY OF THE SPINAL CORD

The major blood supply of the spinal cord is the anterior spinal artery, which is supplied by the vertebral arteries, the artery of Adamkiewicz, and other anterior radiculomedullary arteries.[1] The rostral origin of the anterior spinal artery comes from the V4 (intradural or intracranial) segment of the vertebral arteries, before they join to form the basilar artery on the brainstem.[2] During embryonic development it is supplied caudally, by the 31 pairs of segmental arteries, at each spinal level.[3] An adult has only six to nine radicular arteries at various locations as most of them degenerate. They enter the spinal cord through the intervertebral foramen, along with the nerve roots and become anterior or posterior radicular arteries, or divide to become both.[14] Sulcal penetrating arteries from the anterior spinal network supply the anterior two-thirds of the spinal cord, which includes the anterior horn and anterior portion of the lateral columns.[15]

The "artery of cervical enlargement" and the "artery of Adamkiewicz" are enlarged radicular arteries present at the cervical and lumbar levels, respectively.

The posterior circulation is supplied by a pair of posterior spinal arteries, which arise from the vertebral arteries or posterior inferior cerebellar arteries (PICA).[15] The posterior spinal arteries are not continuous and consist of extensive feeding vessels, anastomoses, interruptions, and irregular pial circumferential arteries. There are about 18–22 small posterior radicular arteries that supply the posterior spinal arteries and this network supplies the posterior columns and posterior horn.[13] At the caudal end, the conus medullaris is supplied by the "arterial basket" comprising the artery of Adamkiewicz, the anterior spinal artery, and the posterior spinal arteries.

The venous circulation of the spinal cord is a valveless system and is autoregulated by hypoxia/hypercapnea and hypocapnia. It occurs from a network that is formed by the median posterior and anterior spinal veins, which drain into the paravertebral and intravertebral plexi and then into the azygous and pelvic systems.[16]

PATHOPHYSIOLOGY AND LEVELS OF SPINAL CORD INFARCTION

Specific neurovascular syndromes occur due to the anatomy of the spinal vascular supply and involvement of specific blood vessels. The most common of spinal neurovascular syndromes is the anterior spinal artery syndrome (ASAS) caused by infarction in the anterior two-thirds of the cord. This syndrome spares the dorsal columns since they are supplied by the posterior spinal arteries.[17] The clinical picture of ASAS varies with the level of ischemia. Symptoms occur very rapidly and are often experienced within 1 hour of the initial damage, which includes the following:

- Complete motor paralysis below the level of the lesion due to interruption of the corticospinal tract
- Loss of pain and temperature sensation at and below the level of the lesion due to interruption of the spinothalamic tract
- Retained proprioception and vibratory sensation due to intact dorsal columns
- Autonomic dysfunction may be present and can manifest as hypotension (either orthostatic or frank hypotension), sexual dysfunction, and/or bowel and bladder dysfunction.
- Areflexia, flaccid internal and external anal sphincter, urinary retention, and intestinal obstruction may also be present in individuals with anterior cord syndrome.

The loss of motor power usually parallels that of pain because of the anatomical proximity of the pyramidal and spinothalamic tracts in the cord. Transient radicular or back pain may herald these findings and spasticity eventually ensues, with exaggerated deep tendon reflexes, Babinski responses, and clonus. But when ischemia involves the anterior horn cells, nerve roots, or the cauda equina, a case of mixed or lower motor neuron deficits may occur.[17]

Autonomic dysfunction may accompany anterior spinal artery infarctions. Lesions that interrupt innervation to the diaphragm via C3–5 segments may compromise respiration. The urological consequences of complete suprasacral lesions usually include detrusor hyperreflexia and striated sphincter dyssynergia and, if above T-6, smooth sphincter dyssynergia may also occur. Orthostatic hypotension may result from lesions superior to the origin of the greater splanchnic nerve at T4–9. In addition to sexual dysfunction, impairment of vasomotor and sudomotor tone and piloerection may occur below the level of the lesion, leading to impaired thermoregulation. Disinhibited sympathetic neurons of the intermediolateral cell column may mount an exaggerated response to mildly noxious stimuli such as a distended bladder, resulting in the paroxysmal, generalized hypersympathetic state known as spinal dysautonomia.[18]

Spinal cord hemisection, or the Brown-Sequard syndrome, sometimes originates from a lesion obstructing the sulcocommissural artery. It causes ipsilateral paralysis and contralateral loss of spinothalamic sensations, while sparing the dorsal columns.[19]

The posterior spinal arteries supply the posterior 20% to 30% of the cord, including the posterior columns, the posterior aspect of the dorsal horns, and a border zone partially involving the corticospinal and anterolateral tracts. The watershed area between the posterior spinal artery and the anterior spinal artery encompasses the anterior dorsal horns and part of the corticospinal and spinothalamic tracts. This vascular anatomy accounts for not only the profound proprioceptive deficits but also the variable degree of weakness and cutaneous sensory loss in the posterior spinal artery syndrome. Weakness can sometimes be found because the corticospinal tracts lie at the border zone between the anterior and posterior spinal artery territories.[20]

Traditional teaching holds that a midthoracic watershed zone near T-4 is especially vulnerable to hypotensive infarction because of the relative hypovascularity of this region of the spinal cord. A minor watershed area in the distribution of cervical radicular arteries at C-4 and the interface of the anterior and posterior spinal artery territories constitutes a potential intrasegmental watershed zone of uncertain clinical significance.[21]

Spinal TIAs typically manifest as painless paraparesis or quadriparesis (drop attacks) that may be sporadic or associated with postural changes but without loss of consciousness or cranial localizing features. This is most likely to occur in patients with foraminal stenosis during cervical or lumbar extension, which maximally compromises the intervertebral foramina through which spinal radicular arteries pass.[22] Table 22.2 summarizes the presentation of spinal cord infarction syndromes according to vascular patterns.

MANAGEMENT OF ACUTE AND CHRONIC SPINAL CORD INFARCTION

There are no guidelines specific to the treatment of spinal cord infarcts, and acute management is best directed by suspected etiology and symptoms. Many tests can be considered as part of the initial investigation to confirm diagnosis and to investigate the cause. This includes imaging, biochemical and immunological studies from CSF and blood, and spinal angiography.[23] MRI can help in the diagnosis by showing abnormalities such as "pencil-like" hyperintensities, best seen on sagittal T2-weighted images.[24] T2 hyperintensity in the vertebral body has been reported in posterior spinal cord syndrome.[25] These abnormalities are not specific for ischemia, however, as inflammatory conditions can have similar findings.[24] Further testing is guided by clinical suspicion. CSF analysis can be helpful if an autoimmune or inflammatory condition is suspected, such as cell count, protein, and electrophoresis.[26] Hematological studies can include syphilis, Lyme, HIV, cytomegalovirus (CMV), herpes simplex virus (HSV), varicella zoster virus (VZV), enterovirus, Coxsackievirus, adenovirus, and Epstein-Barr virus (EBV).[26]

Acute therapies vary and are best directed by suspected etiology. In the case of abdominal

TABLE 22.2. VASCULAR SYNDROMES OF THE SPINAL CORD

Vascular Syndrome	Vascular Lesions	Neuropathology	Symptoms
Anterior spinal artery syndrome	Vertebral, aorta, radicular branches	Anterior spinal cord infarction (corticospinal, spinothalamic, and anterior horn) with sparing of the dorsal columns	Paraplegia, pain and temperature sensory loss, corticospinal tract findings. Proprioception intact. Dysautonomia, bowel and bladder impairment
Posterior spinal artery syndrome	Diffuse posterior anastomotic network, watershed infarction (hypotension)	Dorsal column and variable central cord infarction (anterior dorsal horn, medial corticospinal and spinothalamic tracts)	Sensory ataxia (profound loss of proprioception), variable weakness, dysautonomia, pain and temperature hypesthesia
Hemicord syndrome of Brown-Sequard	Sulcal-commissural arterial occlusion, radicular arteries (thrombotic, embolic)	Ipsilateral infarction of the spinal cord affecting predominantly anterior tracts and gray matter	Ipsilateral weakness and corticospinal findings, contralateral loss of pain and temperature sensation. Proprioception may remain intact.

aorta aneurysm (AAA) repair, CSF drainage via lumbar drain is used to decrease pressure and increase arterial flow.[27] Reports on efficacy vary. Raising blood pressure and increasing oxygen delivery are also often employed concurrently.[27] Cardiovascular issues in acute spinal cord injury, particularly arrhythmias and fluctuating blood pressures, are common and should be addressed.

In one case series, patients were treated with intravenous (IV) corticosteroids or anticoagulation with heparin without improvement.[6] Patients are also sometimes treated with antiplatelet therapy, typically aspirin.[28] Numerous animal investigations have shown some benefit to various agents, including barbiturates, such as thiopental; free radial scavengers, such as allopurinol and superoxide dismutase; ion channel agents, such as NMDA channels blockers; vasodilators, such as prostacyclin; anesthetics, such as sodium nitroprusside or nitroglycerin; and other agents, such as adenosine and naloxone. However, none of these agents have been proven yet to help in the clinical setting.[29]

The management of deficits associated with chronic myelopathies can be equally challenging. Orthostatic hypotension and other signs of reduced cardiac reflexes are commonly seen. Temperature dysregulation in high cervical and high thoracic injuries is due to the loss of sympathetic control, leading to hyperthermia, hypothermia, or poikilothermia.[30] Autonomic dysreflexia is seen with acute and chronic spinal cord injuries at or above the level of T6.[31] Noxious stimuli below the level of injury can trigger an exaggerated sympathetic response, sometimes leading to hypertensive crises that in extreme cases result in intracranial hemorrhage and seizures. Relatively minor noxious stimuli like bladder distension/calculi, bowel impaction, pressure sores, occult bone fractures, visceral disturbances, or sexual activity are documented triggers. Treatment of the inciting stimulus along with use of antihypertensives (short-acting agents, including topical or sublingual nitrates) may be employed.

Cervical and thoracic spinal cord injury affects respiratory muscles, causing pneumonia from impaired cough and reduced ability to mobilize secretions. These patients are at increased risk for obstructive sleep apnea, chronic respiratory failure, and reduced exercise tolerance due to a compromised pulmonary reserve.[32]

Neurogenic bladder is one of the common sequelae of myelopathies, and all patients with spinal cord injury need an emergent urological evaluation. Bladder function is impaired to a varying degree in patients with spinal cord injury. The most common pathology in spinal cord injury is detrusor hyperreflexia (spastic bladder) with or without sphincter dyssynergia, with typical symptoms of urgency, frequency, and episodic incontinence. Injury to the cauda equina or conus medullaris results in chronic urinary retention from an atonic bladder and overflow incontinence from sphincter incompetence. Intermittent catheterization is the cornerstone of treatment.[33] Pharmacological interventions include anticholinergics or tricyclic antidepressants in patients with detrusor hyperreflexia.[34]

Spasticity is commonly seen in patients with chronic spinal cord injury. This will limit the functional capacity of the individual, as severe chronic spasticity results in pain and dystonic posturing of the paretic limbs.[35]

The functional and management goals for spinal cord injury patients should be individualized.[36] Physiotherapeutic approaches such as stretching and weight-bearing exercises may benefit certain individuals. Interventions to prevent development of contractures are unknown. Positioning, range-of-motion exercises, and splinting have been recommended, but of joints for up to 7 months has not demonstrated clinically meaningful short-term or long-term effects.[36] Commonly used oral medications include baclofen (γ-aminobutyric acid [GABA]B receptor agonist), tizanidine (centrally acting α2-adrenergic agonist), and benzodiazepines (allosteric modulators of GABAA receptors).[37-39] For individuals who do not benefit from oral medications, chemodenervation with botulinum toxin injections and intrathecal delivery of baclofen via an implantable pump are additional therapeutic modalities that can be considered.[37-39] Botulinum toxin injection is FDA approved as a treatment for spastic flexor muscles at the elbow, wrists, and fingers, and is also beneficial for spasms of the hip adductor muscles. An intrathecal baclofen pump may be used in patients with refractory spasticity in the trunk and lower extremities. A combined approach of botulinum toxin, intrathecal baclofen, and general rehabilitative measures has been shown to improve the overall function in nontraumatic myelopathies.

Pain is a common symptom seen in both traumatic and nontraumatic spinal cord injury. About 70% of the patients suffering from nontraumatic myelopathies (due to pathologies such as vascular disease, spinal stenosis, malignant or benign tumors, and infections) report that pain is a problem in daily life.[35] Post–spinal cord injury pain can be classified into two types of pain: nociceptive pain (from non-neural tissue irritation and injury) and neuropathic pain. Patients can experience sensory deficits, allodynia, or hyperalgesia. Treatment for neuropathic pain includes tricyclic antidepressants, gabapentin, pregabalin, or mixed serotonin-noradrenaline reuptake inhibitors.[36] A recent study provided class 1 evidence for pregabalin 150 to 600 mg/day in treatment of pain due to spinal cord injury. Other interventions that have been tried in this population include an intrathecal drug delivery system, neurostimulation techniques, and neuroablation procedures.

Pressure sores occur commonly in myelopathies when the skin and subcutaneous tissue are constantly sheared, reducing regional blood circulation. Prevention is the best treatment for pressure ulcers, and patients at risk should be educated about pressure-relief techniques. Adequate care needs to be taken when transferring the patient, to minimize stress on tissue, and wheelchair cushions can be customized to relieve the pressure.[40]

A variety of other issues are important to be aware of and should also be addressed. The consequences of chronic spinal cord injury include immobility and inactivity, causing an increased risk for coronary artery disease.[41] Gastrointestinal complications associated with these lesions produce a characteristic upper motor neuron bowel syndrome. A bowel routine with a convenient time for evacuation should be established. Dietary regulation, oral medications, rectal suppository, or digital stimulation should be used judiciously.[42] Immobility and medications such as steroids can lead to osteoporosis. Calcium, vitamin D, and bisphosphonates can be used.[43]

PREVENTION OF INTRAOPERATIVE SPINAL CORD ISCHEMIA

Paraplegia is one of the devastating complications of complicated surgeries such as open thoracoabdominal aortic aneurysm (TAAA) repair, endovascular repair of thoracic aortic aneurysm (TEVAR), and spinal interventional procedures. Spinal cord ischemia after thoracic aortic occlusion can be caused by an ischemia-reperfusion injury that may progress to infarction. This can be prevented by neuroprotective interventions that prolong ischemic tolerance and improve spinal cord perfusion, thereby reducing paralysis risk.[44]

Optimizing physiological factors that determine tissue oxygen delivery, such as oxygen saturation, hemoglobin concentration, and cardiac index, and reducing spinal cord oxygen demand are important not only during surgery but also in the immediate postoperative period. These interventions will reduce spinal cord ischemia, when the spinal cord circulation adjusts to the circulatory changes imposed by aortic replacement. Hypoxemia, hypotension, and anemia can compromise oxygen delivery and should be avoided in this setting.[45]

Intensive Neuromonitoring of the Spinal Cord

Serial neurological examination to assess the sensory and motor function in proximal and distal groups of muscles of the lower extremity in an awake patient and neuromonitoring with somatosensory-evoked potentials and motor-evoked potentials in the anesthetized patient help in the detection of spinal cord ischemia in the intraoperative period.[46] Intraoperative monitoring of the transcranial motor-evoked potentials (tcMEPs) by tailoring the anesthetic plan to intervene in a timely fashion will enhance spinal cord perfusion and benefit the spinal cord. Depending on changes of the signals, maintaining a high systemic blood pressure, augmented CSF drainage, and red blood cell transfusion for correction of anemia can maximize spinal cord oxygen delivery.[46]

Spinal Cord Perfusion Pressure and Spinal Fluid Drainage

Animal experiments have shown that, as the central venous pressure (CVP) increases, spinal fluid pressure (SFP) also increases. Lowering the SFP with spinal fluid drainage (SFD) in animal studies caused a reduction in paralysis risk after descending thoracic aortic occlusion.[47] Randomized controlled trials of SFD performed in high-grade aneurysm patients have showed its effectiveness, and by the year 2000, SFD had become the standard of care in most centers doing TAAA surgery; statistically significant results were seen in reducing paralysis risk. The complications of CSF catheter insertion and drainage include infection, catheter fracture, CSF leak, abducens nerve palsy, neuraxial hematoma, and bleeding with hematoma, with subsequent potential epidural or subdural hematoma.[48]

Hypothermia

Hypothermia causes a reduction in metabolic rate and oxygen demand in nervous tissues and prolongs ischemic tolerance. It also stabilizes cell membranes, reduces excitatory neurotransmitter release from ischemic neurons, and blunts hyperemic reperfusion injury.[49] Animal studies showed that hypothermic circulatory arrest, spinal cord cooling, and moderate systemic hypothermia reduce paralysis after aortic occlusion.[49] Based on these studies, most centers performing TAAA surgery now use moderate systemic hypothermia of 32°–34°C, which reduces the risk of paralysis.[50] Other centers have used regional spinal cord cooling and hypothermic circulatory arrest (HCA) with encouraging results. The combined approach of SFD and hypothermia prolongs the ischemic tolerance of the spinal cord by increasing spinal cord perfusion and oxygen delivery.[51,52]

Pharmacological Adjuncts

Spinal cord perfusion is improved with intrathecal papaverine, as it dilates spinal arteries, leading to an increase in the spinal cord blood flow.[53] Other drugs used include anesthetics (barbiturates), which reduce oxygen demand; corticosteroids, which decrease inflammation and stabilize membranes; naloxone, which reduces excitatory amino acid released in ischemia; and mannitol, which scavenges free radicals and reduces intracellular edema. These pharmacological adjuncts offer neuroprotection in animal models of spinal cord ischemia, although clinical studies have not proven the effectiveness of drugs in reducing paralysis risk.

Prevention of Complications during Spinal Intervention

The cardinal risk of cervical and lumbar transforaminal steroid injections is intra-arterial injection. Therefore, a test dose of contrast medium is injected to identify any unintended entry into an artery before any other agent is injected. The commonly used particulate steroids are betamethasone (Celestone), methylprednisolone (Depomedrol), and triamcinolone (Kenalog). They can form aggregates and act as emboli in arterioles if injected into a radicular artery by mistake and cause spinal cord infarction.[54] Dexamethasone sodium phosphate has particles that are approximately 10 times smaller than red blood cells, and the particles do not appear to aggregate even when mixed with 1% lidocaine HCl solution and with contrast medium. For this reason, many physicians commonly use dexamethasone for lumbar transforaminal injections, and studies have shown that its effectiveness is not significantly less than that of the particulate steroids.[54]

Digital subtraction imaging (DSI) is sometimes used, as it shows vascular uptake of contrast medium when used in transforaminal injections. One study showed that the sensitivity of DSI is about 60% compared to about 20% with aspiration. However, DSI is not widely available and increases radiation exposure. Most physicians rely on real-time fluoroscopy to view the images during the injection of contrast medium, lest the fleeting appearance of a small artery escapes notice.[55,56]

FUNCTIONAL RECOVERY AND PROGNOSIS

Recovery after spinal cord injury is variable, as it depends a great deal on the severity of the injury. Much research is aimed at improving outcomes, and there are many ongoing clinical trials focused on enrolling patients with acute or chronic spinal cord injury. Cellular injury triggers a cascade that includes membrane breakdown products such as arachidonic acid, leukotrienes, and thromboxane; excitatory amino acids such as glutamate and aspartate; monoamines; neuropeptides; and cations such as calcium.[57] Areas of research include calcium, as it is present in higher concentrations in injured spinal segments and is thought to regulate neuronal excitation, contribute to modulation of multiple enzymes, and serve an important role in cell death. Glutamate is also being studied, as it plays a role in delayed tissue injury. Oxygen free radical species such as peroxynitrite, and antioxidants such as 21-aminosteroid compounds (lazaroids) and tirilizad mesylate are also being investigated[58] Regulating temperature by induced hypothermia is another area of research.[59]

Another important area of focus is CNS plasticity, including neurogenesis, apoptosis, and sprouting. Earlier research suggested that CNS axons have the ability to regenerate under the right conditions and functional recovery has been shown to be achieved with as little as 5% to 10% of spinal axons surviving injury.[57] GM1 ganglioside and transplanting exogenous cells may promote sprouting and synaptic transmission by exerting their effect through releasing trophic factors and enhancing the local environment. Much research is still needed, including timing, duration, and intensity of therapy, before these modalities become standard of care.[57] Dalfampridine, a potassium channel blocker used in multiple sclerosis, has also been shown to increase voluntary motor unit recruitment and decrease spasticity in persons with spinal cord injury.[58]

Pain is another area of investigation, which is especially important since it is often refractory to medications after spinal cord injury. Besides pharmacotherapy, other means of treating chronic pain that have been used include exercise, behavioral therapy, acupuncture, self-hypnosis, transcutaneous electrical nerve stimulation (TENS), and magnetic stimulation.[60]

Current research involves novel therapies to help with motor function, such as using robotics, exoskeleton-assisted walking devices, functional electrical stimulation (FES), repetitive transcranial magnetic stimulation (rTMS), and precision versus endurance training. Body weight supported treadmill training (BWSTT) is a rehabilitation technique that can be used to promote coordination in walking for those without adequate strength to stand. Use of diaphragm pacing, use of autologous human Schwann cells or spinal cord–derived neural stem cells, and motor stimulators are also being studied. Other issues that are under investigation in patients with spinal cord injury include sleep disorders, cardiovascular disease, fatigue, psychosomatic issues, bladder function, and rehabilitation.

GUIDING QUESTIONS

- What are the important features of the anterior spinal cord syndrome?
- How would you manage neuropathic pain and spasticity from spinal cord infarction?
- What are the most important measures one can take to prevent spinal cord infarction?

KEY POINTS

- Spinal cord infarctions are rare, but the consequences are devastating. It is associated with surgical procedures that compromise oxygen supply to the spinal cord, arteriosclerosis, embolism of the spinal cord circulation, or compression of blood vessels of the spinal cord.
- The most common of spinal neurovascular syndromes is the anterior spinal artery

syndrome (ASAS), caused by infarction in the anterior two-thirds of the cord. This syndrome spares the dorsal columns as the posterior one-third of the spinal cord is supplied by a pair of posterior spinal arteries. It is characterized by complete motor paralysis below the level of the lesion; loss of pain and temperature sensation with sparing of proprioception and vibratory sensation; and autonomic dysfunction, such as hypotension, sexual, and bowel and bladder dysfunction.

- MRI imaging, biochemical and immunological studies from CSF and blood, and spinal angiography can be considered to confirm diagnosis and delineate the cause.
- Treatments are directed at managing motor paralysis and spasticity, sensory dysfunction and pain, and autonomic dysfunction that include neurogenic bladder and autonomic dysreflexia. Cervical and thoracic spinal cord injury affects respiratory muscles, causing pneumonia from impaired cough and reduced ability to mobilize secretions, in addition to autonomic dysreflexia.
- Preventive measures in the intraoperative and immediate postoperative period include neuromonitoring of the spinal cord during abdominal aorta aneurysm surgery, spinal fluid drainage, induced hypothermia, and use of pharmacological adjuncts such as intrathecal papaverine. Precautions in using particulate steroids for transforaminal epidural injection for pain management may help reduce the risk of articular embolism in the spinal cord or brainstem.

REFERENCES

1. Sandson TA, Friedman JH. Spinal cord infarction: report of 8 cases and review of the literature. *Medicine.* 1989;68:282–292.
2. Nedeltchev K, Loher TJ, Stepper F, et al. Long-term outcome of acute spinal cord ischemia syndrome. *Stroke.* 2004;35:560–565.
3. Lintott P, Hafez HM, Stansby G. Spinal cord complications of thoracoabdominal aneurysm surgery. *Br J Surg.* 1998;85:5–15.
4. Robertson CE, Brown RD, Wijdicks EFM, Rabinstein AA. Recovery after spinal cord infarcts: long-term outcome in 115 patients. *Neurology.* 2012;78:114–121.

5. Cheung AT, Pochettino A, McGarvey ML, et al. Strategies to manage paraplegia risk after endovascular stent repair of descending thoracic aortic aneurysms. *Ann Thorac Surg*. 2005;80:1280–1288.

6. Kumar N, ed. Spinal cord, root, and plexus disorders. *Continuum: Lifelong Learning Neurol*. 2008;14(3).

7. Duggal N, Lach B. Selective vulnerability of the lumbosacral spinal cord after cardiac arrest and hypotension. *Stroke*. 2002;33:116–121.

8. Rathmell JP, Benzon HT, Dreyfuss P, et al. Safeguards to prevent neurologic complications after epidural steroid injections: consensus opinion from a multidisciplinary working group and national organizations. *Anesthesiology*. 2015;122(5):974–984.

9. Sliwa JA, Maclean IC. Ischemic myelopathy: a review of spinal vasculature and related clinical syndromes. *Arch Phys Med Rehabil*. 1992;73:365–372.

10. Bockenek WL, Bach JR. Fibrocartilaginous emboli to the spinal cord: a review of the literature. *J Am Paraplegia Soc*. 1990;13:18–23.

11. Toro G, Roman GC, Navarro-Roman L, et al. Natural history of spinal cord infarction caused by nucleus pulposus embolism. *Spine*. 1994;19:360–366.

12. Froscher W, Radiation injury to the spinal cord. *Neurol Psychiatr Grenzgeb*. 1976;44(3):94–135.

13. Kreppel D, Antoniadis G, Seeling W. Spinal hematoma: a literature survey with meta-analysis of 613 patients. *Neurosurg Rev*. 2003;26:1–49.

14. Biglioli P, Roberto M, Cannata A. Upper and lower spinal cord blood supply: the continuity of the anterior spinal artery and the relevance of the lumbar arteries. *J Thorac Cardiovasc Surg*. 2004;127:1188–1192.

15. Novy J, Carruzzo A, Maeder P, Bogousslavsky J. Spinal cord ischemia: clinical and imaging patterns, pathogenesis, and outcomes in 27 patients. *Arch Neurol*. 2006;63:1113–1120.

16. Crum B, Mokri B, Fulgham J. Spinal manifestations of vertebral artery dissection. *Neurology*. 2000;55:304–306.

17. Cheshire WP, Santos CC, Massey EW, Howard, JF. Spinal cord infarction: etiology and outcome. *Neurology*. 1996;47:321–330.

18. Foo D, Rossier AB. Anterior spinal artery syndrome and its natural history. *Paraplegia*. 1983;21(1):1–10. doi:10.1038/sc.1983.1.PMID 6835686.

19. Low PA, Dyck PJ. Pathologic studies and the nerve biopsy in autonomic neuropathies. In: Low PA, ed. *Clinical Autonomic Disorders*. Boston: Little Brown; 1993:331–344.

20. Brown-Sequard CE. De la transmission croisee des impressions sensitives par la moelle epiniere. *C R Sac Biol (Paris)*. 1850;2:70.

21. Bergqvist CA, Goldberg HI. Posterior cervical spinal cord infarction following vertebral artery dissection. *Neurology*. 1997;48(4):1112–1115.

22. Ziilch KJ, Kurth-Schumacher R. The pathogenesis of intermittent spinovascular insufficiency (spinal claudication of Dejerine) and other vascular syndromes of the spinal cord. *Vasc Surg*. 1970;4:116–136.

23. De la Barrera SS, Barca-Buyo A, Montoto-Marqués A, Ferreiro-Velasco ME, Cidoncha-Dans M, Rodriguez-Sotilla A. Spinal cord infarction: prognosis and recovery in a series of 36 patients. *Spinal Cord*. 2001;39:520–525.

24. Weidauer S, Nichtweiss M, Lanfermann H, Zanella FE. Spinal cord infarction: MR imaging and clinical features in 16 cases. *Neuroradiology*. 2002;44:851–857.

25. Suzuki T, Kawaguchi S, Takebayashi T, Yokogushi K, Takada J, Yamashita T. Vertebral body ischemia in the posterior spinal artery syndrome: case report and review of the literature. *Spine*. 2003;28:E260–E264.

26. Nedeltchev K, Loher TJ, Stepper F, et al. Long-term outcome of acute spinal cord ischemia syndrome. *Stroke*. 2004;35:560–565.

27. Coselli JS, LeMaire SA, Köksoy C, Schmittling ZC, Curling PE. Cerebrospinal fluid drainage reduces paraplegia after thoracoabdominal arotic aneurysm repair: results of a randomized clinical trial. *J Vasc Surg*. 2002;35:631–639.

28. De Seze J, Stojkovic T, Breteau G, et al. Acute myelopathies: clinical, laboratory, and outcome profiles in 79 cases. *Brain*. 2001;124:1509–1521.

29. Lintott P, Hafez HM, Stansby G. Spinal cord complications of thoracoabdominal aneurysm surgery. *Br J Surg*. 1998;85:5–15.

30. Hagen E, Rekand T, Grenning M, Faerstrand S. Cardiovascular complications of spinal cord injury. *Tidsskr Nor Legeforen*. 2012;132(9):1115–1120. doi:10.4045/tidsskr.11.0551.

31. Furlan JC. Autonomic dysreflexia: a clinical emergency. *J Trauma Acute Care Surg*. 2013;75(3):496–500. doi:10.1097/TA0b013e31829fda0a.

32. Tollefsen E, Fodenes O. Respiratory complications associated with spinal cord injury. *Tidsskr Nor Legeforen*. 2012;132(9):1111–1114. doi:10.4045/tidsskr.10.0922

33. Jamison J, Maguire S, McCann J. Catheter policies for management of long term voiding problems in adults with neurogenic bladder disorders. *Cochrane Database Syst Rev*. 2013;11:CD0004375. doi:10.1002/14651858.CD004375.pub2.

34. Madersbacher H, Murtz G, Stohrer M. Neurogenic detrusor overactivity in adults: a review on efficacy, tolerability and safety of oral antimuscarinics. *Spinal Cord*. 2013;51(6):432–441. doi:10.1038/sc.2013.19.

35. Werhagen L, Hulting C, Molander C. The prevalence of neuropathic pain after non-traumatic spinal cord lesion. *Spinal Cord.* 2007;45(9):609–615. doi:10.1038/sj.sc.3102000.

36. Finnerup NB, Baastrup C. Spinal cord injury pain: mechanisms and management. *Curr Pain Headache Rep.* 2012;16(3):207–216. doi:10.1046/j.1351-5101-2003.2003.00725.x.

37. Elbasiouny SM, Moroz D, Bakr MM, Mushahwar VK. Management of spasticity after spinal cord injury: current techniques and future directions. *Neurorehabil Neural Repair.* 2010;24(1):23–33. doi:10.1177/1545968309343213.

38. Shakespeare DT, Bogglid M, Young C. Antispasticity agents for multiple sclerosis. *Cochrane Database Syst Rev.* 2003;4:CD001332. doi:10.1002/14651858.CD001332.

39. Strommen JA. Management of spasticity from spinal cord dysfunction. *Neurol Clin.* 2013;31(1):269–286. doi:10.1016/j.ncl.2012.09.013.

40. Kruger EA, Pires M, Ngann Y, et al. Comprehensive management of pressure ulcers in spinal cord injury: current concepts and future trends. *J Spinal Cord Med.* 2013;36(6):572–585. doi:10.1179/2045772313Y.0000000093.

41. Nash MS, Cowan RE, Kressler J. Evidence-based and heuristic approaches for customization of care in cardiometabolic syndrome after spinal cord injury. *J Spin Cord Med.* 2012;35(5):278–292. doi:10.1197/2045772312Y.0000000034.

42. Coggrave M, Norton C, Cody JD. Management of faecal incontinence and constipation in adults with central neurological diseases. *Cochrane Database Syst Rev.* 2014;1:CD002115. doi:10.1002/14651858.CD002115.pub3.

43. Battaglino RA, Lassari AA, Garshick E, Morse LR. Spinal cord injury-induced osteoporosis: pathogenesis and emerging therapies. *Curr Osteoporos Rep.* 2012;10(4):278–285. doi:10.1007/s11914-012-0117-0.

44. Wynn M, Acher CW. A modern theory of spinal cord ischemia/injury in thoracoabdominal aortic surgery and its implications for prevention of paralysis. *J Cardiothorac Vasc Anesth.* 2014;28(4):1088–1099.

45. Acher CW, Wynn MM, et al. Cardiac function is a risk factor for paralysis in thoracoabdominal aortic replacement. *J Vasc Surg.* 1998;27:821–828; discussion 829–830.

46 Drenger B, Parker SD, McPherson RW, et al. Spinal stimulation evoked potentials during thoracoabdominal aortic aneurysm surgery. *Anesthesiology.* 1992;76:689–695.

47. Miyamoto K, Ueno A, Wada T, Kimoto S. A new and simple method of preventing spinal cord damage following temporary occlusion of the thoracic aorta by draining the cerebrospinal fluid. *J Cardiovasc Surg.* 1960;1:188–197.

48. Youngblood SC, Tolpin DA, LeMaire SA, Coselli JS, Lee VV, Cooper JR Jr. Complications of cerebrospinal fluid drainage after thoracic aortic surgery: a review of 504 patients over 5 years. *J Thorac Cardiovasc Surg.* 2013;146:166–171.

49. Rokkas CK, Cronin CS, Nitta T, Helfrich LR Jr, Lobner DC, Choi DW, Kouchoukos NT. Profound systemic hypothermia inhibits the release of neurotransmitter amino acids in spinal cord ischemia. *J Thorac Cardiovasc Surg.* 1995;110:27–35.

50. Parrino PE, Kron IL, Ross SD, et al. Retrograde venous perfusion with hypothermic saline and adenosine for protection of the ischemic spinal cord. *J Vasc Surg.* 2000;32:171–178.

51. Conrad MF, Ergul EA, Patel VI, et al. Evolution of operative strategies in open thoracoabdominal aneurysm repair. *J Vasc Surg.* 2011;53:1195–1201:(e1191).

52. Acher CW, Wynn M. A modern theory of paraplegia in the treatment of aneurysms of the thoracoabdominal aorta: an analysis of technique specific observed/expected ratios for paralysis. *J Vasc Surg.* 2009;49:1117–1124; discussion 1124.

53. Lima B, Nowicki ER, Blackstone EH, et al. Spinal cord protective strategies during descending and thoracoabdominal aortic aneurysm repair in the modern era: the role of intrathecal papaverine. *J Thorac Cardiovasc Surg.* 2012;143:945–952.

54. Derby R, Lee SH, Date ES, Lee JH, Lee CH. Size and aggregation of corticosteroids used for epidural injections. *Pain Med.* 2008;9:227–234.

55. Landers MH, Dreyfuss P, Bogduk N. On the geometry of fluoroscopy views for cervical interlaminar epidural injections. *Pain Med.* 2012;13:58–65.

56. Maus T, Scheueler BA, Leng S, Magnuson D, Magnuson DJ, Diehn FE. Radiation dose incurred in the exclusion of vascular filling in transforaminal epidural steroid injections: Fluoroscopy, digital subtraction angiography, and CT/fluoroscopy. *Pain Med.* 2014;15:1328–1333.

57. LiVecchi MA. Spinal cord injury. *Continuum.* 2011;17(3):568–583.

58. de Haan P, Kalkman CJ, Jacobs MJHM. Pharmacology neuroprotection in experimental spinal cord ischemia. *J Neurosurg Anesthesiol.* 2001;13(1):3–12.

59. Dombovy ML. Introduction: the evolving field of neurorehabilitation. *Continuum.* 2011;17(3):443–448.

60. Boldt I, Eriks-Hoogland I, Brinkhof MWG, de Bie R, Joggi D, von Elm E. Non-pharmacological interventions for chronic pain in people with spinal cord injury. *Cochrane Database Syst Rev.* 2014;11:CD009177.

23

Syringomyelia

ASHWIN VARMA, TIMOTHY BEDNAR, AND GULSHAN DOULATRAM

CASE

A 45-year-old woman presents with pain on the right side of the neck and scapular region with radiation to the entire right forearm; she has had this pain for 10 years. She describes the pain as burning and sharp and it is triggered by activity and changes in temperature. In addition to her pain complaint, she also presents with headaches, numbness in her arms, muscle weakness and atrophy, as well as stiffness and spasms in her arms, back, and legs. The patient has experienced significant limitations in activities of daily living and difficulty sleeping as a result of her pain. On examination she has no skin or color changes but has significant allodynia in her right arm and shoulder and in her neck. The patient has a history of Arnold Chiari malformation type 1, for which she underwent cervical decompression surgery 4 years ago. An MRI scan shows syringomyelia in her C5 through T2 spinal cord.

DEFINITION

Syringomyelia is defined as a cavitation of the central canal of the spinal cord. It is most commonly congenital in origin (90%) and associated with type 1 Arnold Chiari malformation. The syrinx is usually located in the lower cervical and upper thoracic spinal cord[1] but can extend to the brainstem (syringobulbia). Type 1 Chiari malformation involves the caudal displacement of the cerebellar tonsils through the foramen magnum with resultant brainstem compression in some individuals. When not congenital, syringomyelia is associated with trauma, infections, and intramedullary spinal cord tumors.[2,3] Traumatic causes of syringomyelia are almost always accompanied by spinal cord injury (SCI).

PATHOPHYSIOLOGY

The syrinx initially develops in the deeper layers of the dorsal horn and progresses outward to the rest of the cord.[4] This damage to the spinal cord causes the neuropathic pain symptomatology of syringomyelia. The imbalance of nociceptive output due to selective injury to different layers of the dorsal horn may explain the neuropathic pain features, including spontaneous and evoked pain so commonly seen in syringomyelia.[5] Anatomical changes in the dorsal horn cause subsequent neurochemical changes[6], including increased expression of substance P, an undecapeptide member of the tachykinin neuropeptide family, in lamina I, II, III, and V, which can cause changes in modulation and perception of pain.[7,8] Inhibitory transmitters such as GABA may be reduced further, causing an imbalance within the dorsal horn toward increased pronociception.[8] Activation of the neuroimmune system through glial cell–mediated production of cytokines such as interleukin 1 is seen in patients with spinal cord injury.[9]

Involvement of the spinothalamic tracts by the syrinx cavity is also thought to be responsible for pain.[8] The size of the syrinx does not correlate to intensity of neuropathic pain. The location of syrinx also does not correlate to the distribution of symptoms. It has been speculated that the extension of syrinx, rather than the size, influences the severity of symptoms. Paracentral extensions always cause more pain, but may be more amenable to spinal cord stimulation due to sparing of central areas. On the other hand, central syringomyelia may preclude placement of leads or catheters because of narrowing of the vertebral canal, as with central spinal stenosis.

Worsening spasticity is attributable to increasing involvement of the descending corticospinal tracts. Atrophy and fasciculations indicate involvement of the anterior horn cell columns by the syrinx. Pain may persist even when spinothalamic functions (pinprick and thermal sensation) have been completely abolished. In an interesting study looking at syringomyelia patients with and without pain, it was found that the extent of thermal sensory loss was not different between patients with and without pain, thus suggesting that a lesion of the spinothalamic system, though it may be necessary, is not sufficient to drive the pain.[8] In the same study, a direct relationship was found between the degree of thermosensory deficit and the intensity of burning pain in patients with syringomyelia, which suggests that deafferentation or loss of input into a central projection territory may be a driving mechanism for the spontaneous pain.

EPIDEMIOLOGY

The prevalence of syringomyelia and syringobulbia is between 3 and 8 per 100,000 persons. A prevalence of 8.2 per 100,000 and higher has been reported for certain ethnic groups, probably because of use of better neuroimaging techniques in these groups.[10]

CLINICAL FEATURES AND DIAGNOSIS OF SYRINGOMYELIA

Central neuropathic pain is considered the most important symptom in syringomyelia.[11] Chronic pain is a common feature in adults diagnosed with syringomyelia. Various pain types have been described, including central, neuropathic, and dysesthetic pain. Dysesthetic pain, often described as burning pain, pins and needles, or stretching of the skin, is a prominent feature seen in nearly half of patients. Most patients have spontaneous pain, although evoked neuropathic pain can also be present.[9] Patients may have sensory loss in dysesthetic areas.[12] Paraplegia or quadriplegia is usually present in patients who have syringomyelia associated with trauma-related spinal cord injury. These patients may also have secondary spasticity, numbness, and atrophy along with severe neuropathic pain. Patients with a cervical syrinx will have burning pain, allodynia, hyperalgesia, and numbness along unilateral or bilateral multiple cervical root distributions. Involvement of the descending trigeminal tract and nucleus by the syrinx will present as ipsilateral neuropathic facial pain. A syrinx in the thoracic spine will present as neuropathic pain in a trunk or abdominal distribution, along with myelopathy, spasticity, and urinary retention. Involvement of the conus medullaris primarily manifests as sacral neuropathic pain and urinary retention. Besides pain,

the other primary symptom in some patients could be myopathy. Electromyography (EMG) shows a mixture of shortened and prolonged action potentials in syringomyelia. Somatosensory-evoked potential (SEP) may be useful in the electrodiagnosis of syringomyelia.[13] Headaches may be present in patients with syringomyelia associated with type 1 Arnold-Chiari malformation. MRI plays a key role in the diagnosis of syringomyelia.

In some isolated cases, temporomandibular joint dysfunction, fibromyalgia, and complex regional pain syndrome can occur and are thought to be due to direct compression of the medulla and altered sensory processing.[14]

TREATMENT

The definitive treatment of syringomyelia is surgical decompression, especially for a progressive or a large syrinx. Surgical treatment of syringomyelia involves neurosurgical drainage of the syrinx or surgical resection of a spinal cord tumor, or both. Syrinx drainage is primarily performed to limit neurological progression, and placement of ventricular shunts may be beneficial in the presence of communicating syringomyelia or secondarily in non-communication disease with cerebrospinal fluid (CSF) obstruction. Persistence of central pain following drainage of the syrinx is very common owing to compromise of the dorsal horn.

Given the complex pathophysiology of this disease, the approach to medical treatment of syringomyelia is multifaceted and relies on medications from various classes and mechanisms. Improved knowledge of the causative factors of syringomyelia and the use of MRI have led to advancements in both the classification of the disease and treatment modalities. Traditionally, treatment has been symptom based, involving medications such as anticonvulsants, antidepressants, and local anesthetics. However, continued advancements in the understanding of spinal cord stimulation and intrathecal drug administration may provide additional methods to treat syringomyelia.[15] Medical treatment of the central neuropathic pain associated with syringomyelia is often associated with only partial efficacy and a high frequency of treatment-refractory cases.

Pharmacological Treatment
Anticonvulsants

These include the traditional agents, such as carbamazepine and valproate, and newer agents, such as gabapentin and pregabalin. Carbamazepine, phenytoin (Dilantin), and valproate are some of the older anticonvulsants that have been used to treat neuropathic pain. There are not too many studies testing these drugs specifically for syringomyelia.[16] Patients should have detailed laboratory tests including blood urea nitrogen, creatinine, transaminase, iron levels, a complete blood count (including platelets), reticulocyte count, and liver function test. Carbamazepine also can cause dermatological reactions, such as toxic epidermal necrolysis and Stevens-Johnson syndrome. In light of the array of adverse effects, newer anticonvulsants are preferred.

Gabapentin and pregabalin are analogs of the neurotransmitter gamma-aminobutyric acid (GABA) and bind the alpha2-delta (a2-d) unit of calcium channels, reducing calcium influx at nerve terminals. This reduces the release of several neurotransmitters, including glutamate, noradrenaline, and substance P. The major side effects reported from gabapentin include sedation and dizziness. The major drawback is the poor bioavailability of the drug, requiring high doses. Pregabalin is usually well tolerated and has a good safety profile. Common side effects include somnolence, dizziness, weight gain, and peripheral edema, which rarely require stopping the medication. Pregabalin has the advantage of improving mood and sleep and thus addresses the interaction of chronic pain, sleep loss, and mood disturbance in patients with syringomyelia.

Antidepressants

Tricyclic antidepressants (TCASs) such as amitriptyline and nortriptyline are effective in treatment of syringomyelia-associated neuropathic pain through their central modulation of inhibitory pathways.[17] They are not tolerated well by patients because of effects on α-adrenergic, H1-histamine, muscarinic cholinergic, and N-methyl-D-aspartate receptors. Some of the adverse effects reported with TCAs include orthostatic hypotension, cardiac arrhythmias, dizziness, and sedation. TCAs are contraindicated in patients with heart failure, arrhythmias, or recent myocardial infarction. Because of the anticholinergic effects of TCAs, physicians should be cautious when prescribing them for patients with narrow-angle glaucoma, benign prostatic hypertrophy, orthostasis, urinary retention, impaired liver function, or thyroid disease. The QTc interval should be assessed because of the risk of torsades de pointes.

Serotonin-norepinephrine reuptake inhibitors (SNRIs), including venlafaxine and duloxetine, are also used in the treatment of neuropathic pain.[17] Both are dual reuptake inhibitors of serotonin and norepinephrine transporters. Duloxetine has been shown to be both effective and well tolerated. Some of the side effects include somnolence, nausea, dizziness, decreased appetite, and constipation. When compared to TCA, duloxetine can be safely prescribed to patients with concomitant cardiovascular problems.

A useful adjunct to antidepressants and anticonvulsants is 5% lidocaine, a sodium channel blocker. It is used for patients with painful sensory neuropathy with allodynia and dysesthesia.

Tramadol and Opioids

Tramadol acts at both the opioid receptor and serotonin/norepinephrine receptor and can be useful in some patients not responding to other treatment. However, tramadol and other opioids should be used only as a second-line drug after first-line treatments either alone or in combination are found to be ineffective.[17] The side effects of tramadol are related to both its opioid and serotonergic effects. Constipation, respiratory depression, lowered seizure threshold, somnolence, and serotonin syndrome, especially in patients taking concomitant antidepressants, can occur.

Nonpharmacological Treatment
Sympathetic Blocks

Given the similarities in features of dysesthetic pain seen in syringomyelia and those of complex regional pain syndrome, sympatholytic treatment has been reported in case reports as a successful alternative treatment in syringomyelia.

Spinal Cord Stimulation

The use of spinal cord stimulation (SCS) in the treatment of syringomyelia is reserved for patients with refractory neuropathic pain.[18] Patient selection and localization of the syrinx are key factors in determining whether SCS could be beneficial. Optimal patients for SCS implantation are those in whom the cavitation is lateralized near a dorsal horn and the vertebral canal is not narrowed. Patients with paracentral and eccentric cavities also tend to have more unilateral neuropathic pain. In carefully selected patients and with optimal placement of the electrodes, SCS has the potential to relieve the central, neuropathic, and dysesthetic pain associated with syringomyelia. Although additional research and further clinical studies are necessary, SCS may prove to be a cost-effective means of reducing pain and increasing patient satisfaction when the pain does not respond to traditional treatment.

Patients with lateralized cavitation to the dorsal horn observed on MRI and with pain concordant with spinal cord level may be ideal candidates for treatment with SCS. However, if central cavitation renders an enlarged spinal cord diameter or if there is a relatively narrow vertebral canal, SCS electrode implantation would be contraindicated.

GUIDING QUESTIONS

- What is syringomyelia, and how it is related to neuropathic pain?
- What are the major pathophysiological changes of syringomyelia?
- How do you manage neuropathic pain in patients with syringomyelia?

KEY POINTS

- Syringomyelia is dilation of spinal canal and can be either congenital or post-traumatic. It is associated with central pain with predominantly neuropathic pain–like qualities. The size of the syrinx does not correlate to the severity of pain.
- Damage to the deeper layers of the dorsal horn causes an imbalance between the inhibitory and excitatory stimuli with upregulation of substance P.
- Medical treatment is multifaceted and can be unsuccessful in treating neuropathic pain. Surgical treatment is the definitive treatment, though symptoms of pain may persist after resection. Spinal cord stimulation may offer relief to some patients and can be considered for treatment as long as the dimensions of the vertebral canal are not significantly compromised.

REFERENCES

1. Milhorat TH, Capocelli AL Jr, Anzil AP, Kotzen RM, Milhorat RH. Pathological basis of spinal cord cavitation in syringomyelia: analysis of 105 autopsy cases. *J Neurosurg.* 1995;82:802–812.
2. Stubbs RS. Definitions and anatomic considerations in Chiari I malformation and associated syringomyelia. *Neurosurg Clin North Am.* 2015; 26(4):487–493.
3. Milhorat TH. Classification of syringomyelia. *Neurosurg Focus.* 2000;8(3):E1.
4. Rusbridge C, Greitz D, Iskandar BJ. Syringomyelia: current concepts in pathogenesis, diagnosis, and treatment. *J Vet Intern Med.* 2006;20(3):469–479.
5. Cronin JN, Bradbury EJ, Lidierth M. Laminar distribution of GABAA- and glycine-receptor mediated tonic inhibition in the dorsal horn of the rat lumbar spinal cord: effects of picrotoxin and strychnine on expression of Fos-like immunoreactivity. *Pain.* 2004;112:156–163.
6. Todor DR, Mu HT, Milhorat TH. Pain and syringomyelia: a review. *Neurosurg Focus.* 2000;8(3):E11. Review.
7. DeLeo, JA, Yezierski, RP, The role of neuroinflammation and neuroimmune activation in persistent pain. *Pain.* 2001;90:1–6.
8. Cronin, JN, Bradbury, EJ, Lidierth, M. Laminar distribution of GABAA- and glycine-receptor mediated tonic inhibition in the dorsal horn of the rat lumbar spinal cord: effects of picrotoxin and strychnine on expression of Fos-like immunoreactivity. *Pain.* 2004;112:156–163.
9. Ducreux D, Attal N, Parker F, Bouhassira D. Mechanisms of central neuropathic pain: a combined psychophysical and fMRI study in syringomyelia. *Brain.* 2006;129:963–976.
10. Brickell KL, Anderson NE, Charleston AJ, Hope JK, Bok AP, Barber PA. Ethnic differences in syringomyelia in New Zealand. *J Neurol Neurosurg Psychiatry.* 2006;77(8):989–991.
11. Attal N, Bouhassira D. Pain in syringomyelia/bulbia. *Handb Clin Neurol.* 2006;81:705–713.
12. Milhorat TH, Kotzen RM, Mu HT, Capocelli AL Jr, Milhorat RH. Dysesthetic pain in patients with syringomyelia. *Neurosurgery.* 1996;38(5):940–946.
13. Wagner W, Perneczky A, Mäurer JC, Hüwel N. Intraoperative monitoring of median nerve somatosensory evoked potentials in cervical syringomyelia: analysis of 28 cases. *Minim Invasive Neurosurg.* 1995;38(1):27–31.
14. Thimineur M, Kitaj M, Kravitz E, Kalizewski T, Sood P. Functional abnormalities of the cervical cord and lower medulla and their effect on pain: observations in chronic pain patients with incidental mild Chiari I malformation and moderate to severe cervical cord compression. *Clin J Pain.* 2002;18(3):171–179.
15. O'Hagan BJ. Neuropathic pain in a cat post-amputation. *Aust Vet J.* 2006;84:83–86.
16. Kremer M, Salvat E, Muller A, Yalcin I, Barrot M. Antidepressants and gabapentinoids in neuropathic pain: mechanistic insights. *Neuroscience.* 2016;338:183–206.

17. Baron R, Binder A, Wasner G. Neuropathic pain: diagnosis, pathophysiological mechanisms, and treatment. *Lancet Neurol.* 2010;9(8):807–819.

18. Campos WK, Almeida de Oliveira YS, Ciampi de Andrade D, Teixeira MJ, Fonoff ET. Spinal cord stimulation for the treatment of neuropathic pain related to syringomyelia. *Pain Med.* 2013;14(5):767–768.

24

Multiple Sclerosis

SAMUEL W. SAMUEL AND JIANGUO CHENG

CASE

A 40-year-old female5 presents for evaluation of her pain and long-term neurological complaints. She has heat intolerance, a stumbling gait, and a tendency to fall. Her visual acuity has changed periodically over the last 4 years. At times, she has significant tremors and severe exhaustion. She also complains of arthralgia on the right and burning pain and pins-and-needle sensation on the left side of her body. She has recently developed a right hemisensory deficit. An MRI scan reveals a multifocal white matter disease—areas of increased T2 signal in both cerebral hemispheres. Spinal tap shows the presence of oligoclonal bands in the cerebrospinal fluid. Visual-evoked response testing is abnormal with slowed conduction in optic nerves.

DEFINITION

Multiple sclerosis (MS) is a chronic, autoimmune inflammatory neurological disease of the central nervous system (CNS).[1,2] MS attacks the myelinated axons in multiple foci of the CNS, destroying the myelin and the axons to varying degrees.[3,4] The course of MS is highly varied and unpredictable. In most patients, the disease is characterized initially by episodes of reversible neurological deficits, which is often followed by progressive neurological deterioration over time. The disease is diagnosed on the basis of clinical findings and supporting evidence from ancillary tests, such as magnetic resonance imaging (MRI) of the brain and spinal cord and examination of the cerebrospinal fluid (CSF).

EPIDEMIOLOGY AND ETIOLOGY

About 2.3 million people have MS in the world, with 250,000 to 350,000 patients in the United States.[5] About 50% of patients will need help walking within 15 years after onset of the disease.[6] Women are affected twice as much as men. Caucasians appear to be at highest risk for MS.[2,7] MS typically presents in adults 20–45 years of age; occasionally, it presents in childhood or in late middle age.[7] Genetic predisposition as well as nongenetic triggers such as viruses and metabolic or environmental factors are proposed as the causation of MS.[7] It is estimated that 75% of patients with MS have experienced pain, which is the most commonly treated symptom in MS patients, accounting for 30% of all symptomatic treatment.[8]

CLINICAL FEATURES AND DIAGNOSIS

MS can be classified into four main categories, based on the clinical features of the disease[2]:

(1) *Relapsing remitting MS* is the most common form, affecting about 85% of patients with MS. It is marked by flare-ups (relapses or exacerbations) of symptoms followed by periods of remission, when symptoms improve or disappear.

(2) *Secondary progressive MS* may develop in some patients with relapsing-remitting disease. For many patients, treatment with disease-modifying agents helps delay the progression. The disease course continues to worsen with or without periods of remission or leveling off of symptoms severity (plateaus).

(3) *Primary progressive MS* affects approximately 10% of patients with MS. Symptoms continue to worsen gradually from initiation of the disease. No relapses or remissions are observed but occasional plateaus are possible. This form of MS tends to be more resistant to treatment.

(4)   *Progressive-relapsing MS* is a rare from, affecting about 5% of patients. It is progressive from the start with intermittent flare-ups of worsening symptoms along the way. There are no periods of remission.

There is no single diagnostic test for MS.[2] The diagnosis is based on evidence of the following:

(1)   At lease two different lesions (plaques or scars) of the CNS (the space dissemination criterion)

(2)   At least two different episodes in the disease course (the time dissemination criterion)

(3)   Chronic inflammation of the CNS, as determined by analysis of the CSF (the inflammatory criterion)

The presence of one or more of these criteria allows for the general diagnosis of MS, which may be further subcategorized depending on the course of the disease. To make an MS diagnosis the physician must[2]

- Find evidence of damage in at least two separate areas of the CNS, which includes the brain, spinal cord. and optic nerve.
- Determine that the damaged areas developed at least 1 month apart.
- Exclude all other possible diagnoses.
- Observe that the symptoms last for more than 24 hours and occur as distinct episodes separated by 1 month or more.
- Obtain MRI evidence of demyelination (plaques).
- Perform a lumbar puncture exam looking for oligoclonal bands.

About 30% of patients with MS have moderate to severe spasticity, mostly in the lower extremity. Initial clinical findings in MS are often sensory disturbances, the most common of which are paresthesias (tingling and numbness) and dysesthesias (burning and "pins and needles"). A common manifestation of MS is unilateral numbness affecting one leg that ascends to the pelvis, abdomen, or thorax. Sensory disturbances usually resolve but sometimes persist as chronic neuropathic pain. Trigeminal neuralgia also occurs.

Another common presenting sign of MS is optic neuritis, presenting as complete or partial loss of vision.[2] Other symptoms include diplopia, ataxia, vertigo, and bladder dysfunction. Bladder dysfunction occurs in more than 90% of patients with MS and results in weekly or more frequent episodes of incontinence in one-third of the patients.[2] At least 30% of patients experience constipation. Fatigue occurs in 90% of patients and is the most common work-related disability associated with MS.[2] Sexual problems are often experienced as well.

MULTIPLE SCLEROSIS AND PAIN

Pain is the most commonly treated symptom in MS patients as 75% of patients present with pain. Pain treatment accounts for 30% of all symptomatic treatment for MS.[8] Pain can generally be classified as nociceptive pain or neuropathic pain.[9] Nociceptive pain occurs as an appropriate encoding of noxious stimuli and represents a physiological response transmitted to a conscious level when nociceptors in bone, muscle, or any body tissue are activated, warning the organism of tissue damage and eliciting coordinated reflexes and behavioral responses. Neuropathic pain is typically initiated by a primary lesion or dysfunction in the somatosensory nervous system, with no biological advantage (such as warning) but causing suffering and damage. Clinical hallmarks of neuropathic pain are burning, dysesthesias, allodynia (painful response to nonpainful stimuli), and/or hyperalgesia (exaggerated pain sensation when noxious stimuli are applied).[9] Pain in MS can be classified into four main categories according to a report in 2008[10]:

1.   Continuous central neuropathic pain
2.   Intermittent central neuropathic pain (trigeminal neuralgia, glossopharyngeal neuralgia, and Lhermitte sign: an intense burst of pain like an electric shock that runs down the back into the arms and legs when patients move their neck. It lasts just a few seconds but can be startling.)
3.   Musculoskeletal pain (painful tonic spasms, pain secondary to spasticity, pain related to being wheelchair-bound)
4.   Mixed neuropathic and non-neuropathic pain (headache)

Prevalence of Pain in Multiple Sclerosis

About 43% of patients with MS experience at least one type of pain[11]; the prevalence can vary from 29% to 86%.[12–20] The presence of pain appears to correlate with disability, disease course, disease duration, and age but not with gender. Interestingly, a study[21] evaluated 771 MS patients and found high prevalence in both MS patients and controls (79.4% vs 74.7%) with no statistical difference between groups, although pain in patients with MS was more severe and more often interfered with daily activities.

Pathophysiology of Central Pain in Multiple Sclerosis

Although not fully understood and poorly defined, the pathophysiology of central neuropathic pain in MS has been studied in animal models. It is thought to be due to demyelination in areas involved in pain processing. A common animal model to study the pathophysiology of MS and related symptoms is experimental autoimmune encephalomyelitis (EAE). It is achieved by injecting various rodent strains with myelin antigens. Although this model is widely used to study MS in animals, there are few reports utilizing this model to study pain. Recently, it has been proposed that MS is an acquired channelopathy.[22] Sodium channel Nav1.8, whose expression is normally restricted to the peripheral nervous system, was found present in the cerebellar Purkinje cells in a mouse model of MS. The ectopic expression of the Na channels contributes to symptom development in that model. Axonal conduction is altered by the altered Na channel expression.[23]

Postmortem examination of MS-affected tissues shows discrete pink or gray areas, which are hard and have a rubbery texture within the white matter. The lesions are composed of areas of myelin and oligodendrocyte loss along with infiltrates of inflammatory cells, including lymphocytes and macrophages.[2] The relative preservation of axons and neurons within these lesions helps to differentiate MS from other destructive pathological processes that involve local inflammation.[2]

Central Neuropathic Pain

Central neuropathic pain is the most common form of pain in MS patients; the prevalence approaches 50% in some reports.[11] Classically, hyperalgesia and allodynia have been reported in 38% of patients with MS, which seems to be less prevalent than in clinical practice, most likely due to patients' difficulty in describing their symptoms.[21] About 40% of patients describe a constant, burning pain in the legs, more frequently distally than proximally, while 30% of patients describe a deep, aching pain.[22] In an attempt to correlate central pain symptoms with locations of the demyelinating lesions, Svensden and colleagues compared 13 MS patients with pain and 10 MS patients without pain and found no correlation between pain and site of demyelination in the CNS.[24]

MANAGEMENT OF PAIN IN PATIENTS WITH MULTIPLE SCLEROSIS

Treatment of the cause of pain is ultimately the ideal treatment of pain. Disease-modifying agents to treat MS will be discussed briefly later in this chapter. Currently, treating pain associated with MS is based primarily on clinical experience, since there are no double-blind studies comparing pain-targeting medications in MS to placebo. There is no specific treatment for MS-related central neuropathic pain, even though tricyclic antidepressants, membrane stabilizers, intrathecally administered baclofen, opioid analgesics, ziconotide, antiarrhythmics, and cannabinoids have all been used with various degrees of success.

Tricyclic Antidepressants

Tricyclic antidepressants (TCAs) are historically considered first-line treatment for MS. This class includes amitriptyline, nortriptyline, desipramine, and clomipramine. They increase serotonin and norepinephrine at the synaptic level. Their applications are limited by their side effects, including but not limited to drowsiness, dry mouth, constipation, and possible extrapyramidal manifestations.[25]

Membrane Stabilizers and Antiepileptics

This class of medications is also considered a mainstay treatment for central neuropathic pain, including central neuropathic pain secondary to MS.[26] Evidence suggests that membrane stabilizers and antiepileptics seem to be a reasonable treatment for MS-related neuropathic pain; their use is usually limited by their side effects.

Carbamazepine

Carbamazepine is a commonly used drug for the treatment of central neuropathic pain.

It is metabolized by the P450 system. It is recommended by the FDA to check *HLA-B1502* allele for patients of Asian descent, owing to recent data implicating the *HLA* allele *B*1502* as a marker for carbamazepine-induced Stevens-Johnson syndrome and toxic epidermal necrolysis in this population. It slows the recovery rate of the voltage-gated Na^+ channels, modulates activated calcium channel activity, and activates the ascending inhibitory modulation system. A starting dose of 100–200 twice daily is commonly used with gradual titration until there is improvement of pain or side effects occur. The average maintenance dose is 600–1200 mg daily in divided doses. Adverse effects include skin rashes, leucopenia, abnormal liver functions, aplastic anemia, and hyponatremia.[27]

Oxcarbazepine

Oxcarbazepine has fewer side effects than carbamazepine and requires less lab testing. It is a 10-keto analog of carbamazepine. Its tolerability is reported to be "good" or "excellent" in 62% compared to 48% of patients receiving carbamazepine. Dose ranges from 900 to 1800 mg/day, with onset of therapeutic effects in 24–72 hours.

Lamotrigine

Lamotrigine has also been tested for neuropathic pain. In an open-label study of 21 patients with neuropathic pain including central neuropathic pain (15 patients), lamotrigine was added as adjunctive therapy to a target dose of 400 mg daily. In 2 of the 15 MS patients the pain was successfully treated, and 6 of 15 patients reported improvement in pain that lasted between 4 months and 1 year. No major side effects were reported.[28] However, a randomized, double-blind, placebo-controlled, crossover study in 12 MS patients, who were treated with a maximum dose of lamotrigine of 400 mg/day, found no difference between the experimental and placebo groups in mean pain intensity.[29]

Gabapentin

Gabapentin was evaluated in an open-label study 25 MS patients; 15 of 22 patients reported moderate to excellent relief of pain at a daily dose of 600 mg.[30] Pain in 15 patients was either improved or resolved. About 50% of patients reported side effects; five patients dropped out of the study because of dyspepsia and somnolence. Other case reports of treating MS central neuropathic pain with gabapentin at doses of 900 mg daily showed dramatic improvement in dysesthetic limb pain without any significant side effects.

Levetiracetam

Levetiracetam was evaluated in a randomized, placebo-controlled study in which 20 MS patients with central neuropathic pain were given a maximum daily dose of 3000 mg.[31] The 12 patients receiving the active treatment reported significant improvement in their pain compared with the placebo group. Side effects occurred in eight patients in the active treatment group and five patients in the placebo group. However, in another double-blind, placebo-controlled study treating 27 MS patients with central neuropathic pain (3000 mg/day for 6 weeks), there were no significant differences between the two groups at the end of the study in terms of pain relief, total pain intensity, or any other outcomes.[32] One exception is that there was a significant improvement in pain in a subgroup of patients with intense pain or without touch-evoked pain.

Pregabalin

Pregabalin was evaluated for treating MS neuropathic pain in an open-label pilot study involving 16 patients; 9 patients reported that the medication was effective (average dose of 154 mg/day). However three patients had to discontinue the medication because of side effects (dizziness in one patient and general malaise in two).[33]

Intrathecal Baclofen

Despite its wide use in MS-related spasticity, only two studies have looked at intrathecal baclofen for the treatment of central neuropathic pain related to MS. Intrathecal baclofen at a daily dose of 50 mcg intrathecally was found to be effective in markedly reducing central neuropathic pain in four patients tested with MS-related spinal cord lesions.[34] Intrathecal baclofen (50–1200 mcg/day) combined with morphine (210–9500 mcg/day) reduced pain in nine patients with MS-related pain, without significant side effects.[35]

Opioid Analgesics

The evidence supporting the use of opioid analgesics in MS patients is very limited despite it's wide use. In one non-randomized, single-blinded, placebo-controlled study of 14 patients with MS-related central neuropathic pain, 4 patients reported more than 50% decrease in their pain scores after treatment with intravenous morphine at a median dose of 0.67 mg/kg body weight.[36] In a randomized, double-blind study, 81 patients with neuropathic pain (some with MS) received either high-strength (0.75 mg) or low-strength (0.15 mg) capsules of the potent mu-opioid agonist levorphanol for 8 weeks.[37] Patients could be titrated up to 21 pills per day. The reduction in neuropathic pain intensity was significantly greater during treatment with higher doses of opioids than with lower doses.

Cannabinoids

Medical and public interest in cannabinoids has increased lately. Cannabinoids are among the most studied drugs in MS. One of the largest studies of cannabinoids, in 630 MS patients, included a 15-week trial with spasticity; pain reduction was a secondary outcome measure. Most patients in the treatment arm reported an improvement in pain; 20% reported worsening pain while receiving treatment with cannabinoids.[38] A trial of delta 9 tetrahydrocannabinol (delta 9 THC) reported benefit with regard to pain intensity in the treatment group, although the treated patients experienced deficits in long-term memory retention.[39] The study was extended in an open-label trial for up to 2 years to determine the long-term tolerability and the effectiveness of delta 9 THC; 28 patients completed the 2-year follow-up. The mean numeric score in the last week of the randomized trial was 2.9 (scale 0–8) compared to 3.8 in the placebo group.[39] In another study, delta 9 THC administered sublingually was compared to placebo in a consecutive series of randomized, double blind, single-subject crossover trials. The study consisted of a 2-week treatment phase followed by a double-blind phase of 6 weeks duration. The active treatment group had improved pain, but the improvement was not significantly different from that in the placebo control group.[40]

Central Intermittent Neuropathic Pain

Intermittent neuropathic pain in MS patients includes primarily trigeminal neuralgia (TN), Lhermitte sign, and glossopharyngeal neuralgia. TN secondary to MS is the most prevalent intermittent central neuropathic pain in this patient population. In fact, 4% of all patients with TN will be diagnosed with MS.[41] The clinical presentation of TN in MS is similar to the idiopathic form of TN, which is discussed in Chapter 33 (please also refer to ICHD beta 3 classification). Interestingly, there is no relationship between the extent of involvement of the trigeminal complex and the clinical symptoms.[42] As with classic TN, the most common presentation is involvement of the V2, V3, or both in 90% of cases, with V1 being the least involved.[43] The pathophysiology of TN in MS patients is thought to be caused by a demyelinated plaque at the trigeminal nerve entry zone in the pons, although vascular compression etiology has also been proposed as a cause for TN in patients with MS. An MRI study[44] found a plaque in the pons in one of seven patients, whereas vascular compression of the nerve by an artery at the root entry zone was demonstrated in five subjects.

TN can significantly affect the quality of life of patients with MS; at one point the condition could be so severe that TN was called the "suicide disease." Various treatment modalities exists to treat TN in patients with MS. Medical management is the primary modality for treatment, consisting of membrane stabilizers acting on voltage-gated sodium channels, namely carbamazepine, oxcarbazepine, and lamotrigine. Other medications used include gabapentin[45] and topiramate.[46]

Multiple interventional and surgical treatments are available to treat TN. Most of the studies done have been primarily directed at classic TN; few studies specifically address MS-related TN. The interventional and surgical treatment modalities are discussed in Chapter 8. Briefly, radiofrequency ablation is less invasive than microvascular decompression and has had excellent outcomes, although studies were not specifically designed for TN secondary to MS.[47] Microvascular decompression (MVD) was previously contraindicated in patients with MS. However, there is a small subset of 35 patients who received 22% fair and 39% excellent long-term pain relief via MVD.[48] In general, patients with MS respond less well to medical and interventional treatments. These patients may require more aggressive treatments than those for patients with classic idiopathic TN.

Lhermitte sign occurs in 40% of patients with MS whereas glossopharyngeal neuralgia is quite rare. Lhermitte sign and glossopharyngeal neuralgia can both be treated with carbamazepine. MVD can also be used to treat glossopharyngeal neuralgia, when indicated.

Pain is a common feature of MS. Multiple treatments are available to manage neuropathic pain secondary to MS, including both medical and interventional treatments. Yet pain can sometimes be quite disabling, persistent, and refractory to currently available treatment modalities. Thus further research into new treatments and compounds is needed that directly targets the pain generators specific to patients with MS.

GUIDING QUESTIONS

- What is multiple sclerosis (MS) and how is it related to neuropathic pain?
- What are the major pathophysiological changes of MS?
- How is neuropathic pain in MS classified?
- How do you manage neuropathic pain in patients with MS?

KEY POINTS

- Multiple sclerosis (MS) is a chronic, autoimmune demyelinating disease of the central nervous system (CNS). MS attacks the myelinated axons in multiple foci of the CNS, destroying the myelin and axons to varying degrees.
- The diagnosis of MS is based on evidence of at lease two different lesions (plaques or scars) in the CNS, at least two different episodes in the disease course, and chronic inflammation of the CNS as determined by analysis of the CSF (oligoclonal bands).
- Central neuropathic pain is the most common form of pain in MS patients, with an estimated prevalence of about 50%. In addition to the classic neuropathic pain features, such as spontaneous pain (dysesthesia and burning) and evoked pain (allodynia and hyperalgesia), patients with MS may also suffer from intermittent neuropathic pain, such as trigeminal neuralgia, Lhermitte sign, and glossopharyngeal neuralgia.
- In addition to disease-modifying therapies of MS, multiple treatments are available to manage neuropathic pain secondary to MS, including medical, interventional, and surgical treatments with varying level of evidence.

REFERENCES

1. Calabresi PA. Diagnosis and management of multiple sclerosis. *Am Fam Physician*. 2004;70:1935–1944.
2. Hauser SL, Goodwin DS. Multiple sclerosis and other demyelinating diseases. In: Fauci AS, Braunwald E, Kasper DL, Hauser SL, eds. *Harrison's Principles of Internal Medicine*, Vol. II, 17th ed. New York: McGraw-Hill Medical; 2008:2611–2621.
3. Weinshenker BC. Epidemiology of multiple sclerosis. *Neurol Clin*. 1996;142:1–308.
4. Olek MJ. Epidemiology, risk factors and clinical features of multiple sclerosis in adults. *UpToDate*. March 15, 2014. http:www.uptodate.com/contents/epidemiology-and-clinical-features-of-multiple-sclerosis-in-adults. Accessed July 21, 2018.
5. Singh VK, Mehrotra S, Agarwal SS. The paradigm of Th1 and Th2 cytokines: its relevance to autoimmunity and allergy. *Immunol Res*. 1999;20:147–161.
6. Navikas V, Link H. Review: cytokines and the pathogenesis of multiple sclerosis. *J Neurosci Res*. 1996;45:322–333.
7. Cree BAC. Multiple sclerosis. In: Brust JCM, ed. *Current Diagnosis and Treatment in Neurology*. New York: Lange Medical Books/McGraw-Hill Medical; 2007.
8. Brochette G, Messmer Uccelli M, Mancardi GL, Solaro C. Symptomatic medication use in multiple sclerosis. *Mult Scler*. 2003;9(5):458–460.
9. Treede RD, Jensen TS, Campbell JN, et al. Neuropathic pain: redefinition and a grading system for clinical and research purposes. *Neurology*. 2008;70:1630–1635.
10. O'Connor AB, Schwid SR, Herrmann DN, Markman JD, Dworkin RH. Pain associated with multiple sclerosis: systematic review and proposed classification. *Pain*. 2008;137:96–111.
11. Solaro C, Brichetto G, Amato MP, et al. The prevalence of pain in multiple sclerosis. A multicenter cross-sectional study. *Neurology*. 2004;63:919–921.
12. Clifford DB, Trotter JL. Pain in multiple sclerosis. *Arch Neurol*. 1984;41:1270–1272.
13. Vermote R, Ketalaer P, Carltonn H. Pain in multiple sclerosis patients: a prospective study using the McGill pain questionnaire. *Clin Neurol Neurosurg*. 1986;88:87–93.
14. Kassirer MR, Osterberg DH. Pain in chronic multiple sclerosis. *J Pain Symptom Manage*. 1987;2:95–97.
15. Moulin DE, Foley KM, Ebers GC. Pain syndromes in multiple sclerosis. *Neurology*. 1988;38:1830–1834.
16. Stenager E, Knutsen L, Jensen K. Acute and chronic pain syndromes in multiple sclerosis. *Acta Neurol Scand*. 1991;84:197–200.
17. Warnell P. The pain experience of a multiple sclerosis population: a descriptive study. *Axon*. 1991;13:26–28.
18. Archibald CJ, McGrath PJ, Ritvo PG, et al. Pain prevalence, severity and impact in a clinical sample of multiple sclerosis patients. *Pain*. 1994;58:89–93.

19. Indaco A, Iachetta C, Nappi C, Socci L, Carrieri PB. Chronic and acute pain syndromes in patients with multiple sclerosis. *Acta Neurol.* 1994;16:97–102.

20. Stenager E, Knudsen L, Jensen K. Acute and chronic pain syndromes in multiple sclerosis. *Ital J Neurol Sci.* 1995;16:629–632.

21. Svendsen KB, Jensen TS, Overvad K, Hansen HJ, Koch-Henriksen N, Bach FW. Pain in patients with multiple sclerosis: a population-based study. *Arch Neurol.* 2003;60:1089–1094.

22. Beiske AG, Pedersen ED, Czujko B, Myhr KM. Pain and sensory complaints in multiple sclerosis. *Eur J Neurol.* 2004;1:479–482.

23. Waxman SG, Dib-Hajj S, Cummins TR, Black JA. Sodium channels and pain. *Proc Natl Acad Sci USA.* 1999;96(14):7635–7639. 6.

24. Svendsen KB, Sørensen L, Jensen TS, Hansen HJ, Bach FW. MRI of the central nervous system in MS patients with and without pain. *Eur J Pain.* 2011;15(4):395–401.

25. Saarto T, Wiffen PJ. Antidepressants for neuropathic pain. *Cochrane Database Syst Rev.* 2007;4:CD005454.

26. Solaro C, Brichetto G, Battaglia MA, Messmer Uccelli M, Mancardi GL. Antiepileptic medications in multiple sclerosis: adverse effects in a three-year follow-up study. *Neurol Sci.* 2005;25:307–310.

27. Killian JM, Fromm GH. Carbamazepine in the treatment of neuralgia: use and side effects. *Arch Neurol.* 2001;19:129–136.

28. Cianchetti C, Zuddas A, Randazzo AP, Perra L, Marrosu MG. Lamotrigine adjunctive therapy in painful phenomena in MS: preliminary observations. *Neurology.* 1999;53:433.

29. Breuer B, Pappagallo M, Knotkova H, Guleyupoglu N, Wallenstein S, Portenoy RK. A randomized double blind, placebo-controlled, two-period, crossover, pilot trial of lamotrigine in patients with central pain due to multiple sclerosis. *Clin Ther.* 2007;29:2022–2030.

30. Houtchens MK, Richert JR, Sami A, Rose JW. Open label gabapentin treatment for pain in multiple sclerosis. *Mult Scler.* 1997;3:250–253.

31. Rossi S, Mataluni G, Codecà C, et al. Effects of levetiracetam on chronic pain in multiple sclerosis: results of a randomized placebo-controlled study. *Eur J Neurol.* 2009;16:360–366.

32. Falah M, Madsen C, Holbech JV, Sindrup SH. A randomized, placebo-controlled trial of levetiracetam in central pain in multiple sclerosis. *Eur J Pain.* 2011;1532–2149.

33. Solaro C, Boemker M, Tanganelli P. Pregabalin for treating paroxysmal symptoms in multiple sclerosis: a pilot study. *J Neurol.* 2009;256:1773–1774.

34. Herman RM, D'Luzansky SC, Ippolito R. Intrathecal baclofen suppresses central pain in patients with spinal lesions. A pilot study. *Clin J Pain.* 1992;8:338–345.

35. Sadiq S, Poopatana C. Intrathecal baclofen and morphine in multiple sclerosis patients with severe pain and spasticity. *J Neurol.* 2007;254:1464–1465.

36. Kalman S, Österbergn A, Sörensenn J, Boivie J, Bertler A. Morphine responsiveness in a group of well-defined multiple sclerosis patients: a study with i.v. morphine. *Eur J Pain.* 2002;6:69–80.

37. Rowbotham MC, Twilling L, Davies PS, et al. Oral opioid therapy for chronic peripheral and central neuropathic pain. *N Engl J Med.* 2003;348:1223–1232.

38. Zajicek J, Fox P, Sanders H, et al. Cannabinoids for treatment of spasticity and other symptoms related to multiple sclerosis (CAMS study): multicenter randomized placebo-controlled trial. *Lancet.* 2003;362:1517–1526.

39. Rog DJ, Nurmikko TJ, Young CA. Oromucosal delta9-tetrahydrocannabinol/ cannabidiol for neuropathic pain associated with multiple sclerosis: an uncontrolled, open-label, 2-year extension trial. *Clin Ther.* 2007;29:2068–2079.

40. Wade DT, Makela P, Robson P, House H, Bateman C. Do cannabis-based medicinal extracts have general or specific effects on symptoms in multiple sclerosis? A double-blind, randomized, placebo- controlled study on 160 patients. *Mult Scler.* 2004;10:434–441.

41. Hooge JP, Redekop WK. Trigeminal neuralgia in multiple sclerosis. *Neurology.* 1995;45:1294–1296.

42. Mills RJ, Young CA, Smith ET. Central trigeminal involvement in multiple sclerosis using high-resolution MRI at 3T. *Br J Radiol.* 2010;83:493–498.

43. Cruccu G, Biasiotta A, Di Rezze S, et al. Trigeminal neuralgia and pain related to multiple sclerosis. *Pain.* 2009;143:186–191.

44. Meaney JFM, Watt JMG, Eldridge PR, Whitehouse GH, Wells JCD, Miles JB. Association between trigeminal neuralgia and multiple sclerosis: role of magnetic resonance imaging. *J Neurol Neurosurg Psychiatry.* 1995;59:253–259.

45. Solaro C, Lunardi GL, Capello E, et al. An open-label trial of gabapentin treatment of paroxysmal symptoms in multiple sclerosis patients. *Neurology.* 1998;51:609–611.

46. Solaro C, Uccelli MM, Brichetto G, Gasperini C, Mancardi GL. Topiramate relieves idiopathic

and symptomatic trigeminal neuralgia. *J Pain Symptom Manage.* 2001;21:367–368.

47. Broggi G, Franzini A. Radiofrequency trigeminal rhizotomy in treatment of symptomatic non-neoplastic facial pain. *J Neurosurg.* 1982;57:483–486.

48. Broggi G, Ferroli P, Franzini A, et al. Role of microvascular decompression in trigeminal neuralgia and multiple sclerosis. *Lancet.* 1999;354:1878–1879.

25

Phantom Pain

JAGAN DEVARAJAN AND BETH H. MINZTER

CASE

A 64-year-old man presents to the pain clinic with pain in his amputated left leg. He had a history of osteosarcoma of the tibia and is status-post above-knee amputation that took place 6 months ago. Now he complains of shooting pain that travels down into his legs. He also feels as though his feet are being crushed with associated throbbing pain. His past medical history includes hypertension and diabetes mellitus. Examination of the amputated leg stump shows normal healing and absence of any discharge or discontinuity. He has been treated with pregabalin, which is not effective.

DEFINITION

Amputation is derived from the Greek word *amputation,* which means "to cut around." There is historical and archeological evidence that amputations were performed as far back as 45,000 years ago.[1] Phantom limb pain (PLP) was identified as early as 1871, when Silas Weir Mitchell coined the term.[2]

Phantom pain is defined as an unpleasant or painful sensation in the distribution of the lost or deafferentiated body part. The absence can be due to a congenitally missing body part or to amputation. Though phantom pain is known to occur most commonly in the extremities, it has also been reported to occur in other missing or amputated body parts, such as the eye,[3] tongue,[4] breast,[5] teeth, nose, penis,[6] or even part of the gastrointestinal (GI) tract. The pathophysiology and management are similar irrespective of body parts. PLP has myriad pathophysiological pathways and various etiologies. The mechanism of origin and precipitating factors are not well defined. We have yet to evolve a standard therapeutic regimen despite having a plethora of studies looking at different options. The onset of phantom pain is variable; in most patients, it

appears within a week's duration, and approximately 50% of patients experience some type of phantom pain as early as within 24 hours.[7]

EPIDEMIOLOGY AND ETIOLOGY

The incidence and prevalence vary depending on patient population, patient comorbidities, etiology, and site of and duration since amputation. The range varies between 42.2% and 78.8%.[8] A study by Desmond and Maclachlan.[9] found the prevalence to be 43% following upper extremity amputation. Two-thirds of patients perceive phantom pain within 6 months, and in up to 60% of patients the pain persists even after 2 years. The cumulative incidence has been reported to be as high as 85%. However, Ephraim and colleagues[10] conducted a survey which showed that 95% of patients with amputation suffer from either phantom sensation or PLP or residual limb pain. Patients have difficulty differentiating between these categories.[11]

The impact of PLP is significant both at the individual and societal levels. It is more common among upper-limb amputees than persons with lower-limb amputations. Females are more likely to and more often suffer from this condition than males.[12] Females also are more prone to suffer severe pain. In addition, pain interferes with their daily activities more commonly than in their male counterparts, and females also show fewer pain-coping strategies and poor adjustment.[13]

Presence of pre-amputation pain and residual limb pain are also considered risk factors. An interesting fact is that bilateral amputation is not a significant risk factor for phantom pain, compared to that of unilateral amputation. Time since amputation determines the incidence and severity of phantom pain.

Phantom pain has two peaks of incidences: the first is within a month and the second is within a year. After the first year, the prevalence is reported to decrease with time after amputation. Psychological factors such as anxiety, stress, and depression precipitate and exacerbate PLP. Patients with depression have more severe PLP than individuals without depression.[14] Some studies have disputed these results, finding that the incidences of anxiety and depression are no higher among amputees than among individuals who have not undergone amputation.[15]

A 78-year-old woman presents with abnormal sensation in her amputated right leg. She is a known patient with peripheral vascular disease who underwent below-knee amputation. She complains of a sensation in which her foot is withdrawn into her leg even though both are absent. She complains of burning and aching pain, which is present throughout the entire day in her missing leg. She suffers from anxiety-depression syndrome. Her medical history includes diabetes, hypertension, and peripheral vascular disease. How would you differentiate her symptoms of phantom pain from residual stump pain and progression of her peripheral vascular disease?

CLINICAL FEATURES

Phantom Sensation

Perception of nonpainful sensations from the amputated body part is known as *phantom sensation*. These are common in the early postoperative period. About one-third of patients perceive these sensations as early as the first 24 hours postoperatively and three-quarters within 4 days.[16] The majority of patients develop phantom sensations within 6 months after surgery. Phantom sensations are not only associated with amputation but also known to occur after brachial plexus injury[17] or spinal cord injury.[18] Phantom sensations are divided into kinetic, kinesthetic, and exteroceptive sensations. *Kinetic movements* refer to perception of gross movements in the amputated limb—for example, flexion and extension of the toes and foot.[19] *Kinesthetic sensations* are distorted sensations with respect to the size and function of the missing body parts—for example, a sensation of twisting of the hand or foot. They are more frequent after mastectomy than extremity amputation. *Exteroceptive sensations* consist of tingling, perception of touch, pressure, or paresthesia in the amputated parts. Phantom sensations occur most commonly in the hands and feet. This is due to a rich innervation of these regions and large topographic representation in cerebral areas.

Quadriplegics and paraplegics, irrespective of etiology, can perceive phantom sensations.

Telescoping

Telescoping is a type of phantom sensation.[16] This occurs in one-fourth to two-thirds of amputees. A patient with telescoping has the perception of shortening of the limb, which results in a sensation that the distal part is very close to the proximal part.[20] This can become so real to patients that they try to perform maneuvers with the absent limb. Although over time the sensations fade away, phantom sensation of a hand or foot attached to a stump may remain for a prolonged period of time.

Phantom Pain

There is no particular characteristic or type of pain that is associated with phantom pain. It can be burning, shooting, sharp or dull, cramping, squeezing, or an electrical sensation. It can vary in character, frequency, duration, and intensity. It can be a transient, painful cramp or a more severe constant, intense perception of a painful limb. Studies have shown that the severity and frequency of attacks slowly decrease with time during the first 6 months, after which they remain constant.[21] The incidence of phantom pain is similar in children and adults.[22] The incidence of phantom pain is about 70%–75% among children.[23] The prevalence decreases to less than 10% after 1 year's duration of amputation.

PATHOPHYSIOLOGY

The exact pathophysiology of phantom pain is not clear.[24] It is now understood that neither a single mechanism nor a single chemical mediator precipitates or is responsible for phantom pain. It is the combination of chemical mediators, which interact with receptors along with peripheral, spinal, and supraspinal sensitization, that are responsible for PLP. Both psychological and neurological factors are involved.[25] The principal factor that contributes to phantom pain is damage to peripheral nerve endings and subsequent nerve ending changes.[7] However, phantom pain has been reported in patients with congenital absence of limbs, which suggests that the central nervous system[26] plays a key role as well.

Changes in Peripheral Nervous System

Patients with residual stump pain and infection and those with pathological changes, which affect the stump, manifest with a higher incidence of phantom pain. This signifies that changes in the peripheral nerves and tissues contribute to phantom pain as well.

Neuroma Formation

After any injury to the nerve, the nerve afferents degenerate. When a receptor or nerve ending is injured, injury, edema, and ischemia occur, which cause degeneration of afferent fibers. The injured axons may regenerate from the cut ending[27]; however, the regeneration is not orderly and thus results in disorganized clumping of A-delta and C fiber endings. This causes both spontaneous ectopic firing and firing in response to mechanical stimulus.[28] There is a significant change in the pattern of afferent transmission of new generating axons. Type C ectopic discharge shows a slow, irregular pattern due to upregulation of sodium channels and downregulation of potassium channels. This results in alteration in transduction, which results in perception of touch as painful, as is evidenced by the creation of a painful response to the injection of gallamine, a sodium channel conductance facilitator.

During surgery, nerve endings are cut and nociceptors are damaged.[14] This causes disorganization of A-delta and C fibers and neuroma formation. The neuromas show increased density and upregulation of sodium channels and demonstrate abnormal spontaneous excitatory action potentials. Rapid spontaneous firing is responsible for the perception of phantom pain. This pain is exacerbated by touch and pressure on neuromas, which causes the repetitive abnormal firing of nerve fibers. A study by Nikolajsen and Jensen shows that there is an inverse relationship between the mechanical threshold of pressure on neuromas and stump and phantom pains.[29] This finding is confirmed by the relief of phantom pain after resection of neuromas and the perineural injection of local anesthetics around a neuroma. Florence and colleagues have shown abnormal sprouting of cut nerve endings causing an excessive volley of aberrant signals.[30]

Although the periphery is the main source of phantom pain, it is not the sole determinant, as neither removal of neuroma nor regional block completely eliminates phantom pain. There are also independent abnormal excitatory potentials arising from the dorsal root ganglion (DRG). Efferent sympathetic neurons play a role in initiating and maintaining the phantom pain. Catecholamines sensitize the severed nerve endings and cause exacerbation of pain.[31]

The spinal cord undergoes structural reorganization in response to peripheral nerve damage.[32] Normally, neurons in lamina 2 of the spinal cord receive input from nociceptors and are involved in the perception of pain. After nerve damage, the central terminals of axonotomized myelinated afferents from A-beta fibers, which normally terminate in laminae 3 and 4, sprout into lamina 2, causing aberrant conduction in afferent fibers. This is explained by the structural damage of a neuron. In addition to peripheral receptors and the DRG, there is a contribution from the central nervous system, as evidenced by the presence of phantom limb pain in patients with paraplegia or who had spinal anesthesia. In fact, spinal anesthesia is known to exacerbate phantom pain.[33] The DRG amplifies the responses, along with the neuroma, and causes cross-excitation and depolarization of neighboring neurons.[10] This results in generalized increased excitability of spinal cord neurons and an expansion of the receptive field of the noxious dorsal horn spinal cord area. Hyperalgesia, which is very common among amputees, is explained by this potentiation of excitability. Excitability of these neurons is chemically mediated by excitatory neurotransmitters such as glutamate and neurokinins. This explains why PLP responds to antiepileptic medication and NMDA-receptor antagonist treatments. Pain is also exacerbated by sympathetically mediated responses and an increase in catecholamines, and is decreased by use of beta-adrenergic blockers and surgical blockade of sympathetic neurons.

Spinal Plasticity

Peripheral nerve injury causes sensitization of neurons in the dorsal horn of the spinal cord. This is characterized by prolonged postsynaptic potentials in the spinal cord in response to short and innocuous stimuli. This phenomenon is due to downregulation of inhibitory processes, which modify the sensory transmission. Primary structural changes include reduction in inhibitory GABAergic, glycinergic interneurons. There is also an increase in brain-derived neurotrophic factor (BDNF), which converts inhibitory neurons to excitatory ones.[32] Downregulation of opioid receptors and upregulation of cholecystokinin-opioid receptor inhibitor receptors also occur.

Supraspinal Plasticity

Similar changes have been reported in the supraspinal structures,[34] including the thalamus and cerebral cortex in both animal models and human patients. For instance, sensory afferent neurons are redistributed from amputated hands to converge on the expansive receptive field representing the forearm. This reorganization was minimal to none in patients with amputation who did not develop phantom pain. There is a strong positive relationship between the development of cortical reorganization and the frequency and severity of PLP. The area corresponding to the stump is also enlarged in both the thalamus and cerebral cortex, and stimulation of both areas results in phantom sensations and PLP. A complex interaction between development or reorganization at different levels and PLP may take place.[35] This is evidenced by the fact that analgesics acting at one level fail to treat PLP. The central reorganization may be independent of any peripheral input that may contribute to the development and maintenance of PLP.[36]

Contribution of Psychological Factors

Certain psychological factors are associated with PLP.[37] Such factors maintain the pain process and subsequently result in resistance to many of the treatment regimens. It is still not known whether they are the main causative factors. Patients with passive coping strategies and catastrophizing behaviors tend to develop PLP more often than patients who have more resilient coping strategies. Psychological studies are retrospective and hence their findings cannot be considered conclusive or causative regarding the role of psychological factors in the development of PLP.[38] Nonetheless, psychological factors such as stress, anxiety, depression, and loss of social support do trigger and exacerbate PLP. Exacerbation by psychological factors indicates that there may be neuroplastic changes in affective areas like the insula, the anterior cingulate gyrus, and the frontal cortex.

In summary, there are multiple pathophysiological changes in response to the loss of body parts. These changes occur not only in the periphery and DRG but also in the spinal cord and brain. The changes are attributed to the damaged neurons and aberrant transmission of regenerative neurons and loss of inhibitory neurons. PLP is mainly explained by neuromas, spinal cord plasticity changes, and reorganization of neural representation of amputated areas in the cerebral cortex. In general, there is increased aberrant excitatory neurotransmission and a decrease in inhibitory neurotransmission.

DIAGNOSIS

The patient's history and physical exam are important in diagnosing PLP as PLP is a diagnosis of exclusion. Duration of pain and quality of pain are needed to differentiate PLP from residual limb pain. As with any assessment of pain, it is important to identify the location, severity, and characteristics of the pain as well as the precipitating, aggravating, and relieving factors of the pain. The degree, frequency, and severity of interference with the quality of daily life need to be assessed. Such assessment not only helps determine how aggressive the treatment approach should be but also allows one to monitor effectiveness of the treatment. Any standard pain rating scale, such as a verbal rating scale (VRS), visual analog scale (VAS), or McGill Pain Questionnaire, can be used.

Initial treatment modalities and therapeutic responses should be taken into consideration as these will guide further treatment options. A psychological and psychosocial evaluation is an important part of the treatment plan. Any psychological or neurological factors such as stress, anxiety, depression, poor social support, and coping strategies should be addressed. It is likely impossible to control PLP without addressing these primary components.

A thorough visual and physical exam of the stump is paramount. PLP should be differentiated from stump pain, and stump pain is one of the most important factors that can lead to PLP. The stump should be examined for any discontinuity in skin, skin abrasions, local sores, and evidence of site infection. One should look for bone exostoses and visible neuromas. Local neuromas may be confirmed by Tinel's sign. One should examine for symptoms and signs of decreased blood flow and ischemia. One of the most common causes of residual limb pain and PLP is continued ischemia. The prosthesis should also be examined. The assessment of appropriateness of size and accuracy of fitting cannot be overemphasized. An ill-fitting prosthesis is another common cause of PLP and back pain. A physiotherapy consult may be needed for proper fitting of orthotics. Other etiologies of local limb pain should be considered, such as complex regional pain syndrome, radicular pain, back pain, and osteoarthritis of local joints such as the hip and knee.

Electromyography and nerve conduction studies may be required to rule out any preexisting neuropathy, nerve entrapment, or radiculopathy. Specialized tests may be required, such as computed tomographic angiography to evaluate blood flow and ischemia, MRI of the joint and synovial fluid analysis to rule out any pathology or infections associated with local joints. Back pain is more common among amputees, and back pain along with radicular pain may mimic PLP,[39] hence it may be useful to obtain an MRI of the lumbar spine if there are any other features suggestive of lumbar spondylosis and radiculitis.

PREVENTION

Given the resistance to treatment and difficulty of managing PLP,[40] it is important and beneficial to make every effort to prevent the development of PLP, which may be related to peripheral sensitization and central reorganization caused by afferent painful stimuli at the time of surgery and thereafter. This provides a target for instituting regimens to prevent the development of PLP altogether, if possible.

Perioperative epidural infusion,[41] initiated preoperatively and continued for 3 days postoperatively, has been shown to reduce the development of PLP. Two studies show impressive results in reducing the incidence from 64% and 75% to 27% and 21%, respectively.[42] However, these results were not reproduced in a study by Nikolajsen et al.[43] Addition of clonidine to the epidural infusion reduced the incidence from 73% to 8%.[21] Similarly, regional analgesia via peripheral nerve catheter has also been shown to reduce the development of PLP.[42] However, continuous transneural administration of local anesthetics using the catheter that was placed during the surgery did not show any beneficial effects in prevention of phantom pain 6 months after amputation. Bupivacaine 0.5% 1 mL/hr infused through a catheter placed adjacent to the cut nerve ending did not provide benefit in either reduction or prevention of phantom pain.[44]

Other techniques have been used during surgery to prevent the development of PLP. Perineuromal lidocaine injection at the time of surgery prevents neuroma pain.[98,99] Targeted nerve reimplantation involves implantation of the proximal amputated nerve stump into a surgically denervated portion of a muscle.[45] This can act as secondary motor point. Pet et al. showed that 11 of 12 patients who underwent targeted nerve implantation developed neither neuromas nor neuroma pain.[46] The other technique used was targeted muscle reinnervation, in which

spare nerve muscle units are transferred to control a myoelectric prosthesis. Targeted muscle innervation prevented neuroma pain in all of the patients.[45] Despite the great success of these procedures, they are not popularly utilized, as there are not many studies involving these procedures. We need more definitive studies before recommending these procedures.

MANAGEMENT OF PHANTOM LIMB PAIN

PLP is difficult to manage because of its varied pathophysiology and complex interaction between different parts of nervous system.[47] It is often resistant to different kinds of treatment and can be a source of frustration to patients and physicians alike. The treatment modalities used are pharmacological, nonpharmacological, noninvasive, minimally invasive, and surgical.

Pharmacological Management
NSAIDs and Acetaminophen

NSAIDs are the most commonly used medications to manage pain. Their efficacy is moderate and less than that of opioids. The efficacy of NSAIDs for PLP is similar to that for neuropathic pain.[48]

Opioids

Opioids are the most commonly used treatment for PLP. Their efficacy is modest. Huse et al. compared the efficacy of oral morphine against placebo in a study involving 12 patients.[49] They did imaging pre- and post-treatment to evaluate whether opioids had any effect on reorganization of somatosensory cortex, electric perception, and pain thresholds as well as any effect on selective activation. Twelve patients received oral morphine ranging from 70 mg/day to 300 mg/day. The pain was reduced by half in 43% of patients and partially in another 25% of patients. The neuromagnetic imaging showed reduced cortical reorganization in three patients who had exhibited significant pain reduction. Pain threshold was not affected, however.

Wu et al. performed a randomized trial involving 32 subjects.[50] They compared IV morphine to lidocaine for 3 consecutive days. Morphine was found to reduce both stump pain and phantom pain and improved patients' satisfaction scores. Lidocaine improved the stump pain but not phantom pain. The same group of investigators also compared morphine against mexiletine, which is an oral sodium channel blocker. The mean percentage of pain reduction was 50% with morphine and 33% for oral mexiletine.

In a systematic neuroanatomical review, McCormick et al. found that IV morphine and IV ketamine showed the best evidence for short-term pain management and oral morphine for long-term pain management.[51]

Methadone has been used to treat phantom pain, as its pharmacokinetic properties and oral bioavailability make it attractive.[52] It is also considered a weak antagonist of NMDA receptors.

Antidepressants

While antidepressants have been found to be effective for neuropathic pain, trials with antidepressants for PLP have shown mixed results. Antidepressants enhance the serotonergic and norepinephrine transmission by blocking their uptake. The side effects are sedation, confusion, and orthostatic hypotension.

Amitriptyline was evaluated using 125 mg/day for 6 weeks in 39 patients in a trial that lasted for 6 months.[53] Amitriptyline was not found to be superior to placebo. Wilder-Smith et al. compared amitriptyline with tramadol and found both to be effective in reducing phantom pain.[54] Tramadol caused more side effects compared to the minor, insignificant side effects with amitriptyline.

The serotonin-norepinephrine reuptake inhibitor (SNRI) milnacipran was found to be effective in reports of case series.[55] It was also shown to be effective in resistant phantom pain unresponsive to paroxetine,[56] another selective serotonin reuptake inhibitor (SSRI) that was shown to be effective in reducing phantom pain by 80%. Mirtazapine, which facilitates both norepinephrine and serotonin, was more effective than SSRIs in a case series.[57] There are case reports involving other drugs, such as nortriptyline, chlorimipramine,[57] and venlafaxine.

Despite the lack of randomized trials with antidepressants for phantom pain, in a survey it was found that the PLP incidence decreases as the incidence of tricyclic antidepressant (TCA) and amitriptyline usage increases.

Anticonvulsants

There is a paucity of randomized studies on PLP regarding different anticonvulsant regimens. Hence the principles used for the treatment of neuropathic pain have been applied to PLP. Their anti-allodynic mode of action is due to the inhibition of ectopic discharge from injured peripheral nerves.

Gabapentin and pregabalin have few pharmacokinetic interactions and minimal side effects. Their main cellular mode of action is inhibition of voltage-gated calcium channels and, to some extent, inhibition of NMDA receptor and enhancement of GABAergic action. The inhibition of calcium channels occurs in the alpha2-delta subunit and prevents release of neurotransmitter. The effectiveness of gabapentin as monotherapy was evaluated for 6 months on phantom pain.[58] Half of the patients treated with gabapentin had reduced VAS scores. Studies on the role of gabapentin in treating post-amputation pain, however, did not report successful results. Pregabalin has been successfully used in a case report of PLP.[51] Pregabalin is structurally related to GABA and blocks calcium channels and, hence, influx of calcium. This in turn decreases the release of glutamate and substance P. Pregabalin has also been shown to decrease spontaneous firing of damaged nerve fibers and adjacent nerve endings in the stump.

Carbamazepine was used at 200 mg 4 times daily for phantom pain following above-elbow amputation and was found to be effective.

Topiramate has been used successfully with a 75% success rate in patients with below-knee amputation. The maximum daily dosage used was 800 mg/day orally.

In summary, anticonvulsants are generally found to be useful adjuncts and they can be used in addition to opioids. No anticonvulsants have been shown to be superior to others; they usually are titrated as tolerated.

NMDA Receptor Antagonists

Ketamine and memantine are the recognized NMDA receptor antagonists commonly utilized in treatment. NMDA receptors are involved in sensitization and maintenance of the increased excitability of neurons. Ketamine has been successfully used to treat PLP in a number of trials. Ketamine infusion was used to prevent the development of PLP in patients with above-knee amputation.[59] An intravenous infusion of ketamine at 0.5 mg/kg/hr was started before surgery and continued for 72 hours after surgery. The development of PLP was reduced from 71% to 47%. In a study of ketamine to prevent phantom pain,[60] a continuous infusion of ketamine was used for 80 minutes and was shown to reduce the phantom pain for 24 hours. Treating phantom pain with oral memantine (30 mg PO daily for 4 weeks) did not result in any benefits.[61] Dextromethorphan is a weak NMDA antagonist and has been shown to minimize phantom pain. It is used at a dose of 90 mg orally twice daily.

Calcitonin

Intravenous calcitonin has been used to successfully treat phantom pain. The mechanism of action is not known; it may involve central serotonergic neurons. It has been shown in rats that activation of calcitonin receptors in peripheral neurons helps to normalize sodium channel expression and thus decreases the excitability of ectopic neurons. Calcitonin receptors are normally dormant; however, they get expressed and activated during nerve injury. Calcitonin infusion at a dosage of 200 IU over an hour achieved a 75% reduction in PLP.[62] These results were not reproduced in a crossover trial involving 20 patients.[63] This study used infusion of calcitonin, ketamine, and a combination of ketamine and calcitonin and placebo and found ketamine to be effective in reducing PLP compared to calcitonin and placebo. Infusion of calcitonin 200 IU produced results similar to that of infusion of placebo. Combined infusion of ketamine and calcitonin showed results similar to those of ketamine.

Noninvasive Treatment
Transcutaneous Electrical Nerve Stimulation (TENS)

Case reports have shown the effectiveness of TENS in reducing both phantom and stump pains.[64] In 10 patients, TENS was applied at the stump and projected toward the phantom pain for 60 minutes. It was utilized successfully with projected phantom pain by applying the electrodes at the site of the transected nerve endings: phantom pain was reduced both at rest and during movement. The study also showed a reduction of phantom sensation and prosthesis embodiment. In another study, TENS was applied on the contralateral side for 60 minutes every day for 3 months, producing 50% improvement of phantom symptoms that lasted up to a year.[65]

Mirror Therapy

The principle behind mirror therapy is that movement of one limb is perceived as movement of the other limb. This improves spatial sensory perception and serves to alleviate phantom pain and promote motor recovery.[66] A mirror is placed in a parasagittal plane at the center of the body. The patient watches the movement of the intact limb in the mirror and perceives it as movement of the injured or amputated limb. Mirror visual feedback increases neural activities in areas of the brain involving attention and cognitive control. The areas are mapped to be dorsolateral prefrontal cortex, posterior cingulate cortex, S1 and S2, or precuneus. Visual input appears to activate sensory neurons of the amputated limb, which[67] in turn reduces the activity of systems that perceive protopathic pain. In addition, the mirror therapy activates areas of the motor cortex.

A randomized trial involving 22 patients showed that mirror therapy for 4 weeks improved phantom pain by 80%. Virtual reality and augmented reality are improved forms of mirror therapies which also have been shown to improve phantom pain.[67] This kind of treatment has been shown to reduce phantom pain in a resistant case unresponsive to a variety of treatment options. This treatment protocol aims to reduce cortical reorganization and establishes enhanced coherence between sensory feedback and motor command by means of virtual reflected imagery.

Some studies have shown significant improvement of PLP with mirror therapy. However, a later study could not reproduce the results and the phantom pain VAS scores were not affected by mirror therapy. Although improvement in phantom sensation has been demonstrated with mirror therapy, at the current time there is no conclusive evidence to support mirror therapy, thus it is not recommended as first-line management of phantom pain. Given its safety and ease of compliance, this therapy is nonetheless widely practiced.

Mirror therapy may interfere with psychological acceptance of and adaptation to the amputated limb and may affect construction of the body image, which would enable use of the prosthetic limb and its function and integration into daily life.

Invasive Treatment Options

The best available evidence for an invasive treatment option is spinal cord stimulation (SCS). SCS involves application of pulsed electrical stimulation at the areas of the dorsal column of the spinal cord by means of placement of epidural electrodes, which are then connected to an internal or external pulse generator. In addition to neuromodulation, it may achieve sympatholysis as well. SCS was trialed for phantom limb pain as early as 1975. Of four patients, three had successful pain relief with subdural electrode placement for SCS.[68] Overall, the success of treatment has been shown to be high initially and then to fade as duration of use is prolonged. The typical success rate in one study was 52.4% at 2 years after SCS implantation and subsequently decreased to 39% at 5 years.[69]

Motor cortex stimulation (MCS) involves stimulation of the prefrontal cortex through surgically implanted epidural electrodes using subthreshold stimulating currents. It was initially used for stroke and trigeminal neuralgia pain and its use has been extended to phantom pain. As in SCS, MCS starts with a trial of stimulation followed by direct implantation and internalization of generator. The trial is considered successful if there is a definite improvement in pain as reflected by a reduction of VAS by more than 30% and patients being comfortable.[70] For phantom pain following upper limb amputation, electrodes are placed on the convex part of the precentral gyrus, whereas for lower limb amputation, interhemispheric leads are preferred. Despite the invasive nature of the procedure, MCS has been shown to be successful in 53% of patients.

Transcranial magnetic stimulation of motor cortex is another commonly used procedure and it has produced long-lasting effects. The mode of action is presumed to be due to elevation of endorphins in the brain.[71]

Deep brain stimulation (DBS) consists of electrical stimulation of stereotactically implanted stick leads into subcortical areas, the thalamus, and basal ganglia areas. DBS has been used for chronic pain conditions and phantom pain patients were included as part of a large trial. DBS was shown to reduce pain by 25% in this study. It also improved patients' quality of life by reducing the amount of opioid intake. More than 75% of patients showed improvement.[72]

Other Invasive Methods

Several other invasive methods have been suggested, but these options should be considered as a last resort. The results are not very impressive, except for peripheral nerve stimulation.[73] Peripheral nerve stimulation is similar to SCS but is confined to the nerve distribution of amputated extremity. It has been shown to be effective.[74] These procedures are done both peripherally and at spinal locations. Intrathecal administration of medication (e.g., a "pain pump") is a rarely used modality for treating phantom pain. Neuroablative neuroma excision was not effective for PLP. Other procedures suggested are dorsal root entry lesioning, anterolateral cordotomy,[75] thalamotomy,[76] and sympathectomy. But these procedures have not been studied specifically for phantom pain.

GUIDING QUESTIONS

- How do you differentiate phantom pain and phantom sensation?
- What are the risk factors associated with development of phantom pain?
- Does phantom pain arise from the peripheral nervous system or central nervous system?
- What is the pathophysiology of phantom pain?
- What are the clinical features of phantom pain?
- What is the differential diagnosis for phantom pain? How does one differentiate it from residual stump pain?
- What are the pharmacological choices for management of phantom pain?
- What are noninvasive treatment options for phantom pain?
- What is the role of spinal cord stimulation in the management of phantom pain?
- Does targeted nerve implantation reduce neuroma pain in amputees?

KEY POINTS

- Phantom pain is defined as an unpleasant or painful sensation in the distribution of the lost or deafferentiated body part. Though phantom pain is known to occur most commonly in the extremities, it has also been reported to occur in other missing or amputated body parts, such as the eyes,[4,5] tongue,[6] breast,[7] teeth, nose, penis,[8] or even part of the GI tract. Incidence of phantom pain varies between 42.2% and 78.8%. Females are more likely to develop and more often suffer from this condition than males. Phantom sensations are divided into kinetic, kinesthetic, and exteroceptive sensations.
- Amputation of the painful limb does not provide a guarantee for relief of the pain. The principal factor contributing

to phantom pain is damage to the nociceptor. Spinal cord plasticity and central nervous system changes also play a role. When nerve endings are cut and receptors are damaged, the arrangement of existing nerve fibers of A-delta and C fibers get disorganized and later grow to form neuromas.

- Psychological factors play a major role in maintenance of the pain. Patients with passive coping strategies and catastrophizing behaviors tend to develop phantom limb pain more often than patients who have better coping strategies. Continuous epidural infusion of local anesthetic initiated before surgery and continued for 72 hours postoperatively has been shown to reduce the development of phantom pain.
- Medications have variable success rates in reducing phantom limb pain. These include NSAIDs, opioids, NMDA receptor antagonists, antidepressants, anticonvulsants, and calcitonin. TENS, mirror therapy, and psychological counseling are some of the noninvasive methods used to manage phantom pain. Spinal cord stimulation has been used successfully to treat phantom limb pain, though the success rate decreases over time.

REFERENCES

1. Padula PA, Friedmann LW. Acquired amputation and prostheses before the sixteenth century. *Angiology.* 1987;38(2 Pt 1):133–141. doi:10.1177/000331978703800207 [doi]
2. Louis ED, York GK. Weir Mitchell's observations on sensory localization and their influence on Jacksonian neurology. *Neurology.* 2006;66(8):1241–1244. doi:66/8/1241 [pii]
3. Soros P, Vo O, Husstedt IW, Evers S, Gerding H. Phantom eye syndrome: Its prevalence, phenomenology, and putative mechanisms. *Neurology.* 2003;60(9):1542–1543.
4. Hanowell ST, Kennedy SF. Phantom tongue pain and causalgia: case presentation and treatment. *Anesth Analg.* 1979;58(5):436–438.
5. Rothemund Y, Grusser SM, Liebeskind U, Schlag PM, Flor H. Phantom phenomena in mastectomized patients and their relation to chronic and acute pre-mastectomy pain. *Pain.* 2004;107(1–2):140–146. doi:S0304395903004159 [pii]
6. Ramachandran VS, McGeoch PD. Occurrence of phantom genitalia after gender reassignment surgery. *Med Hypotheses.* 2007;69(5):1001–1003. doi:S0306-9877(07)00181-8 [pii]
7. Jensen TS, Krebs B, Nielsen J, Rasmussen P. Immediate and long-term phantom limb pain in amputees: incidence, clinical characteristics and relationship to pre-amputation limb pain. *Pain.* 1985;21(3):267–278. doi:0304-3959(85)90090-9 [pii]
8. Richardson C, Glenn S, Nurmikko T, Horgan M. Incidence of phantom phenomena including phantom limb pain 6 months after major lower limb amputation in patients with peripheral vascular disease. *Clin J Pain.* 2006;22(4):353–358. doi:10.1097/01.ajp.0000177793.01415.bd [doi]
9. Desmond DM, Maclachlan M. Prevalence and characteristics of phantom limb pain and residual limb pain in the long term after upper limb amputation. *Int J Rehabil Res Zeitschrift fur Rehabil Int Rech Readapt.* 2010;33(3):279–282. doi:10.1097/MRR.0b013e328336388d [doi]
10. Ephraim PL, Wegener ST, MacKenzie EJ, Dillingham TR, Pezzin LE. Phantom pain, residual limb pain, and back pain in amputees: results of a national survey. *Arch Phys Med Rehabil.* 2005;86(10):1910–1919. doi:S0003-9993(05)00358-8 [pii]
11. Sherman RA, Sherman CJ, Parker L. Chronic phantom and stump pain among American veterans: results of a survey. *Pain.* 1984;18(1):83–95.
12. Hirsh AT, Dillworth TM, Ehde DM, Jensen MP. Sex differences in pain and psychological functioning in persons with limb loss. *J Pain.* 2010;11(1):79–86. doi:10.1016/j.jpain.2009.06.004 [doi]
13. Bosmans JC, Geertzen JH, Post WJ, van der Schans CP, Dijkstra PU. Factors associated with phantom limb pain: a 31/2-year prospective study. *Clin Rehabil.* 2010;24(5):444–453. doi:10.1177/0269215509360645 [doi]
14. Csillik B, Knyihar E, Rakic P. Transganglionic degenerative atrophy and regenerative proliferation in the Rolando substance of the primate spinal cord: discoupling and restoration of synaptic connectivity in the central nervous system after peripheral nerve lesions. *Folia Morphol (Warsz).* 1982;30(2):189–191.
15. Fisher K, Hanspal RS. Phantom pain, anxiety, depression, and their relation in consecutive patients with amputated limbs: case reports. *BMJ.* 1998;316(7135):903–904.
16. Jensen TS, Krebs B, Nielsen J, Rasmussen P. Phantom limb, phantom pain and stump pain in amputees during the first 6 months following limb amputation. *Pain.* 1983;17(3):243–256.

17. Berman JS, Birch R, Anand P. Pain following human brachial plexus injury with spinal cord root avulsion and the effect of surgery. *Pain.* 1998;75(2–3):199–207.

18. Hains BC, Waxman SG. Activated microglia contribute to the maintenance of chronic pain after spinal cord injury. *J Neurosci.* 2006;26(16):4308–4317. doi:26/16/4308 [pii]

19. Melzack R. Phantom limb pain: implications for treatment of pathologic pain. *Anesthesiology.* 1971;35(4):409–419.

20. Schmalzl L, Ehrsson HH. Experimental induction of a perceived "telescoped" limb using a full-body illusion. *Front Hum Neurosci.* 2011;5:34. doi:10.3389/fnhum.2011.00034 [doi]

21. Miles J. Prevention of phantom pain after major lower limb amputation by epidural infusion of diamorphine, clonidine and bupivacaine. *Ann R Coll Surg Engl.* 1995;77(1):71.

22. Madabhushi L, Reuben SS, Steinberg RB, Adesioye J. The efficacy of postoperative perineural infusion of bupivacaine and clonidine after lower extremity amputation in preventing phantom limb and stump pain. *J Clin Anesth.* 2007;19(3):226–229. doi:S0952-8180(07)00035-9 [pii]

23. Krane EJ, Heller LB. The prevalence of phantom sensation and pain in pediatric amputees. *J Pain Symptom Manage.* 1995;10(1):21–29. doi:0885-3924(94)00062-P [pii]

24. Kern U, Busch V, Muller R, Kohl M, Birklein F. Phantom limb pain in daily practice--still a lot of work to do! *Pain Med.* 2012;13(12):1611–1626. doi:10.1111/j.1526-4637.2012.01494.x [doi]

25. Koplovitch P, Minert A, Devor M. Spontaneous pain in partial nerve injury models of neuropathy and the role of nociceptive sensory cover. *Exp Neurol.* 2012;236(1):103–111. doi:10.1016/j.expneurol.2012.04.005 [doi]

26. Reilly KT, Sirigu A. The motor cortex and its role in phantom limb phenomena. *Neuroscientist.* 2008;14(2):195–202. doi:1073858407309466 [pii]

27. Shapira Y, Midha R. Centrocentral Short Circuiting for Management of Stump Neuroma Pain in Amputees. *World Neurosurg.* 2016;86:59–60. doi:10.1016/j.wneu.2015.09.065 [doi]

28. Economides JM, DeFazio M V, Attinger CE, Barbour JR. Prevention of Painful Neuroma and Phantom Limb Pain After Transfemoral Amputations Through Concomitant Nerve Coaptation and Collagen Nerve Wrapping. *Neurosurgery.* 2016;79(3):508–513. doi:10.1227/NEU.0000000000001313 [doi]

29. Nikolajsen L, Jensen TS. Phantom limb pain. *Br J Anaesth.* 2001;87(1):107–116.

30. Florence SL, Garraghty PE, Carlson M, Kaas JH. Sprouting of peripheral nerve axons in the spinal cord of monkeys. *Brain Res.* 1993;601(1–2):343–348. doi:0006-8993(93)91734-A [pii]

31. Fagius J, Nordin M, Wall M. Sympathetic nerve activity to amputated lower leg in humans. Evidence of altered skin vasoconstrictor discharge. *Pain.* 2002;98(1–2):37–45. doi:S0304395901004663 [pii]

32. Saris SC, Iacono RP, Nashold Jr BS. Successful treatment of phantom pain with dorsal root entry zone coagulation. *Appl Neurophysiol.* 1988;51(2–5):188–197.

33. Schmidt AP, Takahashi ME, de Paula Posso I. Phantom limb pain induced by spinal anesthesia. *Clinics (Sao Paulo).* 2005;60(3):263–264. doi:S1807-59322005000300014 [pii]

34. Henry DE, Chiodo AE, Yang W. Central nervous system reorganization in a variety of chronic pain states: a review. *PM R.* 2011;3(12):1116–1125. doi:10.1016/j.pmrj.2011.05.018 [doi]

35. Flor H. Phantom-limb pain: characteristics, causes, and treatment. *Lancet Neurol.* 2002;1(3):182–189.

36. Giummarra MJ, Gibson SJ, Georgiou-Karistianis N, Bradshaw JL. Central mechanisms in phantom limb perception: the past, present and future. *Brain Res Rev.* 2007;54(1):219–232.

37. Frazier SH, Kolb LC. Psychiatric aspects of pain and the phantom limb. *Orthop Clin North Am.* 1970;1(2):481–495.

38. Coffey L, Gallagher P, Horgan O, Desmond D, MacLachlan M. Psychosocial adjustment to diabetes-related lower limb amputation. *Diabet Med.* 2009;26(10):1063–1067. doi:10.1111/j.1464-5491.2009.02802.x [doi]

39. Kulkarni J, Gaine WJ, Buckley JG, Rankine JJ, Adams J. Chronic low back pain in traumatic lower limb amputees. *Clin Rehabil.* 2005;19(1):81–86. doi:10.1191/0269215505cr819oa [doi]

40. Woolf CJ, Chong MS. Preemptive analgesia--treating postoperative pain by preventing the establishment of central sensitization. *Anesth Analg.* 1993;77(2):362–379.

41. Ypsilantis E, Tang TY. Pre-emptive analgesia for chronic limb pain after amputation for peripheral vascular disease: a systematic review. *Ann Vasc Surg.* 2010;24(8):1139–1146. doi:10.1016/j.avsg.2010.03.026 [doi]

42. Schug SA, Burrell R, Payne J, Tester P. Pre-emptive epidural analgesia may prevent phantom limb pain. *Reg Anesth.* 1995;20(3):256.

43. Nikolajsen L, Ilkjaer S, Jensen TS. Effect of preoperative extradural bupivacaine and morphine on stump sensation in lower limb amputees. *Br J Anaesth.* 1998;81(3):348–354.

44. Pinzur MS, Garla PG, Pluth T, Vrbos L. Continuous postoperative infusion of a regional

anesthetic after an amputation of the lower extremity. A randomized clinical trial. *J bone Jt surgeryAmerican Vol.* 1996;78(10):1501–1505.

45. Souza JM, Cheesborough JE, Ko JH, Cho MS, Kuiken TA, Dumanian GA. Targeted muscle reinnervation: a novel approach to postamputation neuroma pain. *Clin Orthop Relat Res.* 2014;472(10):2984–2990. doi:10.1007/s11999-014-3528-7 [doi]

46. Pet MA, Ko JH, Friedly JL, Mourad PD, Smith DG. Does targeted nerve implantation reduce neuroma pain in amputees? *Clin Orthop Relat Res.* 2014;472(10):2991–3001. doi:10.1007/s11999-014-3602-1 [doi]

47. Halbert J, Crotty M, Cameron ID. Evidence for the optimal management of acute and chronic phantom pain: a systematic review. *Clin J Pain.* 2002;18(2):84–92.

48. Alviar MJ, Hale T, Dungca M. Pharmacologic interventions for treating phantom limb pain. *Cochrane database Syst Rev.* 2016;10:CD006380. doi:10.1002/14651858.CD006380.pub3 [doi]

49. Huse E, Larbig W, Flor H, Birbaumer N. The effect of opioids on phantom limb pain and cortical reorganization. *Pain.* 2001;90(1–2):47–55. doi:S0304-3959(00)00385-7 [pii]

50. Wu CL, Tella P, Staats PS, et al. Analgesic effects of intravenous lidocaine and morphine on postamputation pain: a randomized double-blind, active placebo-controlled, crossover trial. *Anesthesiology.* 2002;96(4):841–848. doi:00000542-200204000-00010 [pii]

51. McCormick Z, Chang-Chien G, Marshall B, Huang M, Harden RN. Phantom limb pain: a systematic neuroanatomical-based review of pharmacologic treatment. *Pain Med.* 2014;15(2):292–305. doi:10.1111/pme.12283 [doi]

52. Bergmans L, Snijdelaar DG, Katz J, Crul BJ. Methadone for phantom limb pain. *Clin J Pain.* 2002;18(3):203–205.

53. Robinson LR, Czerniecki JM, Ehde DM, et al. Trial of amitriptyline for relief of pain in amputees: results of a randomized controlled study. *Arch Phys Med Rehabil.* 2004;85(1):1–6. doi:S0003-9993(03)00476-3 [pii]

54. Wilder-Smith CH, Hill LT, Laurent S. Postamputation pain and sensory changes in treatment-naive patients: characteristics and responses to treatment with tramadol, amitriptyline, and placebo. *Anesthesiology.* 2005;103(3):619–628. doi:00000542-200509000-00027 [pii]

55. Sato K, Higuchi H, Hishikawa Y. Management of phantom limb pain and sensation with milnacipran. *J Neuropsychiatry Clin Neurosci.* 2008;20(3):368. doi:10.1176/appi.neuropsych.20.3.368 [doi]

56. Nagoshi Y, Watanabe A, Inoue S, et al. Usefulness of milnacipran in treating phantom limb pain. *Neuropsychiatr Dis Treat.* 2012;8:549–553. doi:10.2147/NDT.S37431 [doi]

57. Kuiken TA, Schechtman L, Harden RN. Phantom limb pain treatment with mirtazapine: a case series. *Pain Pract.* 2005;5(4):356–360. doi:PPR038 [pii]

58. Bone M, Critchley P, Buggy DJ. Gabapentin in postamputation phantom limb pain: a randomized, double-blind, placebo-controlled, cross-over study. *Reg Anesth Pain Med.* 2002;27(5):481–486. doi:S1098733902000184 [pii]

59. Hayes C, Armstrong-Brown A, Burstal R. Perioperative intravenous ketamine infusion for the prevention of persistent postamputation pain: a randomized, controlled trial. *Anaesth Intensive Care.* 2004;32(3):330–338. doi:2003204 [pii]

60. Nikolajsen L, Hansen CL, Nielsen J, Keller J, Arendt-Nielsen L, Jensen TS. The effect of ketamine on phantom pain: a central neuropathic disorder maintained by peripheral input. *Pain.* 1996;67(1):69–77. doi:0304-3959(96)03080-1 [pii]

61. Wiech K, Kiefer RT, Topfner S, et al. A placebo-controlled randomized crossover trial of the N-methyl-D-aspartic acid receptor antagonist, memantine, in patients with chronic phantom limb pain. *Anesth Analg.* 2004;98(2):408–413, table of contents.

62. Jaeger H, Maier C. Calcitonin in phantom limb pain: a double-blind study. *Pain.* 1992;48(1):21–27. doi:0304-3959(92)90127-W [pii]

63. Eichenberger U, Neff F, Sveticic G, et al. Chronic phantom limb pain: the effects of calcitonin, ketamine, and their combination on pain and sensory thresholds. *Anesth Analg.* 2008;106(4):1265–1273, table of contents. doi:10.1213/ane.0b013e3181685014 [doi]

64. Mulvey MR, Radford HE, Fawkner HJ, Hirst L, Neumann V, Johnson MI. Transcutaneous electrical nerve stimulation for phantom pain and stump pain in adult amputees. *Pain Pract.* 2013;13(4):289–296. doi:10.1111/j.1533-2500.2012.00593.x [doi]

65. Carabelli RA, Kellerman WC. Phantom limb pain: relief by application of TENS to contralateral extremity. *Arch Phys Med Rehabil.* 1985;66(7):466–467.

66. Barbin J, Seetha V, Casillas JM, Paysant J, Perennou D. The effects of mirror therapy on pain and motor control of phantom limb in amputees: A systematic review. *Ann Phys Rehabil Med.* 2016;59S:e149. doi:S1877-0657(16)30414-6 [pii]

67. Dunn J, Yeo E, Moghaddampour P, Chau B, Humbert S. Virtual and augmented reality in

the treatment of phantom limb pain: A literature review. *NeuroRehabilitation.* February 2017.
doi:10.3233/NRE-171447 [doi]

68. Nielson KD, Adams JE, Hosobuchi Y. Phantom
limb pain. Treatment with dorsal column stimulation. *J Neurosurg.* 1975;42(3):301–307.
doi:10.3171/jns.1975.42.3.0301 [doi]

69. De Caridi G, Massara M, Serra R, et al. Spinal
Cord Stimulation Therapy for the Treatment of
Concomitant Phantom Limb Pain and Critical
Limb Ischemia. *Ann Vasc Surg.* 2016;32:131.e11–
131.e14. doi:10.1016/j.avsg.2015.10.015 [doi]

70. Lee JH, Byun JH, Choe YR, Lim SK, Lee KY,
Choi IS. Successful Treatment of Phantom Limb
Pain by 1 Hz Repetitive Transcranial Magnetic
Stimulation Over Affected Supplementary
Motor Complex: A Case Report. *Ann Rehabil
Med.*   2015;39(4):630–633.   doi:10.5535/
arm.2015.39.4.630 [doi]

71. Taheri A, Lajevardi M, Arab S, Firouzian A, Sharifi
H. Repetitive Transcranial Magnetic Stimulation
for Phantom Limb Pain: Probably Effective but
Understudied. *Neuromodulation.* 2017;20(1):88–
89. doi:10.1111/ner.12569 [doi]

72. Falowski SM. Deep Brain Stimulation for Chronic
Pain. *Curr Pain Headache Rep.* 2015;19(7):21–27.
doi:10.1007/s11916-015-0504-1 [doi]

73. Deer TR, Mekhail N, Provenzano D, et al. The
appropriate use of neurostimulation of the spinal
cord and peripheral nervous system for the treatment of chronic pain and ischemic diseases: the
Neuromodulation Appropriateness Consensus
Committee. *Neuromodulation.* 2014;17(6):515–
550; discussion 550. doi:10.1111/ner.12208 [doi]

74. Rauck RL, Kapural L, Cohen SP, et al.
Peripheral nerve stimulation for the treatment of postamputation pain--a case report.
Pain Pract. 2012;12(8):649–655. doi:10.1111/
j.1533-2500.2012.00552.x [doi]

75. White JC, Sweet WH. Effectiveness of chordotomy
in phantom pain after amputation. *AMA.archives
Neurol psychiatry.* 1952;67(3):315–322.

76. Jamieson KG. Thalamotomy for Phantom Pain.
Med J Aust. 1965;1(19):687–688.

PART V

Spinal Nerve Root Disease: Radicular Pain

26

Cervical Radiculopathy

SAMUEL W. SAMUEL AND EDUARDO E. ICAZA

CASE

A 45-year-old Caucasian man presents with right-sided neck pain with radiation to his right shoulder and to his right ring and little finger. The pain seems to be positional and worsens when he turns his neck to the right. Turning his neck to the left seems to produce some pain relief. After sleeping for 5 hours, his right arm tingles and it wakens him from sleep. He has tried physical therapy with traction. Ultimately he obtained an MRI of the cervical spine, which showed right C6-7 disc herniation with uncovertebral joint hypertrophy causing moderate to severe right C6-7 foraminal stenosis.

DEFINITION

Cervical radiculopathy is defined by the multidisciplinary North American Spine Society (NASS) as "a pain in a radicular pattern in one or both upper extremities related to compression and/or irritation of one or more cervical roots. Frequent signs and symptoms include varying degrees of sensory, motor and reflex changes as well as dysesthesias and paresthesias related to nerve root(s) without evidence of spinal cord dysfunction (myelopathy)."[1]

EPIDEMIOLOGY AND ETIOLOGY

The incidence of cervical radiculopathy is estimated to be 107.3 per 100,000 for men and 63.5 per 100,000 for women, with a mean incidence of around 83 per 100,000. The age-specific annual incidence per 100,000 population reached a peak of 202.9 for the age group 50–54 years. Cervical radiculopathy is less common than lumbar radiculopathy. C7 monoradiculopathy has the most common incidence, followed by C6 monoradiculopathy. Disc herniation was responsible for symptoms in only 21.9% of cases, whereas cervical spondylosis was responsible for 68.4% of cases. During a mean duration of

4.9 years' follow-up, 31.7% of patients experienced a recurrence, though only 26% required surgical intervention to relieve symptoms.[2]

It is estimated that, in 70% of patients with cervical radiculopathy, the etiology of the pain and the symptoms are secondary to foraminal stenosis. In most cases such symptoms are due to degenerative changes, including decreased disc height or degenerative changes of the uncovertebral joints anteriorly or zygapophyseal joints posteriorly.[2]

Cervical neuroforamina are widest in the upper cervical spine, with the C7–T1 foramina being the narrowest. Hypermobility of the cervical facet joints leads to ligamentous hypertrophy as well as bony hypertrophy. An increase in size of the superior articular process from the distal vertebra causes compression of the nerve root. Cervical disc herniation accounts for 20%–25% of cervical radiculopathy, which may be acute or chronic. Chronic disc herniation results from disc degeneration and desiccation with resultant decrease in disc height and neuroforaminal narrowing. Chronic disc herniation leads to the insidious onset of symptoms. Acute disc herniation, by contrast, results in ischemia and inflammation of the nerve root with acute onset of severe pain.[3] Chronic herniation allows the body to adapt to the changes, and symptoms are usually milder and usually resolve spontaneously.

Asymptomatic neural compression is not uncommon, and compression of the nerve root alone does not necessarily cause pain unless the dorsal root ganglion is involved.[4] In most cases, cervical radiculopathy tends to be self-limiting with spontaneous resolution of symptoms with conservative therapy, although it is hard to define the natural history given the unreported cases of patients who do not seek medical attention.[1]

CLINICAL FEATURES, DIAGNOSIS, AND DIFFERENTIAL DIAGNOSIS

History and physical examination are the most important diagnostic tools in the diagnosis of cervical radiculopathy. In fact, up to 75% of cases can be diagnosed on the basis of history and physical examination; most patients present with classic unilateral symptoms.[5] Classic symptoms include neck pain with arm pain and dysesthesias in a dermatomal/myotomal distribution that correlates with the level of nerve root compression. Pain is often characterized as a sudden, intense shooting or stabbing that is triggered by certain movements. Bilateral symptoms are rare but usually indicate central cervical stenosis. Table 26.1 outlines the level of compression with the corresponding pain pattern, muscles affected, and diminished reflex. Symptoms associated with recent trauma or red flags for malignancy, myelopathy, hematoma, or infection warrant immediate imaging.[3–5]

History should include questions to determine symptoms or signs of myelopathy. Myelopathy symptoms often reported by patients include problems with hand dexterity (difficulty writing or opening jars, buttoning, and using door knobs) as well as gait and/or balance problems. Elderly persons have a higher incidence of myelopathy and require special attention to rule out occult symptoms.[6]

Cervical radicular symptoms can overlap with multiple other clinical entities (Table 26.2). C5 radiculopathy radiates to the shoulder, the anterior arm, and elbow, which can be confused with shoulder impingement. Shoulder impingement is a common condition that presents with painful movement of the shoulder and inability to lie on the affected side. Shoulder-provocative tests, including Hawkin's and empty can sign, should be used to differentiate between the two conditions. Limited cervical range of motion and a positive Spurling's test (extension and lateral rotation/flexion to the affected side) are usually positive in cervical radiculopathy. Spurling's test has been shown to be 93% specific and 30% sensitive.[7,8]

C6 radiculopathy can be confused with carpal tunnel syndrome (CTS). CTS commonly presents with nighttime pain and tingling and numbness in the thumb, index and middle fingers and the lateral aspect of the ring finger. Motor manifestations of CTS include weakness of the abductor pollicis brevis, which is innervated by the recurrent branch of the median nerve (which takes off distal to the transverse carpal ligament). Advanced CTS presents with atrophy of the thenar eminence. Positive Tinel's sign at the wrist, Durken's median nerve test, and wrist flexion will exacerbate CTS symptoms, but not those of cervical radiculopathy.[9] In contrast, a C6 radiculopathy affects the elbow flexors and wrist flexors with a positive Spurling's test. A C7 radiculopathy includes dysesthesias down the posterior arm to the middle finger and can also be confused with CTS. C8 radiculopathy presents with pain down the medial aspect of the arm into the ring and little fingers, potentially confused with ulnar neuropathy. Ulnar neuropathy is reproduced with elbow flexion and may also manifest with a positive Tinel's sign over the cubital tunnel.

Motor examination would show corresponding muscle weakness (see Table 26.1). The upper four cervical nerve roots lack a myotomal correspondence. C5 will result in weakness in

---

TABLE 26.1. DISTRIBUTION OF CERVICAL RADICULOPATHY

Nerve Root	Pain Pattern	Muscles Affected	Reflex
C2	Occipital, eye	N/A	N/A
C3	Neck, trapezius	N/A	N/A
C4	Lower neck, trapezius	N/A	N/A
C5	Neck, shoulder and lateral arm	Deltoid, supraspinatus, infraspinatus	Biceps
C6	Lateral arm, first two fingers	Biceps, brachioradialis, wrist extensors	Brachioradialis
C7	Neck, lateral arm and middle finger	Triceps, wrist flexors, finger extensors	Triceps
C8	Neck, medial forearm, ulnar digits	Finger flexors	N/A

TABLE 26.2. DIFFERENTIAL DIAGNOSIS OF CERVICAL RADICULOPATHY

Cardiac pain	Typically to left upper extremity
Rotator cuff impingement	Pain with shoulder movement, pain at night when sleeping on the symptomatic side, positive shoulder impingement maneuvers
sParsonage-Turner syndrome (acute brachial plexopathy)	Acute onset, usually affecting C5, affecting motor and sensory
Cervical myelopathy	Difficulties with hand dexterity, gait disturbances, hyperreflexia in lower extremities, positive long tract signs
Thoracic outlet syndrome	Usually affecting the lower trunk of brachial plexus, may be accompanied by vascular compression and diminished upper extremity pulses
Malignancy	Weight loss, loss of appetite, e.g., Pancoast tumor
Entrapment syndromes	Median or ulnar nerve compression resulting in motor and sensory deficits in distribution of the peripheral nerve
Complex regional pain syndrome	Pain out of proportion of physical findings, hyperesthesia, sudomotor, vasomotor changes

the deltoid muscle on the affected side, while C6 will show weakness in the biceps and the extensor carpi radialis longus and brevis (wrist extensors). C7 radiculopathy may cause weakness of the triceps and the brachioradialis, and C8 radiculopathy causes weakness of the intrinsic muscles of the hand, which can be evaluated by finger abduction and handgrip. Provocative tests for cervical radiculopathy include the following:

(1) *Spurling's test:* Extension and lateral rotation/flexion to the affected side occur.
(2) *Shoulder abduction test:* The shoulder of the symptomatic side is abducted above the patient's head; a positive test relieves the pain.[8]
(3) *Traction/neck distraction:* The patient lies supine while the examiner cups the occiput while supporting the angle of the mandible. Gentle traction is then applied; pain relief would constitute a positive test. This test has low to moderate sensitivity and high specificity.[1,8]
(4) *Valsalva maneuver:* Exhaling against a closed glottis results in increased intrathoracic pressure and intrathecal pressure; a positive test results in increased pain. This test has low to moderate sensitivity and high specificity.[8]

In addition to the history and physical examination, imaging studies play an important role in diagnosing cervical radiculopathy. Plain anteroposterior and lateral X-rays are useful for demonstrating bony alignment. Flexion and extension films are helpful in diagnosing instability that might not be evident on static films. Magnetic resonance imaging (MRI) is the study of choice for delineation of the soft tissues, nerve roots exiting from the spinal foramen, and morphological changes in the spinal cord. MRI is especially ideal for confirmation of a suspected disc herniation or spondylotic changes. Several studies have correlated MRI findings with postoperative outcome.

Computerized tomography (CT) scans are the most sensitive examination for bony structures. Ossification of the posterior longitudinal ligament resulting in canal stenosis and the bony anatomy of the neuroforamen causing nerve root compression can also be seen. CT scanning is also helpful in surgical planning or appropriate for patients with contraindications to MRI (pacemakers, severe claustrophobia).

Electromyography (EMG) can aid in the diagnosis of cervical radiculopathy; however, EMG has a poor predictive value when used alone. EMG is known to have significant operator variability, and only 42% of patients with a positive EMG finding had compression at the time surgery, whereas 93% of those with a positive MRI finding had pathology. The NASS does not recommend routinely performing EMG if imaging findings do not show any concordant pathology.

TREATMENT

The majority of patients diagnosed with cervical radiculopathy (75%–90%) improve with nonoperative conservative management. Conservative treatment may include physical therapy, oral NSAIDs, membrane stabilizers, osteopathic manipulation, chiropractic manipulation, traction, and steroid injections. Physical therapy accompanied by home exercise for 6 weeks has been shown in a randomized trial to substantially reduce neck and arm pain for patients with cervical radiculopathy.[10] Different physical therapy modalities have been studied, including rest and collar immobilization. Three studies that compared immobilization to active therapy showed no difference in long-term outcome; however, those treated more aggressively tended to improve more quickly. Active intervention is more favored in the literature than prolonged use of collars as the latter leads to deconditioning of the cervical musculature and should generally be avoided.

There is no clear evidence that highlights first-line use of muscle relaxants, corticosteroid tapers, NSAIDs, opioids, or membrane stabilizers over each other. Membrane stabilizers, such as gabapentin and pregabalin, have been extensively studied in treatment of *lumbrosacral* radicular pain. A multicenter double-blinded study comparing gabapentin versus epidural steroid injection found no significant difference at 3 months.[11] Despite the popularity of prescribing oral steroids, there is poor evidence supporting this practice. If there is an associated myofascial component with the radiculopathy, then muscle relaxants are a reasonable therapy. As with starting any new medications, risks and benefits should be carefully weighed and explained to the patient.

Cervical epidural steroid injections, both interlaminar and transforaminal, have long been therapeutic options for various neck pain etiologies, including cervical radiculopathy. Transforaminal approaches remain controversial given their known risk of catastrophic complications, and there are no randomized comparative trials of this approach versus the interlaminar approach. For interlaminar cervical injections, a volume of 2–4 mL is usually adequate to bathe the cervical roots at several levels. A recent systemic review to determine the long-term efficacy of cervical epidural steroids found level II evidence supporting interlaminar cervical epidural steroid injections.[11] Another

randomized controlled study found that 80% of patients received greater than 50% relief from a series of interlaminar cervical epidural steroid injections at 2 years.[12]

Another minimally invasive option is cervical percutaneous epidural neuroplasty, in which the aim is to break down fibrous adhesions in the intervertebral foramina. The clinical effectiveness of cervical percutaneous epidural neuroplasty remains to be thoroughly investigated. A recent study with 80 patients showed improved visual analog scale (VAS) scores for a prolonged period when compared to cervical epidural injections.[13] However, limitations of the study include lack of a control conservative group and inclusion of patients with neck pain with and without radiculopathy, which limit the generalizability of the findings. Furthermore, this procedure is only for single-level cervical disease and is not widely available.

Pulsed radiofrequency is a treatment option that is more commonly used outside the United States. The mechanism of action is theorized to be based on the change in electromagnetic field at temperatures below that of traditional thermocoagulation. One prospective study found comparable outcomes from cervical dorsal root ganglion pulsed radiofrequency to those from transforminal epidural steroid injections.[14] Another smaller study of patients with chronic radiculopathy refractory to transforaminal steroid injections used pulsed radiofrequency of 42°C for 120 seconds and found that 15 of 21 patients (66%) had greater than 50% pain relief at 3 and 12 months.[15] More studies are needed to establish this treatment modality, but it holds promise for future treatment algorithms.

Cervical radiculopathy with myelopathy findings or pain/dysesthesias refractory to conservative therapy and injections should prompt surgical evaluation. Surgical options include anterior cervical decompression and fusion, cervical disc arthroplasty, laminectomy, and posterior foraminotomy. Typically, anterior approaches are preferred for excising lateral disc herniations and osteophytes without having to disrupt the spinal cord. The posterior approaches are favored for performing a laminectomy or foraminotomy. Known surgical complications include infection, hardware failure, worsening compressive symptoms, and nerve damage. Analysis has shown that utilization of surgery for cervical radiculopathy has increased dramatically since 1990.[16] There is evidence that surgery for cervical radiculopathy results in improved short-term pain control, although it does not outperform conservative management at long-term endpoints.[17] Prospective studies comparing surgery versus cervical bracing versus physical therapy found no significant difference in pain, strength, or sensory measures at 1 year.[18] However, the evidence for surgical decompression for myelopathy symptoms is stronger, with one paper reporting neurological improvement in nearly 70% of cases.[19] Overall, the mixed evidence for a variety of outcomes reinforces that physicians, both surgical and nonsurgical, should collaborate to form appropriate treatment plans.[1]

Neuromodulation is a treatment modality that is commonly employed in the treatment of lumbar spine pain conditions, including post-laminectomy syndrome with chronic radicular pain. To date, there have been no extensive studies examining the outcomes for neuromodulation specifically for treatment of cervical radiculopathy. A single-site retrospective review of cervical neuromodulation included six cases with chronic cervical radicular pain.[20] This small sample size found favorable outcomes, although the mean pain relief lasted an average of 3.6 years. This modality also remains controversial as some experts would argue that placing epidural leads may lead to worsening of compressive symptoms.

There are no systemic reviews investigating the outcomes of manipulation or chiropractic therapies in cervical radiculopathy. There are, however, several case reports of serious complications from manipulations. As with all treatments, risks and benefits should be carefully explained to the patient.

GUIDING QUESTIONS
- What are the main pathophysiological causes of cervical radiculopathy?
- How do you approach differential diagnoses of cervical radicular pain?
- How is cervical radiculopathy diagnosed?
- What are the main treatment options for cervical radicular pain?

KEY POINTS
- Cervical radiculopathy is a common painful condition from cervical root compression and/or irritation. There is a peak incidence in males in the fifth decade with a 30% chance of lifetime recurrence.
- A thorough history and physical exam can often diagnose the affected nerve root without the need for reflexive imaging. A series of provocative tests can aid in the differential diagnosis.
- The majority of cases will resolve with conservative management within several weeks of symptom onset. If symptoms include myelopathic symptoms (gait imbalance, lower extremity symptoms, hyperreflexia) or are refractory to 6 to 8 weeks of conservative management, advanced imaging such as MRI should be considered.
- Imaging that reveals a compressive etiology that has failed conservative therapy should trigger a surgical consultation. The North American Spine Society recommends either an MRI or CT be obtained prior to surgical decompression for optimal planning. Evidence-based conservative management includes physical therapy and oral NSAIDs.
- Both interventional and surgical treatments show positive outcomes in the short term but long-term outcomes appear comparable to those with conservative therapies. As with all treatments, appropriate patient selection can lead to more successful outcomes. We recommend pursuing conservative treatment strategies for 6–8 weeks before pursuing procedural or surgical intervention.

REFERENCES
1. Bono CM, Ghiselli G, Gilbert TJ, et al. An evidence-based clinical guideline for the diagnosis and treatment of cervical radiculopathy from degenerative disorders. *Spine J.* 2011;11:64–72.
2. Radhakrishnan K, Litchey WJ, O'Fallon WM, Kurland LT. Epidemiology of cervical radiculopathy. A population-based study from Rochester, Minnesota. *Brain.* 1994;117:325–335.
3. Eubanks J. Cervical radiculopathy: nonoperative management of neck pain and radicular symptoms. *Am Fam Physician.* 2010;81:33–40.
4. Carette S, Fehlings M. Cervical Radiculopathy. *N Engl J Med.* 2005;353:392–399.
5. Polston DW. Cervical Radiculopathy. *Neurol Clin.* 2007;25:373–385.
6. Cohen I, Jouve C. *Cervical Radiculopathy, Essentials of Physical Medicine and Rehabilitation.* 2nd ed. Philadelphia: Elsevier; 2008:17–22.

7. Tong HC, Haig AJ, Yamakawa K. The Spurling test and cervical radiculopathy. *Spine (Phila Pa 1976)*. 2002;27:156–159.

8. Rubinstein SM, Pool JJM, van Tulder MW, Riphagen II, de Vet HCW. A systematic review of the diagnostic accuracy of provocative tests of the neck for diagnosing cervical radiculopathy. *Eur Spine J*. 2007;16:307–319.

9. Diwan SA, Manchikanti L, Benyamin RM, et al. Effectiveness of cervical epidural injections in the management of chronic neck and upper extremity pain. *Pain Physician*. 2012;15:405–434.

10. Kuijper B, Tans JTJ, Beelen A, Nollet F, de Visser M. Cervical collar or physiotherapy versus wait and see policy for recent onset cervical radiculopathy: randomised trial. *BMJ*. 2009;339:b3883.

11. Cohen SP, Hanling S, Bicket MC, et al. Epidural steroid injections compared with gabapentin for lumbosacral radicular pain: multicenter randomized double blind comparative efficacy study. *BMJ*. 2015;350:h1748.

12. Manchikanti L, Cash K a, Pampati V, Wargo BW, Malla Y. A randomized, double-blind, active control trial of fluoroscopic cervical interlaminar epidural injections in chronic pain of cervical disc herniation: results of a 2-year follow-up. *Pain Physician*. 2013;16:465–478.

13. Ji GY, Oh CH, Won KS, et al. Randomized controlled study of percutaneous epidural neuroplasty using Racz catheter and epidural steroid injection in cervical disc disease. *Pain Physician*. 2016;19:39–47.

14. Lee DG, Ahn SH, Lee J. Comparative effectivenesses of pulsed radiofrequency and transforaminal steroid injection for radicular pain due to disc herniation: a prospective randomized trial. *J Korean Med Sci*. 2016;31:1324–1330.

15. Choi G, Ahn S, Cho Y, Lee D. Long-term effect of pulsed radiofrequency on chronic cervical radicular pain refractory to repeated transforaminal epidural steroid injections. *Pain Med*. 2012;13(3):368–375.

16. Patil PG, Turner DA, Pietrobon R. National trends in surgical procedures for degenerative spine disease 1990–2000. *Neurosurgery*. 2005;57:753–758.

17. Nikolaidis I, Fouyas IP, Sandercock PA, Statham PF. Surgery for cervical radiculopathy or myelopathy. *Cochrane Database Syst Rev*. 2010:CD001466. doi:10.1002/14651858.CD001466.pub3

18. Persson LCG, Moritz U, Brandt L, Carlsson CA. Cervical radiculopathy: pain, muscle weakness and sensory loss in patients with cervical radiculopathy treated with surgery, physiotherapy or cervical collar: a prospective, controlled study. *Eur Spine J*. 1997;6:256–266.

19. Pandey AS, Thompson BG. Neurosurgery. In: Doherty GM, ed. *Current Diagnosis and Tteatment: Surgery*. 14 ed. New York: McGraw-Hill; 2015.

20. Chivukula S, Tempel ZJ, Weiner GM, et al. Cervical and cervicomedullary spinal cord stimulation for chronic pain: efficacy and outcomes. *Clin Neurol Neurosurg*. 2014;127:33–41.

27

Thoracic Radicular Pain

VICTOR FOORSOV AND SARAH M. PASTORIZA

CASE

A 37-year-old man presents for evaluation of mid-back and right-sided abdominal pain. The pain started a year ago and had been intermittent. The onset was insidious. The pain is located in the right lower thoracic spine and radiates to the right anterior abdominal wall but does not cross midline. He has generally been avoiding physical activities such as playing tennis as it exacerbates his symptoms. He was seen by a chiropractor with temporary pain relief. He has also tried topical anti-inflammatory medications, physical therapy, acupressure and acupuncture, and massage therapy without clear benefit. Physical examination reveals tenderness of the axial thoracic spine, decreased sensation to light touch along the right T9 dermatome, and right-sided abdominal wall bulging with active thoracic flexion in supine position. Thoracic MRI reveals a T9/10 right paracentral disc herniation abutting the corresponding nerve root. He was started on gabapentin 600 mg three times daily with some pain relief. He underwent a T9/10 interlaminar epidural steroid injection with total solution of 5 cc of lidocaine 1% and triamcinolone 40 mg. He responded with 70% pain reduction for 4 weeks. Repeat injection and physical therapy improved his symptoms, with approximately 80% pain reduction.

DEFINITION

Radiculopathy is described as pain and paresthesia radiating in distribution of the nerve root and is often associated with sensory loss and paraspinal muscle spasm.[1] Thoracic radiculopathy is an uncommon disorder that is often overlooked in clinical practice.[2] Radiculopathy typically originates from mechanical compression of nerve root due to degenerative spine changes, such as disc herniation or spondylosis.[3] The most common etiologies of thoracic radiculopathy are disc disease, osteoporosis leading to vertebral compression fractures, and diabetic neuropathy.[2,4] There have been various case reports describing etiologies such as ossification of the posterior longitudinal ligament and/or the ligamentum flavum, viral infection, metastasis, tumor, scoliosis, tuberculosis, collapsed thoracic vertebral bodies, faulty spinal cord stimulator placement, ischemia, Myodil cyst, and adjacent-level disease after cervical fusion. Thoracic radiculopathies may be confused clinically with intra-abdominal disorders.[3] Given the dermatomal involvement, it is crucial to rule out a chest or intra-abdominal process correlated with various viscerosomatic points throughout the thoracic region (Table 27.1).

PATHOPHYSIOLOGY

The thoracic spine is designed more for protection of the chest and abdominal structures than for movement. It is a kyphotic curve nestled between two lordotic curves. It is unique in that its motions are restricted by the articulations of the rib cage, and its kyphosis is maintained by the shape of the vertebral bodies, not the disc heights as in the cervical or lumbar regions. When compared to the cervical and lumbar spine, the thoracic spine is unique in that mechanical studies have shown that the thoracic intervertebral disks are at high risk for injury with combined torsional and bending loading forces.[5] There are 1–2 degrees of extension at each thoracic segment, giving an overall thoracic extension of 15–20 degrees and a total of 25–45 degrees of side-bending and twisting, which can only occur at the cervicothoracic and thoracolumbar junctions.[2] The spinal cord cross-sectional area narrows while traversing the thoracic region; however, the spinal cord/canal ratio is approximately 40% in the thoracic spine compared with 25% in the cervical spine.[5] This anatomical

TABLE 27.1. THORACIC LEVEL OF SEGMENTAL SYMPATHETIC NERVE SUPPLY (VISCEROSOMATIC REFLEXES)[19]

Thoracic Level	
T1–T5	Heart
T2–T7	Lung
T5–T6	Esophagus
T6–T10	Stomach, spleen, Pancreas, Liver (T6-T9), Gallbladder (T7-T10)
T11–L1	Kidney

variation may be of clinical significance in that small disturbances may be disproportionately potentiated. The most frequent disc herniations occur around T8–T12, with the T11–T12 levels accounting for an incidence of 26%–50%.[2] The combination of the thoracic rib cage, vertically oriented facets at T1–T10, smaller intervertebral discs, and dentate ligament[6] optimizes the stability of the thoracic region. The flexion restraint lessens the potential for intervertebral disk injury in the thoracic region compared to that in the lumbar region.[5]

The incidence of trauma leading to thoracic disc herniation is approximately 20%; degeneration is the prevailing etiology of thoracic disc herniation. Osteoporosis can play a role in vertebral compression fractures of the thoracic spine, which may lead to critical intervertebral foramen narrowing and subsequent nerve root compression. The wedging from a fracture may also lead to disc herniations as a result of the aberrant forces placed on the disc. Most of the thoracic fractures that are associated with neurological injury are due to trauma and may involve the spinal cord and cauda equina. As part of the normal process of aging, the water content within the intervertebral discs decreases, leading to reduced disc height and subsequent impaired ability to absorb the axial loads of the spine.[7] Disc herniations occur 75% of the time below the level of T8, as a result of the increased mobility of these levels and therefore increased exerted forces.[6] Some opine that these lower thoracic levels are also more susceptible to myelopathy owing to increased mobility, delicate vascular supply, and a lack of peripheral white matter surrounding the conus.[8] The most common movement leading to herniations are torsional and hyperextension movements similar to a golf swing.[7]

EPIDEMIOLOGY

The occurrence of symptomatic thoracic disk disease is greatest between the fourth and sixth decade, with peak incidence in the fifth decade[5] in patients with diabetes mellitus, osteoarthritis, degenerative disc disease, compression fractures, structural kyphosis due to Paget's disease, or postural kyphosis. There appears to be a slight male predominance, and there is a small population of adolescents with Scheuermann disease that can present with myelopathy or radicular symptoms of the thoracic region. Symptomatic thoracic disc herniations account for less than 1% of all disc herniations.[3] Analysis of population studies found an incidence of approximately 1 per 1,000,000 patient years.[9]

CLINICAL FEATURES

The presentation of radiculopathy in the thoracic spine is different from that in the lumbar spine, as the spinal cord terminates around L1/L2. The presentation of radicular pain in the thoracic region is more common in the lower thoracic region and with lateral disk herniations often associated with some amount of axial pain.[5] The pain is commonly described as a dermatomal distribution, with T10 being the most common regardless of the level involved.[5] Other symptoms are long track signs, leg weakness, numbness and tingling across chest or abdomen or shoulders, spasticity, and bowel or bladder dysfunction.[9] Gastrointestinal (10%–15% of the time) or cardiopulmonary disturbances also can occur.[6] Reflexes may be retained in thoracic radiculopathy in contrast to decreased or absent in lumbar radiculopathy, and Hoffman's sign is negative, although it can be positive in cervical radiculopathy. Myelopathy is the most worrisome presentation that affects the lower extremities, with positive Babinski sign, sustained clonus, a wide-based gait, and spasticity.[5] Another presenting factor for thoracic radiculopathy is abdominal wall bulging, due to weakness (Beevor's sign, which is the movement of the navel toward the head on flexing the neck, seen in selective weakness of lower abdominal muscles).[10] High thoracic disk herniations (T2–T5) can mimic cervical disk disease and present with symptoms of upper arm pain, radiculopathy, paresthesias, and even Horner's syndrome.[5] Poorly localized visceral pain could be a presenting symptom of mid- to low thoracic radiculopathy.[3]

The muscles for evaluating thoracic nerve involvement on electromyographic (EMG) studies are paraspinals, intercostals, and abdominal muscles.[3] The process of obtaining an EMG in someone with thoracic radiculopathy is difficult as it requires testing bilaterally and multiple levels above and below the suspected area. There is an 8.8% risk of pneumothorax with doing nerve conduction studies for thoracic radiculopathy.[11] EMG in thoracic radiculopathy can reveal fibrillation potentials, positive sharp waves, and bizarre high-frequency discharges, with normal and long-duration polyphasic motor unit potentials in multiple areas such as bilateral lower abdominals, right upper abdominal, left iliopsoas, and right lower thoracic paraspinal muscles. EMG studies of motor, F waves, and H reflexes and sural sensory nerve studies are normal in thoracic radiculopathy.[12] Imaging modalities can also be used for diagnosis. CT myelography had long been the gold standard, but MRI has largely replaced this technique except for in patients with ferromagnetic implants.[3] MRI and CT scanning can be considered precise when signs and symptoms are radicular and pain originates from a compressed nerve root. However, in the absence of objective neurological deficits or EMG findings, the correlation from imaging may not be precise.[3]

TREATMENT

Conservative Treatment

Conservative treatment is recommended for thoracic radicular pain. In the vast majority of patients with thoracic radicular pain, the natural course of the disease process was such that most patients returned to their previous functional level without surgical intervention.[13]

Physical Therapy, Exercise, and Physical Modalities

Exercise has numerous benefits and is the cornerstone of any treatment program to address thoracic radicular pain. Regular exercise optimizes intervertebral disc health as normal compressive forces aid with disc hydration and nutrition because the discs do not have a direct vascular supply. Endogenous endorphin release is an additional benefit and directly reduces pain levels. Specific strengthening exercises such as that of the multifidus muscle and erector spinae group help improve segmental stabilization and proprioception of the vertebral levels while reducing the forces placed on hypermobile and less stabilized segments, such as those of the lower thoracic spine. Typically, extension-based exercises have been advocated, especially for vertebral body compression fractures. However, this form of exercise may prove difficult with intervertebral foraminal stenosis as thoracic extension reduces the size of the foramen.

Transcutaneous electrical nerve stimulation (TENS) is thought to reduce pain by means of the gate control theory[14] and may be of benefit. Other modalities such as therapeutic ultrasound, phonophoresis, and electrophoresis may also be utilized, however evidence of efficacy is weak.

Manual therapy may be of benefit as gentle mobilization of hypomobile thoracic segments may help reduce damaging forces placed on hypermobile symptomatic segments and lead to overall balanced thoracic mobility.

Aquatic therapy may help off-load the disc and temporarily improve radicular symptoms. However, "land-based" exercises are required to place sufficient forces on bone to improve bone density.

Optimization of posture with biofeedback devices and appropriate strengthening of postural muscles minimize aberrant forces placed on the thoracic spine.

Medication Management

Management of thoracic radicular pain is similar to that of cervical and lumbar radicular pain syndrome. Medications widely used include the following:

- Nonsteroidal anti-inflammatories (NSAIDS) to decrease pain and inflammation associated with degenerative disc disease. Acetaminophen may also be used.
- Anticonvulsants (such as gabapentin, pregabalin, topiramate) and tricyclic antidepressants (such as amitriptyline, nortriptyline) may help address the neuropathic pain components.
- Serotonin and norepinephrine reuptake inhibitors such as duloxetine and milnacipran may be utilized to address the central pain components.
- Muscle relaxants such as cyclobenzaprine, methocarbamol, and tizanidine may be utilized to aid with myofascial pain.
- Diabetes oral medications and injectable solutions such as insulin should be utilized to address progression of peripheral

neuropathy pain, in conjunction with anticonvulsants.

- Bisphosphonates, 1500 mg oral calcium, and 400 IU vitamin D supplementation should be taken daily[15] to aid prevention of further osteoporotic fractures leading to neuroforaminal compromise.
- Opiates, although more widely used in the past, have now fallen out of favor as a result of the inherent risks of this class of medication and should be reserved for malignant pain syndromes and, in rare cases, for short-duration acute management of debilitating pain.

Spinal Injections

If conservative measures fail to adequately provide symptom relief, a variety of injections with steroids may be used. To address single-level radicular pain as a result of a herniated disc, a transforaminal epidural steroid injection at the symptomatic level may be effective, because this approach delivers the injectate to the anterior epidural space, precisely the location of the offending disc. Technically, this approach is demanding because of the critical structures that need to be taken into account, namely the lungs and the artery of Adamkiewicz, which is present typically on the left side at the levels ranging from the T6 to L1 neuroforamen.[16] An interlaminar epidural steroid injection may also be used. However, the practitioner should be cautious regarding proximity of the spinal cord to the thoracic epidural space. This approach may not as effectively introduce injectate to the symptomatic disc and lacks nerve root specificity.

Subarachnoid Neurolysis

Subarachnoid neurolysis involves destruction of the dorsal sensory nerve roots while attempting to spare the more anteriorly located motor nerve roots. Alcohol or glycerol may be used, although many clinicians prefer phenol because of the reduced duration of blockage and overall safety with utilization. This procedure has been less used over the years, and practitioners who are able to perform this technique are becoming more difficult to find. This form of neurolytic blockade may be considered for cancer patients whose pain has failed to respond to conventional treatment regimens. Indications include the following:

(1) The diagnosis is well established.
(2) The patient's life expectancy is short, usually 6 to 12 months.
(3) The patient's pain is unresponsive to antineoplastic therapy (chemotherapy, radiation).
(4) All other conventional intervention pain management techniques have been exhausted.
(5) The patient's pain has failed to respond to adequate trials of analgesic agents and adjunctive drugs.
(6) The pain is localized to two or three dermatomes.
(7) The pain is predominantly somatic in origin.
(8) The pain is unilateral (neurolytic blocks for bilateral pain should be staggered).

Spinal Cord Stimulation

Spinal cord stimulation (SCS) involves the epidural percutaneous or surgical placement of leads over the spinal cord and traditionally involves electrical stimulation of the dorsal columns to produce paresthesia and pain reduction in a dermatomal pattern. Traditional indications for SCS include chronic radiculopathy, complex regional pain syndrome (CRPS) (types 1 and 2), and pain due to ischemia.[17] To cover radicular chest wall pain associated with thoracic radiculopathy, leads are implanted in the upper thoracic level to produce paresthesia. New paradigms for stimulation have been growing over the past decade. Dorsal root ganglion stimulation, although approved in Europe for many years, obtained FDA approval for the treatment of CRPS in the United States in February of 2016. In this form of stimulation, electrodes are placed directly over the dorsal root ganglion; it has the advantage of being able to target specific nerve roots. Although not currently approved for treatment of thoracic radiculopathy, one may foresee this new technology eventually being adopted for this purpose, particularly for low thoracic levels.

Surgical Intervention

Indications for surgical intervention are controversial, owing to the fact that all types of symptomatic disc herniations of the thoracic level are the least common and data on the natural history of this pathology are limited. Intervention of this nature is sometimes required more immediately for those who suffer from concerning neurological compromise, such as with myelopathy, as a result of compression from sources such as herniated nucleus pulposus and tumors. If neurological compromise is not immediately evident at the onset of symptoms, surgical intervention is reserved for those patients with pain that has failed initial conservative management and who have persistent pain symptoms. In contrast to myelopathy, which is an indication for surgical intervention, the role of surgery for radicular pain has not been clearly established.

Initially, laminectomy was advocated, but this has fallen out of favor as a result of the high complication rates and unfavorable outcomes.[18] The transpedicular and the transfacet pedicle-sparing approach discectomy have been advocated as they appear to be relatively safe and are most effective for lateral thoracic disc herniations. Central disc herniations may not be amenable to these surgical techniques and are typically addressed by invasive lateral extracavitary (posterolateral approach) or transthoracic (anterolateral approach).[18] Less invasive techniques have also been devised, such as thoracoscopic surgery and transdural approach. Apparently, there is a need for more effective and less invasive treatment of thoracic radicular pain and radiculopathy.

GUIDING QUESTIONS

- Can you describe the pathophysiology of thoracic radiculopathy?
- How can you diagnose thoracic radiculopathy and how does it present differently than cervical and lumbar radiculopathy?
- What are the various treatment options to address thoracic radiculopathy?

PREVENTION

- Regular exercise, stretching, and strengthening optimize conditioning and help stabilize the thoracic spine.
- Patients should optimize the biomechanics of activities and sports that place undue rotational and flexion forces on the thoracic spine; optimization of golf swing is an example.
- Postural education, biofeedback, and workplace or workstation ergonomic optimization may be achieved through physical and occupational therapy.

- Osteoporosis may be prevented with regular and appropriate exercise, nutrition and medication management with bisphosphonates, and oral calcium and vitamin D supplementation.
- Diabetes management should be optimized through good nutrition, exercise, and appropriate medications.
- Smoking cessation improves disc nutrition, vascular supply, and bone health.
- Use of opioid medications should be minimized to prevent opioid-induced hyperalgesia.
- Psychological health should be optimized to minimize catastrophizing and central sensitization.

KEY POINTS

- Thoracic radiculopathy presents an uncommon spinal disorder that can often be overlooked because numerous structures surround the thoracic spine.[2] Radiculopathy typically originates from mechanical nerve root compression due to degenerative spine changes such as disc herniation or spondylosis.[3] The most common etiologies of thoracic radiculopathy are disc disease, osteoporosis and its associated vertebral compression fractures, and diabetic neuropathy.[3]
- The thoracic spine is designed more for protection of the chest and abdominal structures than for movement. The flexion restraint lessens the potential for intervertebral disk injury in the thoracic region in comparison to the lumbar region.[5]
- Degeneration is favored as the prevailing cause of thoracic disc herniation, and the lower thoracic segments are most at risk because of the increased motion present at these levels.[9]
- The presentation of radicular pain in the thoracic region is more common in the upper thoracic region and with lateral disk herniations often associated with some amount of axial pain.[5] Clinical symptoms are leg weakness, numbness and tingling across the chest or abdomen or shoulders, spasticity, and bowel or bladder dysfunction,[9] as well as gastrointestinal symptoms (10%–15% of the time).
- Studies have indicated that in the vast majority of patients with thoracic pain, the

natural course of the disease process was such that most patients returned to their previous functional level without surgical intervention.[13]

- Strengthening, postural optimization, and general exercise and mobility comprise the cornerstone of all treatment and prevention of thoracic radicular pain.
- Medication may include a variety of choices, ranging from NSAIDs to anticonvulsants. Medications to address specific health issues leading to thoracic radiculopathy (diabetes mellitus and osteoporosis) may be of additional benefit.
- Thoracic epidural injections with corticosteroids and local anesthetics may be a treatment consideration.
- Surgical intervention is reserved for those whose pain failed conservative management and who have persistent pain symptoms. Myelopathy is an indication for surgical intervention.
- Subarachnoid neurolysis may be a treatment option for thoracic radicular pain that is unilateral, localized to two or three dermatomes, and typically in cancer patients with short life expectancy (6 to 23 months).
- Spinal cord stimulation may be effective to address chronic radiculopathy in selected patients.

REFERENCES

1. Preston D. *Electromyography and Neuromuscular Disorders*. Philadelphia: Elsevier Saunders; 2013.
2. O'Connor RC, Andary MT, Russo RB, DeLano M. Thoracic radiculopathy. *Phys Med Rehabil Clin N Am*. 2002;13(3):623–644. doi:10.1016/S1047-9651(02)00018-9
3. Derby R, Chen Y, Lee S-H, Seo KS, Kim B-J. Non-surgical interventional treatment of cervical and thoracic radiculopathies. *Pain Physician*. 2004;7(3):389–394.
4. Bastron J, Hames J. Diabetic polyradiculopathy clinical and electromyographic studies in 105 patients. *Mayo Clin Proc*. 1981;56:725–732.
5. Vanichkachorn JS, Vaccaro AR. Thoracic disk disease: diagnosis and treatment. *J Am Acad Orthop Surg*. 2000;8(3):159–169.
6. Shirzadi A, Drazin D, Jeswani S, Lovely L, Liu J. Atypical presentation of thoracic disc herniation: case series and review of the literature. *Case Rep Orthop*. 2013;2013:621476. doi:10.1155/2013/621476
7. Malanga GA, Alladin I, Tai Q. Thoracic discogenic pain syndrome clinical presentation. Medscape. December 23, 2015. http://emedicine.medscape.com/article/96284-clinical.
8. Cornips EMJ, Janssen MLF, Beuls EAM. Thoracic disc herniation and acute myelopathy: clinical presentation, neuroimaging findings, surgical considerations, and outcome. *J Neurosurg Spine*. 2011;14(4):520–528. doi:10.3171/2010.12.SPINE10273
9. Mcinerney J, Ball P. The pathophysiology of thoracic disc disease. *Neurosurg Focus*. 2000;9(4):1–8.
10. Pearce J. Beevor's sign. *Eur Neurol*. 2005;53(4):208–209.
11. Johnson E, Powell J, Caldwell J. Intercostal nerve conduction and posterior rhizotomy in the diagnosis and treatment of thoracic radiculopathy. *J Neurol Neurosurg Psychiatry*. 1974;37:330–332.
12. Liveson JA. Thoracic radiculopathy related to collapsed thoracic vertebral bodies. *J Neurol Neurosurgery, Psychiatry*. 1984;47:404–406.
13. Brown CW, Deffer PAJ, Akmakjian J, Donaldson DH, Brugman JL. The natural history of thoracic disc herniation. *Spine (Phila Pa 1976)*. 1992;17(6 Suppl):S97–S102.
14. Melzack R, Wall PD. Pain mechanisms: a new theory. *Science*. 1965;150(3699):971–979.
15. Kim DH, Vaccaro AR. Osteoporotic compression fractures of the spine; current options and considerations for treatment. *Spine J*. 2006;6(5):479–487. doi:10.1016/j.spinee.2006.04.013
16. Bley TA, Duffek CC, Francois CJ, et al. Presurgical localization of the artery of Adamkiewicz with time-resolved 3.0-T MR angiography. *Radiology*. 2010;255(3):873–881. doi:10.1148/radiol.10091304
17. Slavin KV. Spinal stimulation for pain: future applications. *Neurotherapeutics*. 2014;11(3):535–542. doi:10.1007/s13311-014-0273-2
18. Coppes MH, Bakker NA, Metzemaekers JDM, Groen RJM. Posterior transdural discectomy: a new approach for the removal of a central thoracic disc herniation. *Eur Spine J*. 2012;21(4):623–628. doi:10.1007/s00586-011-1990-4
19. Beal M. Viscerosomatic Reflexes: A review. *Journal of AOA*. 1985;85(12):786–801.

28

Lumbar Radicular Pain

VARUN RIMMALAPUDI AND RADHIKA GRANDHE

CASE

A 58-year-old man presents with right-sided back pain and leg pain that he has had for 2 weeks. He reports shooting pain along the front of his right thigh, knee, and into his medial calf with progressive weakness of his right knee. He rates the pain at 9/10 and describes it as shooting, burning, and tingling in nature. The pain started as he was lifting a heavy tile while at work and has been worsening since. Physical exam revealed diffuse tenderness over the lower lumbar spine, right-sided paravertebral tenderness, and right gluteal tenderness. A passive straight-leg raise (SLR) test was positive at 30 degrees and a crossed SLR was negative. Motor testing showed 4/5 strength upon right knee extension and 5/5 strength elsewhere. Sensory examination showed a deficit with pinprick testing over the anterior thigh and medial calf on the right. Patellar and Achilles reflexes were 1+ bilaterally. An MRI of the lumbar spine was ordered because of the patient's neurological deficits and showed a disc extrusion affecting the right subarticular zone at the L3/4 level with associated compression of the traversing L4 nerve root. A neurosurgical consultation was obtained and after a discussion regarding the natural progression of disease, a decision was made to initiate conservative management measures. With a combination of physical therapy, transcutaneous electrical stimulation (TENS), NSAIDs, and anticonvulsants, the symptoms resolved in 5 weeks.

DEFINITION

The term *lumbar radicular pain* refers pain that is due to a lesion affecting fibers of a lumbar spinal nerve, typically at the nerve roots or dorsal root ganglia. Pain from the lesion may be felt in the corresponding dermatome or a dynatome, an area in which pain is felt due to lesioning of a specific spinal nerve. Dynatomes and dermatomes may overlap, although this might not always be the case.[1] While radicular pain may be associated with paresthesia, the term *lumbar radiculopathy* implies presence of signs of overt nerve root damage such as loss of sensation, motor weakness, or diminished reflexes. Radicular pain and radiculopathy can coexist, but it is important to note that they may also present independently.

ETIOLOGY AND PATHOPHYSIOLOGY

A diverse number of pathological processes can affect the spinal nerve roots leading to lumbar radicular pain, including intervertebral disc lesions, lumbar spinal stenosis, arachnoiditis, degenerative changes of the spine, neoplastic lesions, infections, entrapment neuropathies, and vascular lesions. Systemic conditions such as lupus, diabetic neuropathy, and viral infections may also rarely affect the spinal nerves leading to radicular pain syndromes.

The pathophysiology of lumbar radicular pain involves generation of ectopic impulses along the course of the spinal nerve fibers either at the level of the sensory nerve root or the dorsal root ganglion, which can be perceived as pain, numbness, or tingling in the areas innervated by these nerves. This may be due to either direct mechanical compression of the nerve root or the release of inflammatory mediators at the site of the nerve root, as in case of disc extrusions. Central spinal canal stenosis can cause compression of multiple nerve roots of the spinal cord or cauda equina, and lateral spinal canal stenosis or foraminal stenosis can cause compression of the traversing or exiting spinal nerve root.

EPIDEMIOLOGY

The prevalence and lifetime incidence of low back pain have been variably reported by several sources. A recent review reported that one in four adults suffer from chronic low back pain with over 40% reporting a radicular pain pattern.[2] Intervertebral disc disorders including disc herniation and disc degeneration account for about 20% of the total visits for low back pain and are one of the most common causes of lumbar radicular pain.

CLINICAL FEATURES

It is important for the clinician to distinguish true radicular pain from referred pain. Although pain from sacroiliac joint dysfunction and lumbar facet joint pathology can be referred to the lower extremities, the distribution of such referred pain is typically nondermatomal, often spreading across several dermatomes. A careful neurological evaluation including clinical tests to elicit nerve root irritation, such as straight-leg raise test or SLR (passive elevation of the extended lower extremity), crossed SLR (elicitation of pain in the affected leg when an SLR is performed on the contralateral leg), and the femoral stretch test (bending the knee and extending the hip with the patient prone), must be used to aid differentiation between these entities. The location of disc herniation also affects the location of symptoms. Paracentral disc herniations affect the traversing nerve roots, and far lateral disc herniations affect the exiting nerve roots, causing radicular symptoms in the corresponding pattern. Figure 28.1 depicts MRI images of a left paracentral disc herniation at the L5–S1 level compressing the traversing S1 nerve root.

Clinical features of lumbar radicular pain can vary significantly depending on the etiology. All patients must be assessed for "red flags" in their history and physical exam that indicate the presence of a condition posing an impending or potential threat to life or neurological function such as malignancy, osteomyelitis, cauda equina syndrome, vertebral fractures, or abdominal aortic aneurysm. These red flags can include a history of cancer, unexplained weight loss, persistent fever, immunocompromised state due to HIV or systemic corticosteroid usage, recent trauma, urinary incontinence or retention, saddle anesthesia, major motor weakness, or sensory deficit. If the patient exhibits any of the red flags, the clinician must have a low threshold to obtain further imaging, a neurosurgical evaluation, or both.

Involvement of the L4 nerve root may manifest as radicular symptoms involving the anterior part of the thigh, knee, and the medial calf, weakness in knee extension, and a diminished patellar reflex. Involvement of the L5 nerve root may manifest as radicular pain along the buttock, posterolateral thigh, anterolateral aspect of the leg, and the dorsal surface of the foot, a difficulty in heel walking, and weakness of big toe extension and ankle inversion. Involvement of the S1 nerve root may present as radicular symptoms in the posterior thigh, calf, and the lateral or plantar surface of the foot, difficulty in toe walking, and loss of the Achilles reflex. Saddle anesthesia, autonomic dysfunction, and urinary incontinence may either indicate direct involvement of sacral

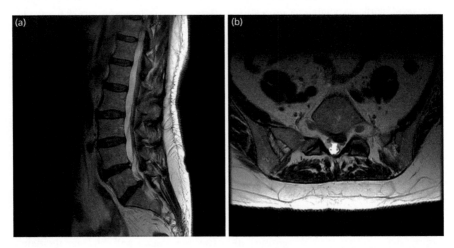

FIGURE 28.1. **A.** Sagittal T2-weighted MRI image showing L5-S1 left paracentral disc herniation. **B.** Axial T2-weighted MRI image showing left paracentral disc herniation compressing S1 nerve root.

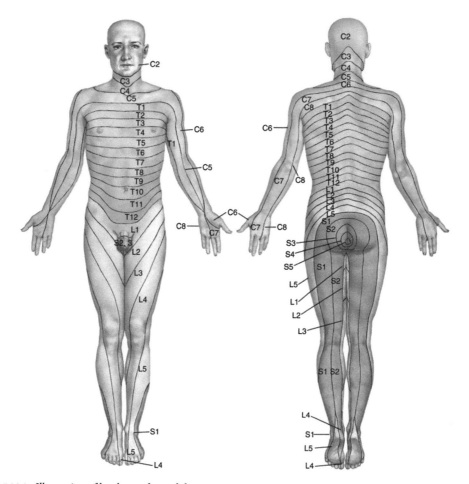

FIGURE 28.2. Illustration of lumbar and sacral dermatomes.

Reused from Netter FH. *Atlas of Human Anatomy*. 6th ed. Philadelphia: Saunders; 2014.

nerve roots or cauda equina syndrome. Figure 28.2 illustrates the typical distribution of lumbar dermatomes.

In addition to the radicular symptoms, patients with lumbar spinal stenosis may exhibit neurogenic claudication. This is typically described as pain radiating to bilateral posterolateral thighs that is worsened with walking and lumbar extension and is relieved upon sitting and leaning forward. As flexion of the spine improves the pain, patients with lumbar spinal stenosis often walk with a stooped gait and report having to use a walker or shopping cart to ambulate comfortably. It is important to distinguish neurogenic claudication from vascular claudication. Unlike neurogenic claudication, the pain of vascular claudication is resolved when the patient rests in a standing position.

MANAGEMENT

Management decisions in patients with lumbar radiculopathy must be made after careful consideration of the etiology, neurological findings or deficits on examination, natural progression of disease, and pertinent imaging findings.

Disc Protrusions and Extrusions

The natural progression of disease is favorable in case of disc disorders and about two-thirds of patients with herniated discs experience resolution of their symptoms in the first few months after onset. Given this favorable natural history, noninvasive modalities are the initial treatments of choice in patients without progressive neurologic deficit or other red flags. Activity as tolerated has been shown to be better than strict bed rest in assisting recovery. Physical therapy and back bracing are also widely used, although the evidence for their use is limited. NSAIDs and muscle relaxants have been shown to have efficacy in the management of acute symptoms in patients with disc disorders. Anticonvulsants and opioids, though widely used, have varying effects.

Epidural steroid injections are also widely used in the management of patients with disc disorders, although the data regarding their efficacy are variable.[3,4] The efficacy of transforaminal steroids may vary depending on the disc pathology. In patients with a contained herniation of the nucleus pulposus, transforaminal injection of steroids has been shown not only to provide relief and reduce the need for home care in the short term but also to reduce the chance of surgical intervention over the next year.[5] However, in patients with disc extrusions, although transforaminal steroid injections have been shown to provide relief and reduce the need for home care in the short term, they have been shown to increase the chance of surgical intervention over the next year. It is therefore very important to categorize the disc pathology using MRI before considering epidural steroids.

Several surgical modalities are in use for management of patients with disc disorders, with procedures varying from traditional laminectomy and removal of the disc fragment to the more recent microdiscectomy and endoscopic discectomy procedures. Although surgical treatment has been shown to be of benefit in the short term, a recent study concluded that the results of surgery deteriorated over time, nullifying the difference between the surgically and nonsurgically treated groups.[6] The decision to undergo surgery might have to be based on the patient's urgency for pain control in the first few weeks after the insult or after failure of conservative management.

Lumbar Spinal Stenosis (LSS)

The nonoperative treatment of radicular pain associated with lumbar spinal stenosis (LSS) is similar to the management of radicular pain due to disc disorders, with a few exceptions.

Calcitonin may be a valuable addition to the medical management of lumbar spinal stenosis, especially in patients with Paget's disease.[7] Flexion-based exercises such as stationary bicycle and inclined treadmill may have a special role in patients with LSS and reduce symptoms by improving the microcirculation and perfusion of previously ischemic neural elements.

Interlaminar epidural steroid injections may be of value in providing symptomatic control of neurogenic claudication, especially in the short term.[8]

Several surgical options are available for the management of LSS, ranging from multilevel laminectomy with spinal fusion to minimally invasive decompression techniques such as laminotomy and laminoplasty. The decision to proceed to surgery has to take into consideration the severity and progression of the patient's symptoms, the response to conservative treatment modalities, and the patient's comorbid conditions.

Other Conditions

Other conditions causing lumbar radiculopathy must be addressed. Patients with cauda equina syndrome must be evaluated thoroughly as compression might occur not only at the lumbar but also at the thoracic or cervical level. These patients require emergency decompressive surgery.

Patients with suspected spinal osteomyelitis must be started on IV antibiotics immediately after blood cultures are obtained, to isolate the pathogen. Noncompressive causes of radicular pain such as diabetic neuropathy, viral infections, and systemic lupus erythematosus must always be ruled out, especially prior to considering interventions for presumed compression of the nerve roots.

In summary, lumbar radicular pain is a syndrome with a wide array of causes. The clinician must rely on astute history taking, serial physical examinations to plot symptom progression, expeditious identification of red flag conditions, review of appropriate imaging, and an understanding of the natural progression of disease in order to provide the appropriate treatment for the patient.

GUIDING QUESTIONS

- What are the important causes of lumbar radicular pain?
- What are the "red flag" signs that must be elicited in the assessment of a patient with lumbar radicular pain?
- What are the key clinical features that distinguish L4 from S1 nerve root involvement?
- How does the management of a contained nucleus pulposus herniation differ from that of a disc extrusion?
- How can the symptoms from a disc herniation in the subarticular zone at the

L3/4 level differ from a disc herniation in the foraminal zone at the same level?

KEY POINTS

- *Lumbar radicular pain* refers to pain along the distribution of a lumbar spinal dermatome or dynatome. *Lumbar radiculopathy* implies occurrence of signs of overt nerve root damage, such as loss of sensation, motor weakness, or diminished reflexes.
- A diverse number of pathological processes can lead to lumbar radicular pain, including intervertebral disc lesions, lumbar spinal stenosis, arachnoiditis, degenerative changes of the spine, neoplastic lesions, infections, entrapment neuropathies, vascular lesions, and systemic neuropathies, among others. Herniated intervertebral discs and lumbar spinal stenosis are the most common causes.
- All patients presenting with lumbar radicular pain must be assessed for red flag signs, including a history of cancer, unexplained weight loss, persistent fever, immunocompromised state, recent trauma, urinary incontinence or retention, saddle anesthesia, and major motor or sensory deficit.
- Management decisions in patients with lumbar radiculopathy must be made after careful consideration of the etiology, location of herniation, neurological findings or deficits on examination, natural progression of disease, and a review of pertinent imaging findings.

REFERENCES

1. Slipman CW, Plastaras CT, Palmitier RA, Huston CW, Sterenfeld EB. Symptom provocation of fluoroscopically guided cervical nerve root stimulation. Are dynatomal maps identical to dermatomal maps? *Spine (Phila Pa 1976)*. 1998;23(20):2235–2242.
2. United States Bone and Joint Initiative. *The Burden of Musculoskeletal Diseases in the United States (BMUS)*, 3rd edition. 2014. Rosemont, IL. Available at http://www.boneandjointburden.org. Accessed June 25, 2016.
3. Vroomen PC, de Krom MC, Slofstra PD, et al. Conservative treatment of sciatica: a systematic review. *J Spinal Disord*. 2000;13:463–469.
4. M. Schaufele, L. Hatch: Interlaminar versus transforaminal epidural injections in the treatment of symptomatic lumbar intervertebral disk herniations. *Arch Phys Med Rehabil*. 2002;83:1661.
5. Karppinen J, Ohinmaa A, Malmivaara A, et al. Cost effectiveness of periradicular infiltration for sciatica: subgroup analysis of a randomized controlled trial. *Spine (Phila Pa 1976)*. 2001;26(23):2587–2595.
6. Atlas SJ, Keller RB, Wu YA, Deyo RA, Singer DE. Long-term outcomes of surgical and nonsurgical management of sciatica secondary to a lumbar disk herniation: 10 year results from the Maine lumbar spine study. *Spine*. 2005;30:927–935.
7. Eskola A, Pohjolainen T, Alaranta H, Soini J, Tallroth K, Slätis P. Calcitonin treatment in lumbar spinal stenosis: a randomized, placebo-controlled, double blind, cross-over study with one year follow-up. *Calcif Tissue Int*. 1992;50:400–403.
8. Benyamin RM, Manchikanti L, Parr AT, et al. The effectiveness of lumbar interlaminar epidural injections in managing chronic low back and lower extremity pain. *Pain Physician*. 2012;15(4):E363–E404. Review.

29

Arachnoiditis

*ZEESHAN MALIK, SHILPADEVI PATIL, SAILESH ARULKUMAR,
AND RINOO V. SHAH*

CASE

A 29-year-old African American woman post-partum 2 months presents with back pain and progressive weakness in her lower extremities. The pain is located in the lower back and referred to the buttocks and is described as numbness and tingling sensation that worsens with exertion. Onset was 1 month prior, and current pain intensity is 7/10. On examination, bilateral lower extremity weakness is noted with uncoordinated strides upon ambulation. Decreased truncal movement is also noted, and she adds that occasionally she urinates on herself. She has decreased sensation on her buttocks and bilateral lower extremities. She also has decreased ability to raise her legs when lying flat. Her past medical history is significant for an epidural placement 2 months prior, which took two attempts. She had been started on Flexeril 5 mg PO BID PRN for pain 1 week prior.

DEFINITION

Arachnoiditis, also known as meningitis serosa, chronic spinal meningitis, spinal fibrosis, and chronic adhesive arachnoiditis, is a rare condition that occurs from insult to the arachnoid layer of the meninges causing inflammation and nerve irritation.[1] Over time, this can cause thickening and scarring of the arachnoid membrane, impinging nerve roots and/or regions of the adjacent spinal cord. Patients may present with symptoms of numbness, tingling, urinary sphincter dysfunction, weakness, and loss of reflexes.[2,3]

PATHOPHYSIOLOGY

In 1978, Burton described arachnoiditis in separate distinct stages.[2] There is an inciting event, such as trauma, back surgery, or infection, which can indicate that the normal structures of the arachnoid layer have been invaded. The arachnoid membrane sits adjacent to the pia mater and below the dura mater. The arachnoid membrane carries a significant amount of blood supply to regions within the spinal cord.[4] The first stage is noted after an insult to the arachnoid layer, where there is inflammation and swelling of the region. The inflammation encompasses nerve roots, which results in adjacent nerve roots and regions of the meninges starting to adhere to each other. In the second stage, over time there is scarring of the membrane layer and extensive collagen deposition, further clumping nerve roots together. In the final stage, blood supply is decreased to the area, with dense collagen deposition and thickening of the arachnoid layer.[4,5] Radiographic imaging reveals progressive atrophy of the nerve roots with resolution of the initial inflammation that was noted. Several different precipitating events have been correlated with arachnoiditis (Table 29.1), although no firm consensus has been formed regarding how long it takes to acquire the condition.[6,7,8]

ETIOLOGY

Several factors have been described in the etiology of arachnoiditis since it was first described in the 1900s. In the first half of the twentieth century, arachnoiditis was initially attributed to infectious causes such as tuberculosis, syphilis, and gonorrhea.[6,9] In the 1940s, blood within the cerebrospinal fluid (CSF), from surgery, or from subarachnoid hemorrhage revealed association with the development of arachnoiditis.[3] Currently, arachnoiditis is seen as a complication of noninfectious origin. While no specific causative agent has been identified for arachnoiditis because of the rarity of the disease, there are various factors

TABLE 29.1. ASSOCIATED CAUSES
OF ARACHNOIDITIS

Blood

Contrast media

Trauma

Neuraxial anesthesia

Contaminants

Local anesthetics

that have been speculated as possible causative factors, such as trauma, post–spinal surgery, mechanical trauma from direct needle or catheter injury, mass lesions, spinal cord ischemia or vascular injury from direct needle or catheter trauma, neurotoxicity from local anesthetics, contrast agents, adjuvants, and antiseptics.[10]

Trauma

Previous spinal surgery has been a well-established risk factor for arachnoidtitis.[6] The nucleus pulposus of the intervertebral disc in monkeys was shown to elicit arachnoidtitis.[11] After having spinal surgery, having a postoperative pain-free period of approximately 6 months followed by onset of lower extremity pain has been postulated as the onset of arachnoiditis.[12] Neuraxial anesthesia, a widely used technique in obstetrics, general surgery, and orthopedics, has also been linked to arachnoiditis.[13] Epidural catheters left within the patient for extended periods of time have been shown to cause an inflammatory reaction within the epidural space. A fibrous sheath formation was noted in rats when the epidural catheter was left in place for a long period of time,[14–16] although, in practice, it is not typical to leave epidural catheters in place for prolonged periods of time. The association of neuraxial anesthesia with arachnoiditis is still weak with no definitive link. Introduction of contaminants, local anesthetics, and blood within the CSF may also play a role.[17]

Blood

Rarely, arachnoiditis can be precipitated by a subarachnoid hemorrhage.[18] As the blood breaks down within the CSF, it forms free radicals, which can cause significant damage to the nerve roots nearby.[19,20] Placing breakdown products of hemoglobin within the CSF of experimental dogs resulted in increased irritation of the meninges

compared to using fresh blood.[19] Placement of autologous blood within the epidural space compared to a direct lumbar puncture showed no discernible difference.[21] A 2-year follow-up study on 118 blood patches revealed no cases of arachnoiditis, 19 cases of persistent back pain, and 2 cases of lower extremity radiculopathy.[22]

Contrast Media

Contrast myelography using the oil-based contrast ethyliophendylate (Pantopaque, Myodil) was associated with the development of arachnoiditis in the 1970s. This previously used ionized fatty-acid contrast agent was highly radio-opaque and had a dose-dependent relationship with the formation of arachnoiditis.[23] In comparison to newer contrast agents, ethyliophendylate had a longer half-life and prolonged excretion time. It was recommended that ethyliophendylate be aspirated and removed after myelography was completed, although no firm evidence suggested a reduction in arachnoiditis cases.[24] The use of oil-based iodine contrast has been abandoned; water-based agents are now used.[25] Water-based agents may also have the capability to produce arachnoiditis, but as of yet no human cases have surfaced. Arachnoiditis in monkeys has been seen with use of extremely high concentrations of water-based contrast agents.[24]

Contaminants

The spinal and epidural space was prone to contaminants used to clean instruments with detergents in the 1950s case by Cope.[26] Chlorhexidine solution used to clean a patient's back before a combined spinal extradural anesthesia (CSE) has also been associated with aseptic meningitis.[27] It has also been postulated that using the needle-through-needle technique with CSE may cause metallic fragments to form; introduced into the intrathecal space can cause an inflammatory reaction.[28]

Local Anesthetics

It has also been proposed that local anesthetics may be implicated in development of arachnoiditis after being injecting into the intrathecal space, although there is no good evidence to support this theory.[29] In animal studies local anesthetics have not been seen to cause meningeal irritation, but supratherapeutic doses have been shown to harm neural issue in laboratory settings.[30–32]

CLINICAL FEATURES OF ARACHNOIDITIS

The diagnosis of arachnoiditis may be difficult to make because of the broad range of symptoms, especially without radiographic evidence. A detailed history and physical exam must be undertaken to evaluate the patient. Common symptoms are back or leg pain that worsen on use; radiculopathy may also be present.[9] Patients may also experience loss of reflexes, bladder symptoms, weakness, back spasms, and paresthesias (Table 29.2). Often arachnoiditis is diagnosed on the basis of radiographic studies, but the patient may remain asymptomatic.[33] Physical exam findings are also nonspecific. Positive straight-leg raise test, sciatic notch tenderness, and decreased truncal mobility are commonly seen,[1] with decreased truncal mobility being most common.[34] The majority of arachnoiditis cases occur in the lumbar region, with back surgery now being more of an associated precursor than neuraxial anesthesia.[35]

RADIOGRAPHIC FEATURES OF ARACHNOIDITIS

Arachnoiditis diagnosis is confirmed with radiographic imaging in addition to clinical findings. Plain radiographs have not shown sufficient evidence to confirm the diagnosis. The current gold standard for arachnoiditis diagnosis is MRI, with a specificity of 100% and sensitivity of 92%.[36] MRI has revealed a common trend: one pattern is the clustering of nerve roots that adhere to the meninges peripherally. Another pattern reveals a higher intensity in the soft tissue region of the thecal sac, with notable deterioration of the central aspect of the subarachnoid space. The third pattern is the clumping of many nerve roots in the center of the thecal sac.[7]

TREATMENT

The treatment options for arachnoiditis are sparse; many severe cases develop long-term disabilities regardless of treatment interventions.[34] Surgical interventions, aimed at decompressive laminectomies, have been used to alleviate symptoms but rarely with any beneficial outcome.[37] Sleep disturbances and depression have also been associated with arachnoiditis; these are typically treated with tricyclic antidepressants and selective serotonin reuptake inhibitors. Neuropathic pain may also be alleviated by use of gabapentin and pregabalin. Spinal cord stimulators have recently shown promise with improved patient functionality and pain relief.[38] Minimally invasive techniques, aimed at adhesiolysis, are also being developed with promising outcomes.[39] With a 48% improvement in pain seen in a study using minimally invasive adhesiolysis with local anesthetics and steroids for arachnoiditis, this procedure may become a more common treatment option.[40]

PREVENTION

A practice advisory for regional anesthesia and pain medicine has several recommendations based on extensive review of research on humans and animal models, case reports, research in pathophysiology, and expert opinion. The advisory, in some cases, especially those associated with neuraxial anesthesia, could help reduce the likelihood of arachnoiditis and other spinal cord complications. Unfortunately, many of these injuries are not predictable. The low incidence of arachnoiditis and the current state of knowledge regarding its causal factors make the likely prevention of this complication very difficult.[41,10]

TABLE 29.2. COMMON CLINICAL SIGNS AND SYMPTOMS OF ARACHNOIDITIS

Back pain increased with activity

Leg pain (often bilateral)

Hyporeflexia

Limited trunk mobility

Sensory abnormality

Urinary sphincter dysfunction

Lower extremity motor weakness

Positive straight-leg test

Sciatic notch tenderness

Paravertebral muscle spasm

GUIDING QUESTIONS

- What are the clinical features of arachnoiditis?
- How do you diagnose arachnoiditis?
- What are the risk factors and pathophysiology of arachnoiditis?
- What are the treatment options for arachnoiditis?

KEY POINTS

- Arachnoiditis is a debilitating condition characterized by back pain, paresthesias, decreased truncal movement, lower extremity weakness, and decreased reflexes. It is the inflammation of the arachnoid layer with swelling and scarring from collagen deposition over time.

- The diagnosis is confirmed with radiographic imaging in addition to clinical findings. The currently gold standard for arachnoiditis diagnosis is MRI, with a specificity of 100% and sensitivity of 92%.[36]
- Possible causative factors of the condition include trauma, post-spinal surgery, mechanical trauma from direct needle or catheter injury, mass lesions, spinal cord ischemia or vascular injury from direct needle or catheter trauma, neurotoxicity from local anesthetics, contrast agents, adjuvants, and antiseptics.
- Tricyclic antidepressants and selective serotonin reuptake inhibitors may improve sleep disturbances and depression associated with arachnoiditis. Gabapentinoids may alleviate neuropathic pain. Spinal cord stimulation may improve patient functionality and provide pain relief.[38] Minimally invasive techniques, aimed at adhesiolysis, are being developed with promising outcomes.[39] Adhesiolysis with local anesthetics and steroids, for example, may achieve significant improvement in pain.[40]

REFERENCES

1. Rice I, Wee M, Thomson K. Obstetric epidurals and chronic adhesive arachnoiditis. *Br J Anaesth.* 2004;92:109–120.
2. Burton CV. Lumbosacral arachnoiditis. *Spine.* 1978;3:24–30.
3. Weston-Hurst E. Adhesive arachnoiditis and vascular blockage caused by detergents and other chemical irritants: an experimental study. *J Pathol Bacteriol.* 1955;70:167–178.
4. Shantha TR, Evans JA. The relationship of epidural anesthesia to neural membranes and arachnoid villi. *Anesthesiology.* 1972;37:543–557.
5. Ransford AO, Harris BJ. Localised arachnoiditis complicating lumbar disc lesions. *J Bone Joint Surg.* 1972;54:656–665.
6. Heary RF. Northrup BE, Baronet G. Arachnoiditis. In: Benzel EC, eds. *Spine Surgery*, 2nd ed. Philadelphia: Elsevier; 2005:2004–2013.
7. Delamarter R, Ross J, Masaryk T, et al. Diagnosis of lumbar arachnoiditis by magnetic resonance imaging. *Spine.* 1990;:304–310.
8. Reigel D, Bazmi G, Shih S, Marquardt M. A pilot investigation of poloxamer 407 for the prevetion of leptomeningeal adhesions in the rabbit. *Pediatr Neurosurg.* 1993;19:250–255.
9. Poon TL, Ho WS, Pang KY. Tuberculosis meningitis with spinal tuberculosis arachnoiditis. *Hong Kong Med J.* 2003;9:59–61.
10. Kok AJ, Verhagen WI, et al. Spinal arachnoiditis following subarachnoid hemorrhage: report of two cases and review of literature. *Acta Neurochir.* 2000;142:794–800.
11. Hauton VM, Nguyen CM, Ho KC. The etiology of focal spinal arachnoiditis: an experimental study. *Spine.* 1993;18:1193–1197.
12. Carroll SE, Wiesel SW. Neurologic complications and lumbar laminectomy: a standardized approach to the multiple-operated lumbar spine. *Clin Orthop Rel Res.*1992;284:14–23.
13. Aroma U, Landensuu M, Cozanitis D. Severe complications associated with epidural and spinal anesthesia in Finland 1987–1993. Study based on patient insurance claims. *Acta Anaesthesiol Scand.* 1997;41:445–452.
14. Kane RE. Neurologic deficits following epidural or spinal anesthesia. *Anesth Analg.* 1981;60:150–160.
15. Kytta J, Rosenburg PH, Wahlstrom T. Long term epidural bupivicaine in pigs. *Acta Anesthesiol Scand.* 1985;29:114.
16. Durant P, Yaksh T. Epidural injections of bupivicaine, morphine, fentanyl, lofentanil and DADL in chronically implanted rats: a pharmacologic and pathologic study. *Anesthesiology.* 1986;64:43–53.
17. Killeen T, Kamat A, Walsh D, Parker A, Aliashkevich A. Severe adhesive arachnoiditis resulting in progressive paraplegia following obstetric spinal anesthesia: a case report review. *Anaesthesia.* 2012;67:1386–1394.
18. Kok A, Verhagen W, Bartels R, Van Dijk R, Prick J. Spinal arachnoiditis following subarachnoid haemorrhage: report of two cases and review of literature. *Acta Neurochir.* 2000;142:795–799.
19. Jackson IJ. Aseptic hemogenic meningitis. *Arch Neurol Radiol.* 1990;155:873–890.
20. Renk H. Neurological complications of central nerve blocks. *Acta Anaesthesiol Scand.* 1995;39:859–868.
21. Digiovanni AJ, Galbert MW, Whale WM. Epidural injection of autologous blood for postlumbar puncture headache. Additional clinical experiences and laboratory investigation. *Anesth Analg.* 1972.;51:226–232.
22. Abouleish E, Dela Vega S, Bledinger I, Tio T-O. Long term follow up of epidural blood patch. *Anesth. Analg.* 1975;54:2856–2863.

23. Shaw M, Russell JA, Grossart KW. The changing pattern of spinal arachnoiditis. *J Neurol Neurosurg Psychiatry*. 1978;41:97–107.

24. Junck L, Marshall WH. Neurotoxicity of radiological contrast agents. *Ann Neurol*. 1983;13:469–484.

25. Howland WJ, Curry JL. Pantopaque arachnoiditis: experimental study of blood as a potentiating agent and corticosteroids as an ameliorating agent. *Acta Radiol*. 1966;5:1032–1041.

26. Cope RW. The Woolley and Roe case. *Anaesthesia*. 1954;9: 249–270.

27. Harding S, Collis RE, Morgan BM. Meningitis after combined spinal extradural anaesthesia in obstetrics. *Br J Anaesth*. 1994;73:545–547.

28. Eldor J, Brodsky V. Danger of metallic particles in the spinal epidural spaces using the niddle-through-needle approach. *Acta Anaesthesiol Scand*. 1991;35:461–463.

29. Aldrete J. Neurologic deficits and arachnoiditis following neuraxial anesthesia. *Acta Anaesthesiol Scand*. 2003;47:3–12.

30. Lambert L, Lambert D, Strichartz G. Irreversible conduction block in isolated nerve by high concentrations of local anesthetics. *Anesthesiology*. 1994;80:1082–1093.

31. Kitsou M, Kostapanagiotou G, Klimeris K, et al. Hitopathological alterations after single epidural injection of ropivicaine, methylprednizolone acetate, or contrast material in swine. *Cardiovasc Intervent Radiol*. 2011;34:1288–1295.

32. Nguyen C, Ho K, Haughton V. Effect of lidocaine on the meninges in an experimental animal model. *Invest Radiol*. 1991;26:745–747.

33. Grahame R, Clark B, Watson M, Polkey C. Toward a rational therapeutic strategy of arachnoiditis. A possible role for d-penicillamine. *Spine*. 1991;16:172–175.

34. Guyer DW, Wiltse LL, Eskay ML, Guyer BH. The long range prognosis of arachnoiditis. *Spine*. 1989;12:1332–1342.

35. Aldrete JA. Diagnosis: the symptoms. In: Arachnoiditis: The Evidence Revealed. Mexico City: Corpus; 2010:443.

36. Ross J, Masaryk T, Modic M. MRI imaging of lumbar arachnoiditis. *Am J Neuroradiol*. 1987;149:1025.

37. Dolan R. Spinal adhesive arachnoiditis. *Surg Neurol*. 1993;39: 479–484.

38. North R, Ewend M, Lawton M. Failed back surgery syndrome: 5 year follow up after spinal cord stimulator implantation. *Neurosurgery*. 1991;28:692–699.

39. Warnke J Mourgela S. Endoscopic treatment of lumbar arachnoiditis. *Minim Invasive Neurosurg*. 2007;50:1–6.

40. Manchikanti L, Boswell M, Rivera J. A randomized, controlled trial of spinal endoscopic adhesiolysis in chronic refractory low back and lower extremity pain. *BMC Anesthesiol*. 2005;5:10.

41. Neal JM1, Kopp SL, Pasternak JJ, Lanier WL, Rathmell JP. Anatomy and pathophysiology of spinal cord injury associated with regional anesthesia and pain medicine: 2015 update. *Reg Anesth Pain Med*. 2015;40(5):506–525. doi: 10.1097/AAP.0000000000000297

PART VI

Neuropathic Pain of the Head and Neck

30

Trigeminal Neuralgia

RADHIKA GRANDHE, ELI JOHNSON HARRIS, AND EUGENE KOSHKIN

CASE

A 65-year-old woman is referred to the pain clinic for left-sided facial pain. Onset of pain was about 6 months ago and the patient denies any preceding event. The pain seems to be progressively worsening. She rates the pain at 8/10 and describes it as sharp and lancinating in nature. In the patient's words, "it takes my breath away." The pain is located over the left forehead, orbit, cheek, and nose. She states that the pain is intermittent and she experiences 10–20 random episodes in a day. Chewing and brushing can provoke her episodes, too. These episodes of pain last about 30–60 seconds at a time. Her spouse also has noted that she is more depressed, eating less, and is losing weight. The patient's primary care physician had been prescribing oxycodone without noticeable benefit. Physical exam reveals no gross facial deformities. Her left eye appears more congested. She appears apprehensive and is reluctant to allow the examiner to touch her face. Cranial nerve exam is normal except for hypersensitivity to touch over the left cheek and forehead. The rest of the neurological exam reveals no deficits. An MRI of brain with and without contrast is ordered. No evidence of demyelinating disease is found. No neurovascular compression is evident on the MRI. Baseline blood work is ordered for complete blood count, basic metabolic panel, and liver function tests, which are all within normal range. Carbamazepine is started at 100 mg twice daily and her blood counts and sodium level are monitored. During a follow-up visit 8 weeks later, the patient reports marked improvement of symptom severity. She has been eating better and the weight has stabilized.

DEFINITION

Trigeminal neuralgia (TN), also known as tic douloureux, is a pain disorder affecting the trigeminal nerve. It is characterized by brief episodes of pain following the distribution of one or more divisions of the trigeminal nerve. The pain is characterized as unilateral, lancinating in nature, and abrupt in onset and termination.[1,2] It is often accompanied by facial spasm or tic. TN causes distress and isolation because attacks are triggered by activities involving facial movements, such as chewing, talking, smiling, drinking fluids, blowing the nose, or even just encountering cold air.[3]

ANATOMY

The trigeminal nerve, or fifth cranial nerve, provides sensory supply to the face and sensory and motor supply to the muscles of mastication. The nerve has three major divisions: ophthalmic (V1), maxillary (V2), and mandibular (V3) (Figure 30.1). The ophthalmic and maxillary nerves are sensory only, while the mandibular nerve has sensory and motor functions. The trigeminal nerve enters and exits the brain at the mid-pons level, called the root entry zone.[3] Its sensory ganglion, the Gasserian ganglion, is located in Meckel's cavity. Meckel's cavity is a fossa of the petrous bone, which is part of the temporal bone. The ophthalmic nerve exits the cranium through the superior orbital fissure, the maxillary nerve exits through the foramen rotundum, and the mandibular nerve exits through the foramen ovale.

The Gasserian ganglion and rootlets of the trigeminal nerve are surrounded by subarachnoid space, called the trigeminal nerve cistern. The trigeminal nerve cistern is a middle fossa extension of subarachnoid space around the trigeminal nerve.[4]

PATHOPHYSIOLOGY

Most cases of TN are caused by compression of the nerve root at the root entry zone. Eighty to 90% of cases of pain in the trigeminal distribution

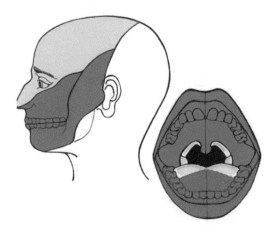

FIGURE 30.1. Innervation of facial and intraoral structures by trigeminal branches. Areas colored yellow represent innervation by ophthalmic branch, green represents maxillary branch, and orange represents mandibular branch innervation.

Courtesy: Cruccu G, Finnerup NB, Jensen TS, et al. Trigeminal neuralgia: new classification and diagnostic grading for practice and research. *Neurology*, 2016;87(2):220–228.

are due to vascular compression on the nerve.[3] One study identified that 64% of the compressing vessels were arterial, most commonly the superior cerebellar artery (81%), while 36% of the compressing vessels were venous.[5]

Other etiologies include herpes zoster and postherpetic neuropathy, trauma, tumors, chronic meningeal inflammation, demyelination from multiple sclerosis, lesions in the pons at the root entry zone, or other vascular lesions.[1,3,6] Tumors that cause TN include acoustic neurinomas, chordomas, pontine gliomas or glioblastomas, epidermoids, metastases, and lymphomas.[1,3] Other vascular lesions that cause TN include pontine infarcts, arteriovenous malformations, or aneurysms near the nerve.[3] These etiologies are relevant to treatment options.[8]

Compression on the nerve leads to local demyelination.[3,7] This leads to ephaptic transmission, in which neural impulses are transmitted to adjacent nerves through direct electrical conduction rather than normal neurotransmission.[7] This communication between the nerve fibers responsible for light touch and pain explains why pain responses are often triggered by innocuous stimuli in patients with TN.[3]

EPIDEMIOLOGY

TN is a rare condition with an annual incidence of 4.3 per 100,000, with women having a slightly higher incidence than men (5.9 vs. 3.4 per 100,000).[8] The incidence increases with age; 90% of idiopathic cases begin after age 40. Pediatric TN is rare. Hypertension may be considered a risk factor for TN.[9] Rare familial cases have also been reported, but TN is almost always a sporadic disorder.

CLINICAL FEATURES

TN is characterized by paroxysms of sharp, stabbing unilateral facial pain along the distribution of one or more divisions of the trigeminal nerve usually triggered by innocuous stimuli.[3]

Triggers of the pain are as follows[3]:

- Chewing, talking, smiling, or grimacing
- Drinking fluids, cold or hot
- Touching, shaving, applying makeup, brushing teeth, blowing nose
- Exposure to cold air, e.g., from a car window

Pain has the following characteristics[1,3,10]:

- Paroxysmal, severe, lancinating
- Usually begins with electric shock–like sensation
- Short-acting pain, usually lasts from 1 to several seconds
- Refractory period in which paroxysm cannot be initiated
- Pain ablates between attacks in classical TN, but often persists in classical TN with concomitant persistent facial pain
- Usually occurs repetitively

Location of the pain[1,6,11]

- Typically unilateral
- Can be bilateral, but rarely on both sides simultaneously. Never crosses the face.

V1	4%	V1 + V2	14%
V2	17%	V2 + V3	32%
V3	15%	V1 + V2 + V3	17%

Associated symptoms are as follows[1,3,12]:

- Often see facial muscle spasms, and attacks may provoke grimacing or wincing; hence the term *tic douloureux*
- May be associated with mild autonomic symptoms of lacrimation, conjunctival injection, and/or rhinorrhea

- Over time, the pain attacks can result in psychosocial dysfunction and significantly impaired quality of life
- Patients with TN likely have a higher rate of suicide than those with other pain disorders
- Over time, TN often leads to weight loss
- Patients avoid touching face, in contrast to other pain syndromes, in which patients use massage, heat, or ice
- Typically does not wake patients up at night
- May be preceded by pretrigeminal neuralgia, which is characterized by a dull, aching pain that evolves over time into TN

DIAGNOSIS AND CLASSIFICATION

Various classification systems have been proposed for trigeminal neuralgia/neuropathy and the terminology used can be confusing. The International Classification of Headache Disorders, 3rd edition (ICHD-3) and the American Academy of Neurology 2016 classification will be discussed here.

The ICHD-3[1] lists the following diagnostic criteria:

A. At least three attacks of unilateral facial pain fulfilling criteria B and C
B. Occurring in one or more divisions of the trigeminal nerve, with no radiation beyond the trigeminal distribution
C. Pain has at least three of the following four characteristics:
    1. Recurring in paroxysmal attacks lasting from a fraction of a second to 2 minutes
    2. Severe intensity
    3. Electric shock–like, shooting, stabbing, or sharp in quality
    4. Precipitated by innocuous stimuli to the affected side of the face
D. No clinically evident neurological deficit
E. Not better accounted for by another ICHD-3 diagnosis

The ICHD-3 diagnostic criteria for classical TN with concomitant persistent facial pain are as follows:

A. Recurrent attacks of unilateral facial pain fulfilling criteria for classical trigeminal neuralgia

B. Persistent facial pain of moderate intensity in the affected area
C. Not better accounted for by another ICHD-3 diagnosis

The American Academy of Neurology has recommended the following classification[10]:

Etiological classification of trigeminal neuralgia:

- Idiopathic TN: no identifiable apparent cause
- Classical TN: caused by vascular compression
- Secondary TN: caused by major central nervous system abnormality

Each of these etiological types may be associated one of the clinical phenotypes of either purely paroxysmal pain or TN with continuous pain.

No laboratory, electrophysiological, or radiographic testing is necessary for the diagnosis of TN; treatment may be initiated in patients based on history along with a normal neurological exam. However, imaging, preferably MRI with and without contrast, should be performed to exclude secondary causes.[1] MRI can also detect neurovascular compression in one-third of patients. More advanced MRI techniques can identify morphological changes of flattening or compression within the root entry zone even in the absence of close contact with vascular structures.[10]

TREATMENT

Pharmacological therapy is the initial treatment for patients with TN. Classical TN is usually initially responsive to pharmacological therapy, especially carbamazepine or oxcarbazepine.[1] A recent systematic review and practice parameter from the American Academy of Neurology and the European Federation of Neurological Societies outlined the evidence classification for the treatment options of TN.[12] Treatment should start with carbamazepine (level A) or oxcarbazepine (level B). Baclofen, lamotrigine, and pimozide may be considered (level C).[12] Other medications have been studied but limited data about effectiveness exist. These medications include clonazepam, gabapentin, pregabalin, topiramate, levetiracetam, phenytoin, tocainide, tizanidine, lidocaine, and valproate.[6,12]

There is limited evidence to support pharmacological alternatives in patients refractory to first-line medical therapy. Gabapentin, lamotrigine, topiramate, baclofen, and tizanidine have been used as supplemental therapy. Intravenous phenytoin, fosphenytoin, and lidocaine have been used to attempt to alleviate pain while oral medications are titrated.

There is moderate evidence to suggest that botulinum toxin A injections into the skin or mucosa in the affected areas of the face has some benefit for patients with TN and postherpetic neuralgia.[13]

Surgical and interventional modalities should be considered for patients who have failed an adequate trial of a single first-line agent. There are no studies comparing medical and procedural treatment[8]. Percutaneous procedures, Gamma Knife surgery, and microvascular decompression may be considered if medical management fails (level C).[12]

No placebo-controlled trials have been conducted to evaluate treatment for secondary TN. Treatment of the underlying condition is recommended, along with the same medications recommended for classical TN.[1]

Classical TN with concomitant persistent facial pain is poorly responsive to medical or interventional treatment and often requires multiple pharmacological treatment trials or a combination of medications.[1]

PHARMACOLOGICAL THERAPY

Carbamazepine

Carbamazepine is the only drug that is FDA approved for treatment of TN.[14] Treatment response is excellent for classical TN, with adequate pain control achieved in 58% to 100% of patients. The number needed to treat is less than 2 with the outcome as significant pain relief. However, patients often experience significant side effects, with the number needed to harm for minor adverse events of 3 and for serious adverse events of 24.[12]

Dosing is as follows[8]:

- Start at 200–400 mg daily divided in two doses.
- Dose can be increased in increments of 200 mg daily or every other day as tolerated until significant pain relief is achieved.
- Slow titration to minimize side effects.
- Typical dose is 600–800 mg daily, given in two divided doses.

- Maximum suggested daily dose is 1200 mg daily.

Side effects and adverse events include the following[8]:

- 6%–10% of patients cannot tolerate carbamazepine because of side effects
- Drowsiness
- Dizziness
- Ataxia
- Diplopia
- Nausea and vomiting
- Leukopenia is common but usually benign
- Aplastic anemia is rare
- Hyponatremia
- Hepatotoxicity
- Stevens-Johnson syndrome and/or toxic epidermal necrolysis (see other considerations, next)

Other considerations to note[8]:

- Carbamazepine induces hepatic enzymes.
- The FDA recommends obtaining blood count, sodium level, and liver function tests before starting therapy and within several weeks of initiating treatment.
- Screen for the allele HLA-B*1502 before starting therapy in patients with Asian ancestry, as the allele has been associated with an increased risk of Stevens-Johnson syndrome and/or toxic epidermal necrolysis. If at least one copy of this allele is present, avoid carbamazepine.

Oxcarbazepine

Pooled analysis of randomized controlled trials (RCTs) comparing oxcarbazepine to carbamazepine showed equal effectiveness between the two drugs, with greater than 50% of reduction in incidence of attacks in 88% of the study patients. The evidence for carbamazepine as treatment for TN is stronger than that for oxcarbazepine, but oxcarbazepine has a better safety profile.[8]

Dosing is as follows[8]:

- Start at 300–600 mg daily, divided in two doses.
- Increase as tolerated in 300 mg daily increments every third day.
- Typical maintenance dose is 600–1200 mg daily.

- Total dose is 1200–1800 mg daily, divided in two doses.

Side effects include the following[15]:

- Hypersensitivity
- Hyponatremia
- Risk of Stevens-Johnson syndrome and or toxic epidermal necrolysis

Other considerations to note[8,15]:

- Rapid titration is possible, unlike with carbamazepine.
- Oxcarbazepine is a weak inducer of hepatic enzymes.
- Measure serum sodium level after initiation of oxcarbazepine.
- Screen for HLA-B*1502 allele; if present, do not start oxcarbazepine.

Baclofen

Limited evidence shows that baclofen is helpful in treating TN. In one study, treatment of daily doses of 40–80 mg resulted in reduced incidences of attacks in 7 out of 10 patients with classical TN, compared with 1 out of 10 taking placebo.[8] The drug has been recommended for patients with multiple sclerosis who develop TN.[16] Dosing is as follows[16]:

- Goal dose is 40 mg to 80 mg daily, divided in three doses

Side effects include the following:

- Sedation
- Dizziness
- Dyspepsia
- Loss of muscle tone

Other considerations to note[16]:

- Discontinue slowly to avoid withdrawal symptoms of seizures and hallucinations.

Lamotrigine

Lamotrigine has been tested both as an adjunct and as sole therapy. As an adjunct, a double-blind study found that the addition of lamotrigine at a daily dose of 400 mg to either carbamazepine or phenytoin in patients who have not responded to the single agent alone showed an improvement in pain.[17] As a single agent, lamotrigine was shown to be beneficial in an open-label study, with improvement in pain outcomes in 11 out of 15 patients at a total daily dose of 400 mg.[18] Lamotrigine is recommended as a second-line treatment, either as an adjunct or sole agent.[8] Slow titration helps to decrease incidence of side effects, but patients often don't accept the long titration phase.

Dosing for patients not already taking an anticonvulsant is as follows:

- Start at 25 mg daily for 2 weeks, then increase to 50 mg daily for weeks 3 to 4.
- After 4 weeks, titrate dose to effect.
- Increase by 50 mg daily every 1–2 weeks.
- Target dose is usually 200–400 mg daily.

Dosing for patients taking other anticonvulsants that are enzyme inducers (carbamazepine, phenytoin, primidone) is as follows[8]:

- Start at 50 mg daily.
- Titrate to 100 mg daily at week 3, 200 mg daily at week 5, 300 mg daily at week 6, and 400 mg daily at week 7.

Dosing for patients taking valproate is as follows[8]:

- Start at 12.5 mg to 25 mg every other day.
- Increase by 25 mg every 2 weeks as needed.
- Maximum of 400 mg daily

Side effects include the following:

- Dizziness
- Nausea
- Blurred vision
- Ataxia
- Skin rash in 7%–10% of patients, usually resolves with continued treatment in 4–8 months
- Stevens-Johnson syndrome; if it occurs, discontinue immediately

Other considerations to note:

- Lamotrigine needs to be titrated over many weeks, so clinical utility is questionable.

Pimozide

Pimozide was shown to be more effective than carbamazepine for refractory TN in a double-blind RTC of 48 patients.[19] However, it is rarely used because of the serious side effects.

Dosing is as follows:

- Start at 1–2 mg daily.
- Increase by 1–2 mg every other day.
- Maximum of 10 mg daily

Side effects include the following[8,19]:

- Sedation
- Arrhythmias
- Anticholinergic effects
- Extrapyramidal symptoms, either acute or long term
- Parkinsonism

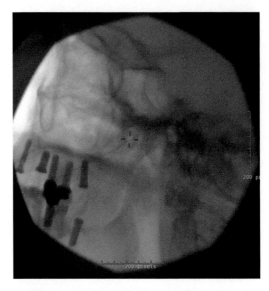

FIGURE 30.2. Submental view, percutaneous approach to foramen ovale for trigeminal nerve block.

SURGICAL AND PROCEDURAL THERAPY

A surgical or procedural therapy should be considered in patients who have trialed an adequate dose of a single first-line agent and continue to experience significant pain.[18] The decision regarding which procedure should be performed should rely on clinical findings and discussion with the patient.[8]

Recommended treatment options include percutaneous procedures (rhizotomy), Gamma Knife surgery, and microvascular decompression.[8] Neuromodulation and peripheral neurectomy are other procedures attempted for TN.

There is no definitive evidence to suggest superiority of one intervention to another. Microvascular decompression likely has a longer duration of pain control, although it is more invasive.[12] Feared procedural complications include CSF leak, infarct, hematoma, aseptic meningitis and facial numbness. Facial numbness is more common with rhizotomy procedures than with Gamma Knife surgery or microvascular decompression.

Rhizotomy

The procedure is conducted as follows[20,21]:

- Rhizotomy is performed by passing a percutaneous cannula through the foramen ovale and lesioning the Gasserian ganglion using radiofrequency thermocoagulation, balloon compression, or percutaneous glycerol rhizolysis (Figures 30.2 and 30.3).

- Radiofrequency thermocoagulation creates a lesion through application of heat.
- In balloon compression, one mechanically compresses the ganglion using a small balloon, which is introduced into Meckel's cavity using a needle. It is technically easier to perform than radiofrequency thermocoagulation or percutaneous glycerol rhizolysis.
- Percutaneous glycerol rhizolysis creates a lesion through injection of 0.1 to 0.4 mL of glycerol into the trigeminal cistern.

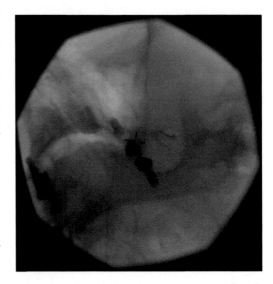

FIGURE 30.3. Lateral view, percutaneous approach to foramen ovale for trigeminal nerve block.

Pain relief outcomes are as follows[8]:

- Initial pain relief: 90%
- Pain-free at 1 year: 68–85%
- Pain-free at 3 years: 54–64%
- Pain-free at 5 years: 50%

Adverse events and complications to note:

- Meningitis, mainly aseptic: 0.2%
- Postoperative dysesthesia (burning, heavy, aching or tired feeling): 6%–12%
- Long-term sensory loss: 50%
- Anesthesia dolorosa: 4%
- Corneal numbness with risk of keratitis: 4%

Gamma Knife Surgery

The procedure involves a focused beam of radiation aimed at the trigeminal nerve in the posterior fossa.[22]

Pain relief outcomes are as follows[8,22]:

- Pain relief (usually delayed for 10 days to 1 month post-procedure): 91.8%
- Pain-free at 1 year: 69%
- Pain-free at 3 years: 52%
- Pain-free 5 years or beyond: unknown, estimated at 45%–60%
- Deafferentation pain is rare.

Adverse events and complications to note[8,22]:

- Facial numbness: 9%–37%; improves over time. One study reports very bothersome facial numbness rates as low as 0.6%.
- Paresthesias: 6%–13%

Other considerations[8,22]:

- High treatment expense; limits widespread usage.
- Usually reserved for patients who cannot undergo craniotomy, but being considered as an initial procedure of choice by some.

Microvascular Decompression

The procedure is conducted as follows[8,23]:

- This is major surgery involving a craniotomy to reach the trigeminal nerve in the posterior fossa (Figure 30.4).
- Veins in contact with the root entry zone are coagulated.
- Arteries are separated from the nerve using a sponge or felt.

Pain relief outcomes are as follows[8]:

- Initial pain relief: 90%
- Pain-free at 1 year: 80%
- Pain-free at 3 years: 75%
- Pain-free at 5 years: 73%

Adverse events and complications to note[8,23]:

- Mortality: 0.2%–0.9%
- Major complications in up to 4% of patients: cerebrospinal fluid (CSF) leak, infarction, hematoma, stroke
- Aseptic meningitis: 11%
- Sensory loss: 7%
- Hearing loss: 10%

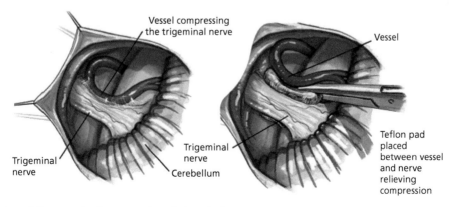

FIGURE 30.4. Microvascular decompression of trigeminal nerve.

Courtesy: Netter.

Other considerations to note[23]:

- Microvascular decompression is often considered early in young patients with TN because of the long treatment effect.
- There are no significant difference in efficacy between young and elderly patients, but elderly patients have higher rates of serious complications.

Peripheral Neurectomy

The procedure involves the following:

- It is performed at branches of the trigeminal nerve: supraorbital, infraorbital, alveolar, and lingual nerves.
- Expose nerve with incision, then lesion the targeted nerve.
- Lesioning includes alcohol injection, radiofrequency lesioning, and cryotherapy.

The surgical techniques described here and percutaneous destructive procedures may be repeated for recurrent neuralgia but the risk of deafferentation pain increases with every repeat procedure.

NEUROMODULATION

Studies in small groups of patients with craniofacial pain using newer technologies such as trigeminal and sphenopalatine ganglion stimulation and peripheral nerve field stimulation have shown promise.[24]

PROGNOSIS

The course of TN is variable, usually waxes and wanes in severity and frequency of attacks, and recurrence is common. Episodes may last weeks to months, followed by intervals without symptoms. Some patients have persistent background pain, while most have complete remission between attacks. TN by itself is not fatal.

GUIDING QUESTIONS

- How can you differentiate classical trigeminal neuralgia from atypical facial pain?
- How would you work up a patient with unilateral facial pain?
- Discuss conservative management options for trigeminal neuralgia. What is the typical first-line treatment?

- What are the risks associated with interventional and surgical approaches to treatment of trigeminal neuralgia?

KEY POINTS

- Trigeminal neuralgia (TN) is a rare condition characterized by brief, electric shock–like sensations within the distribution of trigeminal nerve branches, the fifth cranial nerve. It is typically unilateral and may be associated with facial spasms.
- Classical TN is caused by vascular compression at the nerve root entry zone in the majority of cases. Criteria for diagnosis include brief paroxysms of pain with absence of pain between episodes and absence of neurological deficits.
- Secondary TN may be related to postherpetic neuropathy, trauma, demyelinating diseases, vascular lesions, or tumors in the pons or root entry zone. These patients may have constant facial pain in the background.
- The diagnosis of classic TN is largely based on clinical history and exam findings. Other workup, such as brain MRI and evoked potential testing, may be ordered to rule out secondary etiologies.
- Medical management is the preferred first line of treatment. Carbamazepine and oxcarbazepine have level A evidence for efficacy in the treatment of TN. However, these drugs can cause serious adverse effects and need close monitoring. Other drugs that may be beneficial are baclofen, tizanidine, lamotrigine, and lidocaine.
- Surgery or interventional procedures are considered in patients who have failed pharmacological therapy with at least three agents. Nonablative therapy is microvascular decompression and has the best record for long-term success.
- Ablative procedures include percutaneous balloon compression, radiofrequency thermocoagulation, Gamma Knife surgery, and glycerol rhizolysis. They all carry the risk of anesthesia dolorosa.

REFERENCES

1. Headache Classification Committee of the International Headache Society (IHS). The international classification of headache disorders (beta version). *Cephalalgia*. 2013l;33(9):629–808.

2. Van Kleef M, van Genderen WE, Narouze S, et al. 1. Trigeminal neuralgia. *Pain Pract.* 2009;9(4):252–259.

3. Love S, Coakham HB. Trigeminal neuralgia. *Brain.* 2001;124(12):2347–2360.

4. Kaufman B, Bellon EM. The trigeminal nerve cistern. *Radiology.* 1973;108(3):597–602.

5. Anderson VC, Berryhill PC, Sandquist MA, Ciaverella DP, Nesbit GM, Burchiel KJ. High-resolution three-dimensional magnetic resonance angiography and three-dimensional spoiled gradient-recalled imaging in the evaluation of neurovascular compression in patients with trigeminal neuralgia: a double-blind pilot study. *Neurosurgery.* 2006;58(4):666–673.

6. Zakrzewska JM, Linskey ME. Trigeminal neuralgia. *BMJ.* 2014;348: g474.

7. Devor M, Amir R, Rappaport ZH. Pathophysiology of trigeminal neuralgia: the ignition hypothesis. *Clin J Pain.* 2002;18(1):4–13.

8. Obermann M. Treatment options in trigeminal neuralgia. *Ther Adv Neurol Disord.* 2010;3:107–115.

9. Pan SL, Yen MF, Chiu YH, Chen LS, Chen HH. Increased risk of trigeminal neuralgia after hypertension, a population-based study. *Neurology.* 2011;77(17):1605–1610.

10. Cruccu G, Finnerup NB, Jensen TS, et al. Trigeminal neuralgia: new classification and diagnostic grading for practice and research. *Neurology.* 2016;87(2):220–228.

11. Rozen TD. Trigeminal neuralgia and glossopharyngeal neuralgia. *Neurol Clin.* 2004;22(1):185–206.

12. Gronseth G, Cruccu G, Alksne J, et al. Practice parameter: The diagnostic evaluation and treatment of trigeminal neuralgia (an evidence-based review). Report of the Quality Standards Subcommittee of the American Academy of Neurology and the European Federation of Neurological Societies. *Neurology.* 2008;71(15):1183–1190.

13. Shackleton T, Ram S, Black M, et al. The efficacy of botulinum toxin for the treatment of trigeminal and postherpetic neuralgia: a systematic review with meta-analyses. *Oral Surg Oral Med Oral Pathol Oral Radiol.* 2016;22(1):61–71.

14. CenterWatch. FDA Approved Drugs for Neurology. https://www.centerwatch.com/drug-information/fda-approved-drugs/therapeutic-area/10/neurology. Accessed 5/2/2016. Updated 2016.

15. Chong DJ, Lerman AM. Practice update: review of anticonvulsant therapy. *Curr Neurol Neurosci Rep.* 2016;16(4):1–14.

16. Zakrzewska JM, Linskey ME. Trigeminal neuralgia. *BMJ.* 2015;;350:h1238. doi: 10.1136/bmj.h1238.

17. Zakrzewska JM, Chaudhry Z, Nurmikko TJ, Patton DW, Mullens EL. Lamotrigine (lamictal) in refractory trigeminal neuralgia: results from a double-blind placebo controlled crossover trial. *Pain.* 1997;73(2):223–230.

18. Lunardi G, et al. Clinical effectiveness of lamotrigine and plasma levels in essential and symptomatic trigeminal neuralgia. *Neurology.* 1997;48(6):1714–1717.

19. Zhang J, Yang M, Zhou M, He L, Chen N, Zakrzewska JM. Non-antiepileptic drugs for trigeminal neuralgia. *Cochrane Database Syst Rev.* 2013;12:CD004029.

20. Lopez BC, Hamlyn PJ, Zakrzewska JM. Systematic review of ablative neurosurgical techniques for the treatment of trigeminal neuralgia. *Neurosurgery.* 2004;54(4):973–983.

21. De Córdoba JL, García Bach M, Isach N, Piles S. Percutaneous balloon compression for trigeminal neuralgia: imaging and technical aspects. *Reg Anesth Pain Med.* 2015;40(5):616–622.

22. Régis J, Tuleasca C, Resseguier N, et al. Long-term safety and efficacy of Gamma Knife surgery in classical trigeminal neuralgia: a 497-patient historical cohort study. *J Neurosurg.* 2016;124(4):1079–1087.

23. Phan K, Rao PJ, Dexter M. Microvascular decompression for elderly patients with trigeminal neuralgia. *J Clin Neurosci.* 2016;29:7–14.

24. Maniam R, Kaye AD, Vadivelu N, et al. Facial pain update: advances in neurostimulation for the treatment of facial pain. *Curr Pain Headache Rep.* 2016;20 (4):24.

31

Glossopharyngeal Neuralgia

GEORGE C. CHANG CHIEN, ANDREA M. TRESCOT, AND AGNES R. STOGICZA

CASE

A 65-year-old woman with a past medical history of trigeminal neuralgia presents with a report of episodes of pain in her left throat, jaw, and ear. These attacks are excruciating and described as sharp, stabbing, and "shocks of electricity," lasting up to 30 seconds. She reports that these episodes began 3 weeks ago, and they are unlike her previous episodes of trigeminal neuralgia, which was successfully treated with Gamma Knife surgery. These attacks are triggered when she is swallowing food, yawning, coughing, or laughing. This has resulted in a fear of eating because of the pain. During one episode, she reports feeling light-headed and fainting. Her past medical history is also significant for multiple sclerosis. A fluoroscopically guided glossopharyngeal nerve block was performed, which confirms the diagnosis.

INTRODUCTION

Glossopharyngeal neuralgia (GPN), or Weisenburg-Sicard-Robineau syndrome, was first described by the American neurologist T.H. Weisenburg in 1910 in a patient with a case of facial pain secondary to a cerebellopontine tumor misdiagnosed as tic douloureux (trigeminal neuralgia).[1] Although the French neurologists Jean-Anathase Sicard and Maurice Robineau also published cases in 1920, treating atypical facial pain by resection of the ninth cranial nerve, it was the British neurologist Wilfred Harris who coined the term "glossopharyngeal neuralgia," in 1921.[2]

GPN is characterized by unilateral paroxysmal pain in the oropharynx, nasopharynx, larynx, base of the tongue, tonsillar region, and lower jaw (Figure 31.1). Pain can also radiate to the ipsilateral ear. These attacks are excruciatingly painful and typically described as sharp, stabbing, "shocks of electricity" that can last from seconds to minutes. These painful attacks can be triggered by stimulation to the oropharynx, such as mechanical swallowing, yawning, coughing, laughing, and chewing, and sensory stimulation, such as cold, salty, acidic, or bitter foods.

GPN may mimic trigeminal neuralgia (TN). Both may present with facial/jaw pain elicited by the same mechanical and sensory mechanisms. Cases may be difficult to differentiate in patients who complain of pain in the region of the tragus or deep to the angle of the jaw. However, compared to TN, GPN is relatively rare (and milder),[3] although dual diagnosis has been reported.[3]

GPN has also been referred to as *stylalgia* or *Eagle's syndrome*; these names describe the enlarged or elongated styloid process that can be one of the causes of GPN (Figure 31.2). Eagle described two types of GPN—the *classic styloid syndrome* that occurs primarily after tonsillectomy, and the *stylocarotid syndrome*, caused by stimulation of the fifth, eighth, ninth, and tenth

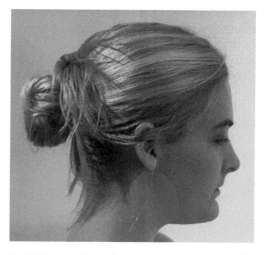

FIGURE 31.1. Pattern of pain associated with glossopharyngeal neuralgia.

Image courtesy of Andrea Trescot, MD.

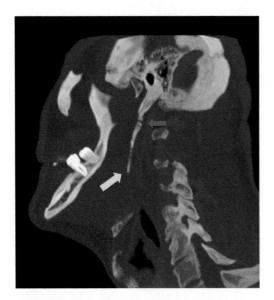

FIGURE 31.2. CT scan showing elongated styloid process (white arrow); note fracture line (blue arrow).

Image courtesy of Christ DeClerck, MD; General Hospital Sint-Jan, Bruges, Belgium, with permission.

cranial nerves by the styloid.[4] Other rare features include tinnitus, vomiting, vertigo, swelling sensation, and involuntary movements.[5]

Because the vagus and glossopharyngeal nerve travel together at the level of the styloid, another name for GPN is *vagoglossopharyngeal neuralgia* (VGPN).[6] Many patients have been described in the literature with asystole, convulsions, and syncope associated with VGPN.[7,8]

EPIDEMIOLOGY

The incidence of GPN increases with age and most often affects persons older than 50 years; however, in patients with multiple sclerosis, GPN tends to occur at a younger age.[9] In 217 cases of GPN seen at the Mayo Clinic,[3] 57% of the cases were in patients greater than 50 years old, while 43% were between the ages of 18 and 50. Twelve percent of these patients had bilateral involvement, but a frequency of bilateral involvement as high as 25% has been reported. Additionally, 12% of the patients exhibited both glossopharyngeal and trigeminal neuralgia. The right side of the face is more associated with TN than GPN.[3] A greater prevalence in males than females has been reported by some authors, while no difference in prevalence by gender has been reported by others.[10]

Although considered "uncommon," Singh et al.[11] felt that GPN was "not as uncommon as has been reported in the literature," but rather

was underdiagnosed because of the variety of presentations, as well as unawareness of the disease. The incidence is 0.7/100,000/year according to Manzoni and Torelli.[12] Katusic et al.[3] compared the epidemiological incidence of TN with that of GPN; they found an annual incidence of 4.7 per 100,000 persons for TN in contrast to 0.8 per 100,000 persons for GPN.

ANATOMY

The glossopharyngeal nerve exits the skull with the vagus and spinal accessory nerves through the jugular foramen, descends through the narrow space between the transverse process of the atlas (C1) and the styloid (Figure 31.3), passes anterior to the carotid artery and deep to the styloid, and then turns to the tongue where it passes through the tonsillar fossa to enter the pharynx. The glossopharyngeal nerve is a mixed cranial nerve with sensory, motor, and autonomic components.

Sensory innervation includes the eustachian tube, middle ear, and mastoid; the oropharynx; the posterior third of the tongue (including taste); the vallecula; the anterior surface of the epiglottis (lingual branch); the walls of the

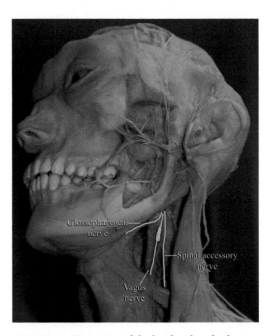

FIGURE 31.3. Dissection of the head and neck, showing the relationship between the spinal accessory nerve, the glossopharyngeal nerve, and the vagus nerve in the neck next to the carotid artery.

Image modified from an image from *Bodies, The Exhibition*, with permission. Image courtesy of Andrea Trescot, MD.

pharynx (pharyngeal branch); and the tonsils (tonsillar branch). Therefore, it is part of the gag reflex.[13] Motor innervation includes the striated stylopharyngeus muscle. The autonomic innervation includes the secretomotor parasympathetic fibers to the parotid gland, the carotid body, and carotid sinus.[14]

PATHOPHYSIOLOGY

Although most cases are categorized as "idiopathic," the majority of GPN cases are currently believed to be caused by vascular compression of the glossopharyngeal nerve. Kawashima et al. studied 14 cases of idiopathic GPN; in all of the cases, vascular compression on the glossopharyngeal nerve was found at surgery.[15] Most commonly, the vascular compression is caused from the posterior inferior cerebellar artery (PICA), followed by the anterior-inferior cerebral artery (AICA). Other causes of GPN include tumors with local invasion, parapharyngeal abscess, trauma, multiple sclerosis, carotid puncture, styloid elongation (Eagle syndrome), adhesive arachnoiditis, and C1 (Jefferson) fractures.

Eagle's syndrome, or stylalgia, is felt to be due to an entrapment of the glossopharyngeal nerve at the elongated styloid process. Eagle himself described entrapment of the GPN at the tip of the styloid from scarring after a tonsillectomy.[16]

CLINICAL FEATURES AND DIAGNOSIS

The pain distribution may be either mainly in the tympanic or in the oropharyngeal region. The patient will describe GPN triggers in several ways: the *oropharyngeal type* is triggered mainly by swallowing, talking, and yawning, whereas the *tympanic type* is provoked by loud sounds or tactile sensations at the outer auditory canal. According to Harris,[17] "repeated coughing or clearing the throat during the pain is suggestive" of GPN. Diagnosis is typically based on clinical presentation, physical examination, imaging studies, and diagnostic blocks.

Physical Exam

Physical exam yields minimal information; history and clinical symptoms aid more in suggesting the diagnosis. The styloid process can be found by creating an imaginary line from the mastoid to the angle of the mandible; the styloid should be found halfway between these two

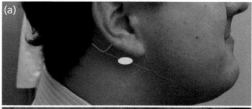
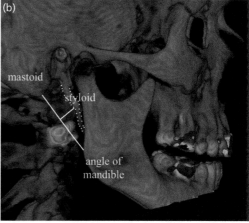

FIGURE 31.4. Surface anatomy (**A**) and 3D X-ray image (**B**) of the styloid process (outlined). **A.** The styloid process (yellow oval) is typically found equidistant between the mastoid process (red line) and the ipsilateral angle of the mandible (blue line) (image courtesy of George C. Chang Chien, DO). **B.** Imaginary line is drawn from the mastoid to the angle of the mandible; styloid process will be found at the halfway point of this line (image courtesy of Andrea Trescot, MD).

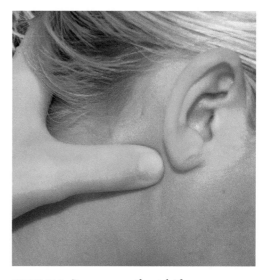

FIGURE 31.5. Pressure over the styloid process may reproduce the pain of glossopharyngeal entrapment.

Image courtesy of Andrea Trescot, MD.

structures (Figure 31.4A and B). Pressure over the styloid process (Figure 31.5) may provoke a pain attack or replicate the pain, but it is not a necessary criterion of GPN.

Imaging

High-resolution magnetic resonance imaging (MRI)[18] or computed tomography (CT)[19] of the head may reveal tumor, bony erosion, multiple sclerosis plaques, abscess, or infection. 3D visualizations of the brainstem[19,20] or magnetic resonance angiography (MRA) may help identify neurovascular compression or arteriovenous malformation (AVM). Visualization of the offending vessel was better in cases of compression from the PICA than from the AICA. Kawashima et al.[15] felt that patients would most likely respond to microvascular decompression (MVD) if the radiological images show a high origin of the PICA, with the PICA making an upward loop, and the PICA coursing over the supraolivary fossette. Similarly, Hiwatashi et al.[18] noted that if the offending vessel was the PICA, a loop formation at the supraolivary fossette was always seen, whereas if it was the AICA, GPN vascular compression was difficult to diagnose before surgery.

Balloon Occlusion Test

Hasegawa et al.[21] reported a case where MRI suggested that the right vertebral artery (VA) was pressing on the glossopharyngeal nerve. Balloon test occlusion of the VA was used to confirm the cause of the neuralgia. The neuralgia disappeared and reappeared with balloon inflation and deflation. Balloon test occlusion may be useful in the diagnosis of GPN and the selection of the most appropriate surgical treatment.

TREATMENT

Medical Treatment

Medical treatment of GPN is similar to treatment for other forms of neuropathic pain, including trigeminal neuralgia. Antiepileptic drugs (AEDs) and tricyclic antidepressants (TCAs) alone or in combination have been studied with variable efficacy. There is also a case report of GPN refractory to AEDs that responded well to opioids.[22] AEDs that have been used include carbamazepine, lamotrigine, diazepam, and gabapentin; TCAs such as amitriptyline and nortriptyline have been used as well.

Surgical Treatment

The treatment of GPN includes the treatment of the secondary causes of GPN, such as tumor resection, AV malformation embolization, styloid resection, and MVD.

Soh[16] stated that the elongated styloid was the most important cause of secondary GPN, and stylectomy should be considered before intracranial neurosurgical procedures. Shin and colleagues[23] described surgical resection in seven patients with an elongated styloid, using a lateral transcutaneous approach; all had "complete" relief for at least 12 months.

More recently, MVD has become popular, mirroring the surgical treatment of TN. Kawashima et al.[15] studied 14 cases of idiopathic GPN; vascular compression on the nerve was found at surgery in all of the cases, which was performed via a transcondylar fossa approach, and 13 of 14 had "complete" relief after surgery. Resnic et al.[24] noted that MVD provided "complete relief" in 76% of the cases and a "substantial improvement" in an additional 16%. Sampson et al.[25] noted pain relief 10 years after MVD.

Injection Techniques

Glossopharyngeal nerve blocks (GNBs) can give rapid relief and confirm the diagnosis of GPN.[26] The injections can be done with or without corticosteroid. Techniques for extraoral, intraoral, fluoroscopic, or ultrasound-assisted procedures have been described. Compared to ultrasound-assisted intervention, the use of fluoroscopy allows real-time imaging of the contrast media and may help minimize intravascular injection in case the needle tip has penetrated either the carotid or jugular vessels. Injections of local anesthetic with or without corticosteroids, chemical neurolysis, cryoneuroablation, and radiofrequency ablation are all options in management of glossopharyngeal nerve dysfunction.

Indications for GPN Injection or Neurolysis

- Glossopharyngeal neuralgia
- Post-tonsillectomy pain control
- Cancer pain
- To reduce gag reflex for awake endotracheal intubation[13]
- Singultus (hiccups)[27,28]
- Carotid sinus syndrome
- Patients who are poor candidates for microvascular decompression[29]

Patients need to be monitored for a minimum of 30 minutes following the block to verify that there has been no systemic response to the injected local anesthetic solution. Even taking these precautions and using fluoroscopic or ultrasound guidance does not completely eliminate the possibility of local anesthetic spillover onto the vagus nerve (with resultant ipsilateral vocal cord paralysis) or onto the spinal accessory nerve (with weakness of the trapezius muscle). An obtunded gag reflex is an indicator of successful GNB. There is a strong relationship between the extent of the obtunded gag reflex and the extent of post-tonsillectomy pain relief.[13]

Styloid (Proximal) Glossopharyngeal Nerve Injection Techniques

Since some entrapment of the glossopharyngeal nerve appears to occur at the styloid, injection at that site can confirm the diagnosis and potentially provide therapeutic relief.

Peristyloid Landmark Technique

If the styloid process is palpable (Figure 31.5), it may be reasonable to attempt a landmark-guided injection of the glossopharyngeal nerve, with a clear understanding of the anatomy. Since the carotid artery is directly behind the styloid process, there is a significant risk of vascular injection and bleeding. With the patient positioned supine and the head turned slightly away, the non-injecting fingers straddle the styloid, which is about 2 cm posterior from the angle of the mandible, slightly anterior and 1–2 cm caudad to the mastoid (Figure 31.6). The needle is advanced onto the styloid process (usually about 3 cm in depth) and then redirected slightly posteriorly. After careful

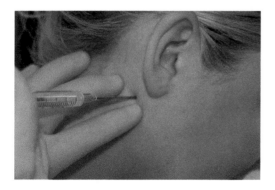

FIGURE 31.6. Landmark-guided glossopharyngeal nerve block.

Image courtesy of Andrea Trescot, MD.

aspiration, 1 to 2 mL of lidocaine at 1% concentration with or without corticosteroid is injected. Because this is a highly vascular area, a nonparticulate steroid should be considered.

Peristyloid Fluoroscopy Technique

The patient is placed supine with the head maintained midline, to overlap the bilateral styloid processes. The styloid process is used to identify the course of the GPN. Once identification of the mastoid process and the ipsilateral angle of the mandible is performed, the styloid process can be found equidistant between these structures (Figure 31.4B).

The skin overlying the styloid process should be prepped and draped in sterile fashion. A small skin wheal is made over the styloid process using a 25 gauge, 1.5 inch needle and 3–4 mL of 1% plain lidocaine. A 22 gauge, 1.5 to 2 inch blunt-tipped needle may be advanced perpendicular to the skin toward the process, aiming for its posterior aspect. Although the styloid process should be met at a depth approximating 1.5 cm to 4 cm, switching between anteroposterior (AP) and lateral imaging as the needle is advanced is necessary to confirm trajectory and depth. Once the styloid process is encountered (Figure 31.7A and B), the needle is slightly withdrawn and "walked off" posteriorly. Aspiration should be performed to ensure that there is no blood or cerebrospinal fluid. About 1 mL of water-soluble, iodinated contrast medium is incrementally injected under live continuous fluoroscopy. Then, barring any intravascular spread, a short-acting, preservative-free anesthetic (1 to 2 mL of 1% lidocaine) is incrementally injected in divided doses. Non-particulate corticosteroid (dexamethasone) may be added to the injectate.

Peristyloid Ultrasound and Combined Ultrasound/Fluoroscopy Techniques

Bedder and Lindsay[30] described an ultrasound approach to the glossopharyngeal nerve in 1989 to treat pain from cancer of the throat and tongue. The linear ultrasound probe is placed obliquely between the mastoid and the angle of the jaw on the lateral neck (Figure 31.8), which allows observation of the blood vessels to facilitate avoidance during in-plane injection.[31] The styloid target is seen as a linear hyperechoic structure with a bone shadow slightly deep to the mastoid (Figure 31.9). A combined ultrasound- and fluoroscopic-directed injection might combine the best of both techniques, allowing for

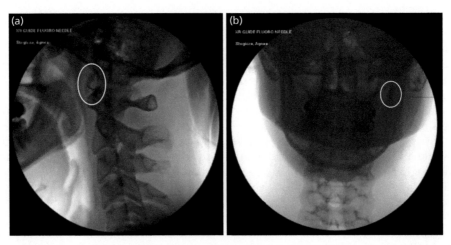

FIGURE 31.7. Fluoroscopy-guided injection of glossopharyngeal nerve. Lateral view shows the needle placed onto the styloid process. White circle identifies the styloid process. **A.** Lateral view. **B.** Anterioposterior view. After bony contact the needle is walked off posteriorly to reach the target area for the glossopharyngeal nerve.

Image courtesy of Agnes Stogicza, MD.

easier identification of the styloid (fluoroscopy) while identifying the nearby vascular structures with ultrasound (Figure 31.10).

Intraoral (Distal) Glossopharyngeal Nerve Techniques

These injections were initially developed for awake oral anesthetic intubations, but they can be useful to break the reflex spasm of hiccups and to provide pain relief from oral cancers.

Anterior Tonsillar Pillar (ATP) Method

The patient is asked to open the mouth widely (Figure 31.11). The operator may choose to anesthetize the tongue to facilitate the procedure.

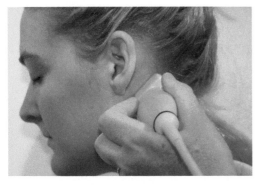

FIGURE 31.8. Location of ultrasound probe for the peristyloid glossopharyngeal nerve injection.

Image courtesy of Andrea Trescot, MD.

The tongue is swept to the opposite side with a tongue depressor, laryngoscope blade, or gloved fingers. A 25 gauge, 3.5 inch spinal needle is inserted 0.5 cm deep, just lateral to the base of the ATP (Figure 31.12). Use of a longer needle is advantageous for visualization of the tonsillar pillars by keeping the syringe out of the patient's mouth. The injection is submucosal, at a depth of about 0.5 cm, and care must be taken to avoid the tonsillar artery. After careful aspiration for blood or cerebrospinal fluid, 2 mL of local anesthetic or local anesthetic plus non-particulate steroid is injected. The advantages of this method are that the ATP is easily identified and exposed, and the tongue movement does not trigger the gag reflex. Local anesthetic spray is recommended to decrease the gag reflex. Note that this injection does not anesthetize the tympanic branch of the glossopharyngeal nerve (GPN), and therefore may not address ear pain.

Posterior Tonsillar Pillar (PTP) Method

The patient is asked to open the mouth widely. The tongue is depressed down with a laryngoscope blade (if done in the operating room) or a tongue blade. A 22 gauge, 3.5 inch spinal needle bent 1 cm from the distal end is directed laterally into the submucosa along the caudal aspect of the PTP, also known as the *palatopharyngeal fold*. After careful aspiration for blood and cerebrospinal fluid, 2 mL of local anesthetic and/

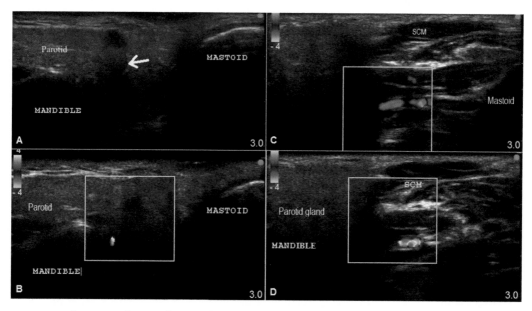

FIGURE 31.9. Composite ultrasound image of the landmarks used for a glossopharyngeal injection at the styloid. **A.** Initial ultrasound image when the linear probe is placed between the angle of the mastoid process and mandible showing the styloid shadow (arrow). **B.** Parotid gland and retromandibular vein identified. **C.** Slight rotation of the ultrasound probe allows visualizing the mastoid, the SCM and the carotid artery underneath. Mandible is not in view. **D.** Slight rotation of the ultrasound probe in the opposite direction of that in C allows visualizing the mandibular angle and the carotid under the SCM. Mastoid is not in view.

Image courtesy of Agnes Stogicza, MD.

or steroid is injected. The PTP method becomes more difficult in patients with large tongues or small oral opening and may cause greater gag reflex.

Neurolytic Techniques

If the diagnostic injections give good but only temporary relief, there are a variety of neurolytic techniques available.

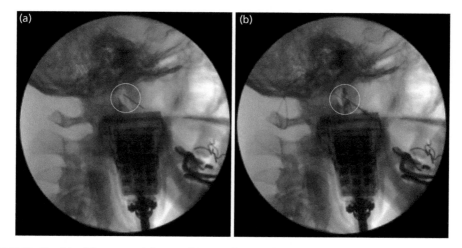

FIGURE 31.10. Combined fluoroscopy/ultrasound images showing the glossopharyngeal nerve injection, with needle seen within the white circle. **A.** Needle placement. **B.** Injection of contrast.

Image courtesy of Christ DeClerck, MD; General Hospital Sint-Jan, Bruges, Belgium, with permission.

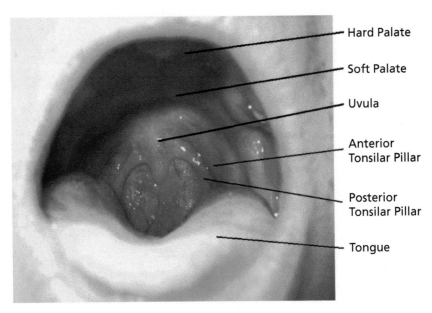

FIGURE 31.11. Anatomy for intraoral glossopharyngeal nerve injection.

Image courtesy of George C. Chang Chien D.O.

Cryoneuroablation

Cryoneuroablation at the styloid process is not recommended because of the proximity of the carotid artery (and the potential for puncturing the carotid artery with a large-gauge introducer) and the lack of visualization of the target itself. In addition, the vagus and spinal accessory nerve pass through this area, and it would be difficult to avoid lysis of these nerves.

As a result, the usual site for cryoneuroablation is at the tonsillar fossa. The patient is placed

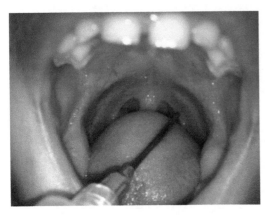

FIGURE 31.12. Tonsillar glossopharyngeal nerve intraoral injection (anterior tonsillar pillar method).

Image courtesy of Agnes Stogicza, MD.

supine and the tongue retracted medially. The nerve is located at the inferior portion of the ATP. The mucosa is anesthetized with a topical spray or pledget, and 1 mL of saline with epinephrine is infiltrated for hemostasis, looking as well for intravascular response to the epinephrine. The 12 gauge introducer is then advanced subcutaneously, and the 2 mm probe is advanced through the catheter. The newer 20 gauge cryo probes may be used with a smaller introducer to lower procedural risks. Sensory stimulation should refer to the ear and throat, and there may be a throat motor stimulation. Care must be used to avoid the palatine artery. This may be done most easily at surgical tonsillectomy, when the nerve is exposed and can be lesioned under direct vision.

Pulsed Radiofrequency Lesioning

Pulsed radiofrequency (PRF) lesioning can be performed either at the styloid level or at the tonsillar fossa. The needle approach is the same as described for the peristyloid fluoroscopy technique, but, before lesioning, the target nerve must be identified by nerve stimulation and must refer sensation to the ear or throat. PRF ablation is then performed at 42°C for up to 10 minutes. Mollinedo et al.[32] described the use of PRF to treat a patient with bilateral GPN.

Phenol

Funasaka and Kodera[33] in 1977 described the injection of 5% phenol in glycerin into the tonsillar pillar for pain relief from GPN.

Potential Complications and Side Effects

Potential undesirable side effects of GNB may include the following:

- Dysphagia secondary to weakness of the stylopharyngeus muscle
- Upper airway obstruction or loss of protective reflexes secondary to bilateral nerve block
- Ecchymosis/hematoma—trauma to the internal carotid artery, the internal jugular vein, or both
- Infection
- Trauma to the nerve
- Toxicity due intravascular injection of local anesthetic
- Tachycardia from vagus nerve block
- Hoarseness or dysphonia secondary to vagus nerve block, and paralysis of the ipsilateral vocal cord
- Post-procedure dysesthesias or anesthesia dolorosa
- Cardiovascular complications resulting in acute-onset hypotension with right bundle branch block secondary to dissection of the uppermost rootlets of the vagus nerve
- Block of the hypoglossal nerve with resultant tongue weakness (CN XII)
- Trapezius muscle weakness secondary to inadvertent block of the spinal accessory nerve (CN XI)

GUIDING QUESTIONS

- Can you describe the pathophysiology of glossopharyngeal neuralgia?
- How do you diagnose glossopharyngeal neuralgia?
- How do you manage glossopharyngeal neuralgia?
- What are treatment options for glossopharyngeal neuralgia?

KEY POINTS

- Glossopharyngeal neuralgia (GPN) is characterized by unilateral paroxysmal pain in the oropharynx, nasopharynx, larynx, base of the tongue, tonsillar region, and lower jaw. Pain can also radiate to the ipsilateral ear. These attacks are excruciatingly painful and typically described as sharp, stabbing, "shocks of electricity" that can last from seconds to minutes.
- GPN attacks are triggered by stimulation to the oropharynx, such as swallowing, yawning, coughing, laughing, and chewing, and sensory stimulation such as cold, salty, acidic, or bitter foods.
- The incidence of GPN increases with age and most often affects persons older than 50; however, in patients with multiple sclerosis, GPN tends to occur at a younger age.
- Physical exam yields minimal information; history and clinical symptoms aid more in suggesting the diagnosis.
- Medical treatment of GPN is similar to treatment for other forms of neuropathic pain, including trigeminal neuralgia.
- Techniques for cervical, extraoral, intraoral, fluoroscopic, or ultrasound-assisted glossopharyngeal nerve block have been described.

SUGGESTED READING

Ferrante L, Artico M, Nardacci B, Fraioli B, Consentino F, Fortuna A. Glossopharyngeal neuralgia with cardiac syncope. *Neurosurgery.* 1995;36: 58–63.

Katusic S, Williams DB, Beard CM, Bergstralh E, Kurland LT. Incidence and clinical features of glossopharyngeal neuralgia, Rochester, Minnesota, 1945–1984. *Neuroepidemiology.* 1991;10:266–275.

Reddy GD, Viswanathan A. Trigeminal and glossopharyngeal neuralgia. *Neurol Clin.* 2014;32:539–552.

Rushton JG, Stevens JC, Miller RH. Glossopharyngeal (vagoglossopharyngeal) neuralgia: a study of 217 cases. *Arch Neurol.* 1981;38:201–205.

Singh PM, Kaur M, Trikha A. An uncommonly common: glossopharyngeal neuralgia. *Ann Indian Acad Neurol.* 2013;16(1):1–8.

Soh KB. The glossopharyngeal nerve, glossopharyngeal neuralgia and the Eagle's syndrome—current concepts and management. *Singapore Med J.* 1999;40:659–665.

REFERENCES

1. Weisenburg TH. Cerebello-pontine tumor diagnosis for six years as tic douloureux: the symptoms of irritation of the ninth and twelfth cranial nerves. *JAMA.* 1910;54:1600–1604.
2. Harris WR. *Neuritis and Neuralgia.* Oxford, UK: Oxford University Press; 1926.

3. Katusic S, Williams DB, Beard CM, Bergstralh EJ, Kurland LT. Epidemiology and clinical features of idiopathic trigeminal neuralgia and glossopharyngeal neuralgia: similarities and differences, Rochester, Minnesota, 1945–1984. *Neuroepidemiology.* 1991;10(5–6):276–281.

4. Eagle WW. Symptomatic elongated styloid process: report of two cases of styloid process—carotid artery syndrome with operation. *Arch Otolaryngol.* 1949;49:490–503.

5. Bohm E, Strang RR. Glossopharyngeal neuralgia. *Brain.* 1962;85:371–388.

6. Rushton JG, Stevens JC, Miller RH. Glossopharyngeal (vagoglossopharyngeal) neuralgia: a study of 217 cases. *Arch Neurol.* 1981;38(4):201–205.

7. Chen J, Sindou M. Vago-glossopharyngeal neuralgia: a literature review of neurosurgical experience. *Acta Neurochir (Wien).* 2015;157(2):311–321; discussion 321.

8. Ferrante L, Artico M, Nardacci B, Fraioli B, Cosentino F, Fortuna A. Glossopharyngeal neuralgia with cardiac syncope. *Neurosurgery.* 1995;36(1):58–63; discussion 63.

9. Carrieri PB, Montella S, Petracca M. Glossopharyngeal neuralgia as onset of multiple sclerosis. *Clin J Pain.* 2009;25(8):737–739.

10. Bruyn GW. Glossopharyngeal neuralgia. *Cephalalgia.* 1983;3(3):143–157.

11. Singh PM, Kaur M, Trikha A. An uncommonly common: glossopharyngeal neuralgia. *Ann Indian Acad Neurol.* 2013;16(1):1–8.

12. Manzoni GC, Torelli P. Epidemiology of typical and atypical craniofacial neuralgias. *Neurol Sci.* 2005;26(2):s65–s67.

13. Park HP, Hwang JW, Park SH, Jeon YT, Bahk JH, Oh YS. The effects of glossopharyngeal nerve block on postoperative pain relief after tonsillectomy: the importance of the extent of obtunded gag reflex as a clinical indicator. *Anesth Analg.* 2007;105(1):267–271.

14. Ong CK, Chong VF. The glossopharyngeal, vagus and spinal accessory nerves. *Eur J Radiol.* 2010;74(2):359–367.

15. Kawashima M, Matsushima T, Inoue T, Mineta T, Masuoka J, Hirakawa N. Microvascular decompression for glossopharyngeal neuralgia through the transcondylar fossa (supracondylar transjugular tubercle) approach. *Neurosurgery.* 2010;66(6 Suppl Operative):275–280; discussion 280.

16. Soh KB. The glossopharyngeal nerve, glossopharyngeal neuralgia and the Eagle's syndrome—current concepts and management. *Singapore Med J.* 1999;40(10):659–665.

17. Harris WR. *The Facial Neuralgias.* Oxford, UK: Oxford University Press; 1937.

18. Hiwatashi A, Matsushima T, Yoshiura T, et al. MRI of glossopharyngeal neuralgia caused by neurovascular compression. *Am J Roentgenol.* 2008;191(2):578–581.

19. Kent DT, Rath TJ, Snyderman C. Conventional and 3-dimensional computerized tomography in Eagle's syndrome, glossopharyngeal neuralgia, and asymptomatic controls. *Otolaryngol Head Neck Surg.* 2015;153(1):41–47.

20. Gaul C, Hastreiter P, Duncker A, Naraghi R. Diagnosis and neurosurgical treatment of glossopharyngeal neuralgia: clinical findings and 3-D visualization of neurovascular compression in 19 consecutive patients. *J Headache Pain.* 2011;12(5):527–534.

21. Hasegawa S, Morioka M, Kai Y, Kuratsu J. Usefulness of balloon test occlusion in the diagnosis of glossopharyngeal neuralgia. Case report. *Neurol Med Chir (Tokyo).* 2008;48(4):163–166.

22. Kouzaki Y, Takita T, Tawara S, Otsuka T, Hirano T, Uchino M. [Opioid effectiveness for neuropathic pain in a patient with glossopharyngeal neuralgia]. *Rinsho shinkeigaku.* 2009;49(6):364–369.

23. Shin JH, Herrera SR, Eboli P, Aydin S, Eskandar EH, Slavin KV. Entrapment of the glossopharyngeal nerve in patients with Eagle syndrome: surgical technique and outcomes in a series of 5 patients. *J Neurosurg.* 2009;111(6):1226–1230.

24. Resnick DK, Jannetta PJ, Bissonnette D, Jho HD, Lanzino G. Microvascular decompression for glossopharyngeal neuralgia. *Neurosurgery.* 1995;36(1):64–68; discussion 68–69.

25. Sampson JH, Grossi PM, Asaoka K, Fukushima T. Microvascular decompression for glossopharyngeal neuralgia: long-term effectiveness and complication avoidance. *Neurosurgery.* 2004;54(4):884–889; discussion 889–890.

26. Dach F, Eckeli AL, Ferreira Kdos S, Speciali JG. Nerve block for the treatment of headaches and cranial neuralgias—a practical approach. *Headache.* 2015;55 Suppl 1:59–71.

27. Gallacher BP, Martin L. Treatment of refractory hiccups with glossopharyngeal nerve block. *Anesth Analg.* 1997;84(1):229.

28. Babacan A, Ozturk E, Kaya K. Relief of chronic refractory hiccups with glossopharyngeal nerve block. *Anesth Analg.* 1998;87(4):980.

29. Yue WL, Zhang Y. Peripheral glycerol injection: an alternative treatment of children with glossopharyngeal neuralgia. *Int J Pediatr Otorhinolaryngol.* 2014;78(3):558–560.

30. Bedder MD, Lindsay D. Glossopharyngeal nerve block using ultrasound guidance: a case report of a new technique. *Reg Anesth*. 1989;14(6): 304–307.

31. Gervasio A, D'Orta G, Mujahed I, Biasio A. Sonographic anatomy of the neck: The suprahyoid region. *J Ultrasound*. 2011;14(3):130–135.

32. Mollinedo FT, Esteban SL, Vega CG, Orcasitas AC, Maguregi AA. Pulsed radiofrequency treatment in a case of Eagle's syndrome. *Pain Pract*. 2013;13(5):399–404.

33. Funasaka S, Kodera K. Intraoral nerve block for glossopharyngeal neuralgia. *Arch Otorhinolaryngol*. 1977;215(3–4):311–315.

32

Persistent Idiopathic Facial Pain

TREVOR VAN OOSTROM

CASE

A 65-year-old woman presents with left-sided facial pain she has had for 2 years. The pain is located in the left mandible and cheek and is present for most of the day. She describes the pain as a deep, pulling sensation and her current pain intensity is 6 on a 10-point scale. The pain started 2 years ago following a tooth extraction and has been persistent. Her dentist has excluded other dental problems as the cause of her pain. Her past medical history reveals fibromyalgia and depression. On examination, there are no neurological findings or sensory changes in the painful area. Given the severity and chronicity of her pain, an MRI is ordered, which is normal. She was already taking over-the-counter pain medications such as acetaminophen and ibuprofen with little effect. She is started on oral amitriptyline 10 mg HS and gabapentin, which is titrated up to 300 mg TID. Her pain decreases slightly but is still bothersome. A sphenopalatine ganglion block with lidocaine and dexamethasone is performed, which does not help her pain. She is referred to a psychologist for evaluation of her depression and for cognitive-behavioral therapy to help control her pain.

DEFINITION

In the late 1800s, most of the focus in addressing facial pain was on the trigeminal nerve, and sectioning of the nerve for treatment of facial pain was commonly performed by neurosurgeons at that time. The modern term, *persistent idiopathic facial pain* (PIFP), can be traced back to two pioneering neurosurgeons, Frazier and Russell, who recognized a distinct group of patients from those with typical trigeminal neuralgia.[1] Rather than the sudden paroxysmal pain, "tic douloureux," these patients had a continuous deep, pressure-like pain that did not follow the distribution of the trigeminal nerve. They found

that surgery may worsen their pain and that the pain may spread to districts outside of trigeminal nerve innervation or even across to the other side of the face. Because of the peculiar nature of the pain they called the ailment "atypical neuralgia." The more modern term is *atypical facial pain*. It has also been called psychogenic facial pain given the lack of physical findings and frequent association with psychiatric comorbidities.

In 2004, the term *atypical* was dropped by the International Classification of Headache Disorders (ICHD) and the condition was renamed *persistent idiopathic facial pain* (PIFP). The new name is a welcome change and more informative as the term *idiopathic* implies something unknown rather than just different from the typical neuralgias.[2] Furthermore, the term *atypical* implies that the frequency of occurrence is very low, which, as we will see later in this chapter, is not correct. The most recent criteria for PIFP are listed in Table 32.1 as presented by the ICHD 3rd edition (beta).[3]

PATHOPHYSIOLOGY

The underlying pathophysiology of PIFP is largely unknown. Given that the topographic location of the pain may not necessarily follow the distribution of the trigeminal nerve and that the clinical neurological examination is normal, it is less likely related to disorders of the peripheral nervous system. However, some studies have found quantitative sensory testing changes in a portion of patients with PIFP consistent with a subclinical trigeminal neuropathy.[4,5] Other studies examining quantitative sensory functions and somatotopy of the primary somatosensory cortex have found no changes.[6] In fact, the ICHD-3 (beta) recognizes that a continuum may exist between PIFP induced by minor trauma and painful post-traumatic trigeminal neuropathy induced by major damage to the trigeminal

TABLE 32.1. INTERNATIONAL
CLASSIFICATION OF HEADACHE
DISORDERS (ICHD) 3RD ED. (BETA)
DIAGNOSTIC CRITERIA FOR PERSISTENT
IDIOPATHIC FACIAL PAIN (PIFP)[3]

A. Facial and/or oral pain fulfilling criteria B and C

B. Recurring daily for >2 hours per day for >3 months

C. Pain has both of the following characteristics:

    1. Poorly localized, and not following the distribution of a peripheral nerve

    2. Dull, aching, or nagging quality

D. Clinical neurological examination is normal

E. A dental cause has been excluded by appropriate investigations

F. Not better accounted for by another ICHD-3 diagnosis

nerve.[3] Thus, in some patients with PIFP, there may be involvement of peripheral sensitization.[7,8]

In many patients with PIFP, a deficient habituation of the blink reflex is seen, which suggests an increase in neuronal excitability at the brainstem or disturbance of inhibitory functions.[9,10] This has been confirmed by altered positron emission tomography (PET) scanning of cerebral blood flow[11] and dopamine receptor binding in the basal ganglia and striatal dopaminergic system.[12,13] These findings confirm the theory that central sensitization plays a role in the pathophysiology of PIFP.[7,8]

The trigger for these pathophysiological changes remains to be determined. Direct injury to the trigeminal sensory system or basal ganglia,[5,13] brain atrophy with aging and loss of inhibitory gray matter,[14] and autoimmune-mediated neural injury[15] have all been proposed triggers.

EPIDEMIOLOGY

Although trigeminal neuralgia is the most frequent type of facial pain presenting to general practitioners and tertiary care centers, PIFP is the next most common facial pain, at an incidence of around 4 per 100,000 person-years.[16,17] There is a threefold increase in incidence in women compared to that in men, and the overall incidence rises steadily with age. PIFP generally does not occur in children.

Since the pain is in the topographic area of the teeth and sinuses, many patients initially present to the dentist or otolaryngologist with this condition.[18,19] It is not uncommon for patients to describe in their history that they underwent a dental extraction or some other intervention prior to the development of pain. Others undergo these procedures because of the pain. Indeed, the ICHD diagnostic criteria recognizes that atypical odontalgia, defined as persistent pain after tooth extraction, may be a subform of PIFP.[3]

PIFP is highly associated with other unexplained syndromes, such as fibromyalgia, irritable bowel syndrome, and chronic fatigue. Moreover, patients with PIFP often have comorbid psychological factors such as high stress levels, anxiety, depression, sleep disturbance, somatization, and catastrophization.[20]

CLINICAL FEATURES AND DIAGNOSIS

Chronic facial pain remains a diagnostic challenge and patients may present with multiple overlapping symptoms and a confusing history. Given the diverse nature of symptoms and uncertainty of diagnosis in many patients with orofacial pain, some authors have called for the expansion of the ICHD classification system to include more orofacial syndromes or even a combination classification systems to include more diagnoses.[21,22] In surveys of orofacial pain clinics, up to a third of patients could not be classified in any category of orofacial pain using only ICHD criteria.[17] In addition, PIFP is not a very specific diagnosis and may be overly broad. Like many poorly understood pain conditions with broad diagnostic criteria, PIFP may represent various pain syndromes that have yet to be diagnosed. Some authors have called for further subtyping of the condition based on topographic location.[23] In the future, more concrete data and advanced studies such as functional imaging may help further categorize PIFP.

Given that the presentation of PIFP has considerable overlap with many other diseases, it is important to consider and rule out other causes of facial pain. Therefore, PIFP remains somewhat a diagnosis of exclusion. However, one of the main features of PIFP is the lack of findings on neurological exam. A detailed neurological exam is essential. Any motor or sensory changes should prompt a search for other causes of facial pain. Imaging such as an X-ray and MRI should also be considered. Although PIFP usually presents with unilateral facial pain, over time, the topographic location of PIFP may spread and the pain may become bilateral. Table 32.2 presents a list of differential diagnoses of unilateral facial pain without an immediate identifiable cause that should be considered when one is presented with a patient with suspected PIFP.[24-27] However, there are also many rare cases in the literature where patients have presented initially with PIFP, only later to discover that the pain was a harbinger of a bony cancer,[28] intracranial tumor,[29] lung cancer,[30,31] aneurysm,[32] ischemic cardiac disease,[33] or even sarcoidosis.[34] Thus, although it is extremely rare, it is important to at least consider a search for more rare causes of facial pain should there be a change in presentation in a patient with previously diagnosed PIFP.

TREATMENT

There are only a few poorly controlled studies that examine the use of medications in the treatment of PIFP. The strongest evidence is in the tricyclic antidepressant (TCA) class of medications, such as amitriptyline and nortriptyline.[35] Anticonvulsant medications such as gabapentin, Lyrica, carbamazepine, and topiramate have been reported to improve pain in PIFP.[36] Serotonin-norepinephrine reuptake inhibitors (SNRIs) such as duloxetine have also been shown to be effective.[37,38] Analgesics such as Tylenol and NSAIDs and topical agents may also be tried. Opioids should generally be avoided given that they carry significant risks with long-term use. There are no FDA-approved medications specifically to treat PIFP.

In refractory cases, sphenopalatine ganglion injections have occasionally been shown to be effective.[39-41] In those that respond to injections, a trial of pulsed radiofrequency stimulation may be performed for longer-lasting relief.[42] There are case reports of neuromodulation techniques being effective, such as peripheral nerve field stimulation,[43,44] sphenopalatine ganglion stimulation,[43,45,46] and spinal cord stimulation.[47] However, there is insufficient evidence at this time to recommend neuromodulation as an approach, as these treatments are costly and not without risk. At least one study has shown that deep brain stimulation is not effective for the treatment of PIFP.[48]

There is some evidence to suggest that psychological techniques such as counseling, hypnosis, and cognitive-behavioral therapy are effective in the treatment of PIFP.[49,50] Psychological referral should be considered in the treatment of PIFP, especially if there is coexisting depression and anxiety.

GUIDING QUESTIONS

- List the diagnostic criteria for persistent idiopathic facial pain (PIFP) according to the International Classification of Headache Disorders, 3rd edition (beta).
- What are the proposed pathophysiological mechanisms of PIFP?
- What other conditions are associated with PIFP?
- List the differential diagnosis for unilateral facial pain.
- What are the treatment options for PIFP?

KEY POINTS

- Persistent idiopathic facial pain (PIFP) is a poorly localized, dull, aching facial pain that recurs daily for more than 2 hours and has persisted for more than 3 months.
- There are no sensory changes on physical exam.
- Peripheral sensitization and central sensitization have been proposed as pathophysiological mechanisms in PIFP.
- PIFP is commonly associated with other unexplained syndromes, such as fibromyalgia, irritable bowel syndrome, and chronic fatigue. Comorbid psychological problems such as stress, anxiety, depression, and sleep disturbances are also common.
- PIFP is a diagnosis of exclusion and appropriate tests (e.g., imaging, blood work) should be performed.
- Consider dental, neurological, vascular, and other rare disorders in the differential diagnosis of PIFP.
- A number of medications have been used to treat PIFP, all of which have been shown to be unreliable in effectiveness. TCAs, anticonvulsants, and SNRIs are all appropriate medications to trial in the treatment of patients with PIFP.
- Consider interventional procedures such as sphenopalatine ganglion injection and pulsed radiofrequency in refractory cases. There is insufficient evidence at this time to support sphenopalatine ganglion, dorsal column, or deep brain stimulation.
- Psychological referral is often appropriate for counseling, treatment of comorbid psychological conditions, and cognitive-behavioral therapy.

TABLE 32.2. DIFFERENTIAL DIAGNOSIS OF UNILATERAL OROFACIAL PAIN WITH NO IMMEDIATELY IDENTIFIABLE CAUSE

Condition	Prevalence	Location	Timing	Character	Provoking Factors	Associated Factors
Dental						
Cracked tooth	Common	Localized to tooth	Seconds	Sharp	Biting	Rebound pain
Pulpitis or periodontitis	Common	Poorly localized intraoral	Hours	Throbbing	Cold, heat	Carries
Osteomyelitis	Rare	Mandible	Continuous	Throbbing, severe	Biting	Pyrexia, malaise, trismus, swelling
Temporomandibular joint (TMJ) disorders	Common	Jaw, mandible, preauricular	Minutes	Dull, stabbing	Biting, palpation	Trismus, clicking
Neurological						
Trigeminal neuralgia (TN)	Rare	Trigeminal area	Seconds to minutes	Sharp, shooting	Light touch	Trigger zones
Atypical TN	Rare	Trigeminal area	Continuous with attacks	Dull, sharp	Light touch	Trigger zones
Trigeminal neuropathy	Very rare	Trigeminal area	Continuous	Dull, sharp	Light touch	Sensory loss, swelling
Glossopharyngeal neuralgia	Very rare	Intraoral	Seconds to minutes	Sharp, burning	Swallowing	No deficits
Postherpetic neuralgia	Rare	Trigeminal area	Continuous	Sharp, tingling	Allodynia	Herpes zoster
Vascular						
Cluster headache	Rare	Orbital, supraorbital, temporal	Hours	Hot, searing, severe	Vasodilators	Autonomic symptoms
SUNCT*	Very rare	Ocular, periocular	Minutes	Burning, stabbing	Neck movement	Autonomic symptoms
Chronic paroxysmal hemicrania	Very rare	Eye, forehead	Minutes	Stabbing, throbbing, boring	Head movements	Responds to indomethacin

	Frequency	Location	Continuity	Quality	Triggers	Associated features
Giant cell arteritis	Rare	Temporal area	Continuous	Aching, throbbing	Chewing	Jaw claudication, diagnosis with biopsy
Carotidynia	Very rare	Face, ears, jaw, neck	Continuous	Throbbing	Compression of carotid	
Other						
Persistent idiopathic facial pain (PIFP)	Rare	Variable, moves	Continuous	Dull, pulling, throbbing	Stress, weather, movement	Depression, fibro-myalgia, anxiety
Atypical odontalgia	Rare	Intraoral, moves	Continuous	Dull, throbbing	Stress, hot, cold, pressure	Tooth extraction
Tolosa-Hunt syndrome	Very rare	Retro-orbital	Continuous	Aching, severe	—	Ophthalmoplegia, ptosis, sensory loss
Raeder paratrigeminal syndrome	Very rare	Fronto-temporal, maxilla	Continuous	Deep, severe, lancinating	—	Ptosis, miosis
Orofacial tumors	Very rare	Variable	Variable	Severe	Jaw movement	Neurological signs, white blood cell (WBC) abnormalities

*SUNCT, shorter-lasting, unilateral neuralgiform, conjunctival injection and tearing.

284   NEUROPATHIC PAIN OF THE HEAD AND NECK

REFERENCES

1. Frazier CH, Russell EC. Neuralgia of the face: an analysis of seven hundred and fifty-four cases with relation to pain and other sensory phenomena before and after operation. *Arch Neurol Psychiatr.* 1924;11:557–563.
2. Bussone G, Tullo V. Reflections on the nosology of cranio-facial pain syndromes. *Neurol Sci.* 2005;26:S61–S64.
3. Headache Classification Committee of the International Headache Society. The International Classification of Headache Disorders, 3rd edition (beta version). *Cephalalgia.* 2013;33:629–808.
4. List T, Leijon G, Svensson P. Somatosensory abnormalities in atypical odontalgia: a case-control study. *Pain.* 2009;139:333–341.
5. Forsell H, Tenovuo O, Silvoniemi P, Jaaskelainen SK. Differences and similarities between atypical facial pain and trigeminal neuropathic pain. *Neurology.* 2007;69:1451–1459.
6. Lang E, Kaltenhauser M, Seidler S, Mattenklodt P, Neundorfer B. Persistent idiopathic facial pain exists independent of somatosensory input from the painful region: findings from quantitative sensory functions and somatotopy of the primary somatosensory cortex. *Pain.* 2005;118:80–91.
7. Sessle BJ. Mechanisms of oral somatosensory and motor functions and their clinical correlates. *J Oral Rehab.* 2006;33:243–261.
8. Forssell H, Jaaskelainen S. List T, Svensson P, Baad-Hansen L. An update on pathophysiological mechanisms related to idiopathic oro-facial pain conditions with implications for management. *J Oral Rehab.* 2015;42:300–322.
9. Jaaskelainen SK, Forssell H, Tenovuo O. Electrophysiological testing of the trigeminofacial system: aid in the diagnosis of atypical facial pain. *Pain.* 1999;80:191–200.
10. Leonard G, Goffaux P, Mathieu D, Blanchard J, Kenny B, Marchand S. Evidence of descending inhibition deficits in atypical but not classical trigeminal neuralgia. *Pain.* 2009;147:217–223.
11. Derbyshire SWG, Jones AKP, Devani P, et al. Cerebral responses to pain in patients with atypical facial pain measured by positron emission tomography. *J Neurol Neurosurg Psychiatry.* 1994;57:1166–1172.
12. Hagelberg N, Forssell H, Aalto S, et al. Altered dopamine D2 receptor binding in atypical facial pain. *Pain.* 2003;106:43–48.
13. Dieb W, Ouachikh O, Durif F, Hafidi A. Lesion of the dopaminergic nigrostriatal pathway induces trigeminal dynamic mechanical allodynia. *Brain Behav.* 2014;4:368–380.
14. Schmidt-Wilcke T, Hierlmeier S, Leinisch E. Altered regional brain morphology in patients with chronic facial pain. *Headache.* 2010;50:1278–1285.
15. Schleifer SJ, Marbach J, Keller SE. Psychoneuroimmunology: potential relevance to chronic orofacial pain. *Anesth Prog.* 1990;34:93–98.
16. Koopman JS, Dieleman JP, Huygen FJ, de Mos M, Martin CG, Sturkenboom MC. Incidence of facial pain in the general population. *Pain.* 2009;147:122–127.
17. Zebenholzer K, Wober C, Vigl M, Wessely P, Wober-Bingol C. Facial pain in a neurological tertiary care centre—evaluation of the International Classification of Headache Disorders. *Cephalalgia.* 2005;25:689–699.
18. Wirz S, Ellerkmann RK, Buecheler M, Putensen C, Nadstawek J, Wartenberg HC. Management of chronic orofacial pain: a survey of general dentists in German university hospitals. *Pain Med.* 2010;11:416–424.
19. Ullas G, McClelland L, Jones NS. Medically unexplained symptoms and somatisation in ENT. *J Laryngol Otol.* 2013;127:452–457.
20. Aggarwal VR, McBeth J, Zakrzewska JM, Lunt M, Macfarlane GJ. The epidemiology of chronic syndromes that are frequently unexplained: do they have common associated factors? *Int J Epidemiol.* 2006;35:468–476.
21. Benoliel R, Birman N, Eliav E, Sharav Y. The International Classification of Headache Disorders: accurate diagnosis of orofacial pain? *Cephalagia.* 2008;28:752–762.
22. Zebenholzer K, Wober C, Vigl M, Wessely P, Wober-Bingol C. Facial pain and the second edition of the International Classification of Headache Disorders. *Headache.* 2006;46:259–263.
23. Pareja JA, Cuadrado ML, Porta-Etessam J, et al. Idiopathic opthalmodynia and idiopathic rhinalgia: two topographic facial pain syndromes. *Headache.* 2010;50:1286–1295.
24. Agostoni E, Frigerio R, Santoro P. Atypical facial pain: clinical considerations and differential diagnosis. *Neurol Sci.* 2005;26:S71–S74.
25. Zakrzewska JM. Diagnosis and differential diagnosis of trigeminal neuralgia. *Clin J Pain.* 2002;18:14–21.
26. Zakrzewska JM. Multi-dimensionality of chronic pain of the oral cavity and face. *J Headache Pain.* 2013;14:37–46.
27. Ailani J. A practical approach to autonomic dysfunction in patients with headache. *Curr Neurol Neurosci Rep.* 2016;16:41–46.
28. Friedrich RE. Long-term follow-up control of pedunculated orbital floor osteoma becoming symptomatic by atypical facial pain. *In Vivo.* 2009;23:117–122.

29. Moazzam AA, Habibian M. Patients appearing to dental professionals with orofacial pain arising from intracranial tumors: a literature review. *Oral Med.* 2012;114:749–755.

30. Ruffatti S, Zanchin G, Maggioni F. A case of intractable facial pain secondary to metastatic lung cancer. *Neurol Sci.* 2008;29:117–119.

31. Pembroke CA, Byrne A, Lester JF, Button M. Persistent unilateral facial pain in lung cancer patients with mediastinal nodal involvement. *Lung Cancer.* 2013;82:173–175.

32. Stone SJ, Paleri V, Staines KS. Internal carotid artery aneurysm presenting as orofacial pain. *J Laryngol Otol.* 2012;126:851–853.

33. Lopez-Lopez J, Garcia-Vicente L, Jane-Salas E, Estrugo-Devesa A, Chimenos-Kustner E, Roca-Elias J. Orofacial pain of cardiac origin: review literature and clinical cases. *Med Oral Patol Oral Cir Bucal.* 2012;17:e538–e544.

34. Smith L, Osborne RF. Facial sarcoidosis presenting as atypical facial pain. *Ear Nose Throat J.* 2006;85:574,578.

35. Brown RS, Bottomley WK. The utilization and mechanism of action of tricyclic antidepressants in the treatment of chronic facial pain: a review of the litterature. *Anesth Prog.* 1990;36:223–229.

36. Volcy M, Rapoport AM, Tepper SJ, Sheftell FD, Bigal ME. Persistent idiopathic facial pain responsive to topiramate. *Cephalalgia.* 2006;26:489–491.

37. Ito M, Kimura H, Yoshida K, Kumura Y, Ozaki N, Kurita K. Effectiveness of milnacipran for the treatment of chronic pain in the orofacial region. *Clin Neuropharm.* 2010;33:79–83.

38. Nagashima W, Kimura H, Ito M, et al. Effectiveness of duloxetine for the treatment of chronic nonorganic orofacial pain. *Clin Neuropharm.* 2012;35:275–277.

39. Voenkamp KE. Inteventional procedures for facial pain. *Curr Pain Headache Rep.* 2013;17:308–314.

40. Cornelissen P, van Kleef M, Mekhail N, Day M, van Zundert J. Evidence-based pain medicine according to clinical diagnosis: persistent idiopathic facial pain. *Pain Pract.* 2009;9:443–448.

41. Piagkou M, Demesticha T, Troupis T, et al. The pterygopalatine ganglion and its role in various pain syndromes: from anatomy to clinical practice. *Pain Pract.* 2012;12:399–412.

42. Bayer E, Racz G, Miles D, Heavner J. Sphenopalatine ganglion pulsed radiofrequency treatment in 30 patients suffering form chronic face and head pain. *Pain Pract.* 2005;5:223–227.

43. Maniam R, Kaye AD, Vadivelu N, Urman RD. Facial pain update: advances in neurostimulation for the treatment of facial pain. *Curr Pain Headache Rep.* 2016;20:24–29.

44. Yakovlev AE, Resch BE. Treatment of chronic intractable atypical facial pain using peripheral subcutaneous field stimulation. *Neuromodulation.* 2010;13:137–140.

45. William A, Azad TD, Brecher E, et al. Trigeminal and sphenopalatine ganglion stimulation for intractable craniofacial pain—case series and literature review. *Acta Neurochir.* 2016;158:513–520.

46. Elahi F, Reddy CG. Sphenopalatine ganglion electrical nerve stimulation implant for intractable facial pain. *Pain Phys.* 2015;18:E403–E409.

47. Neuman SA, Eldrige JS, Hoelzer BC. Atypical facial pain treated with upper thoracic dorsal column stimulation. *Clin J Pain.* 2011;27:556–558.

48. Broggi G, Franzini A, Leone M, Bussone G. Update on neurosurgical treatment of chronic trigeminal autonomic cephalalgias and atypical facial pain with deep brain stimulation of posterior hypothalamus: results and comments. *Neurol Sci.* 2007;28:S138–S145.

49. Nguyen CT, Wang MB. Complementary and integrative treatments: atypical facial pain. *Otolaryngol Clin N Am.* 2013;46:367–382.

50. Abrahamsen R, Baad-Hansen L, Svensson P. Hypnosis in the management of persistent idiopathic orofacial pain—clinical and psychosocial findings. *Pain.* 2008;136:44–52.

33

Occipital Neuralgia

ARMIN DEROEE AND JIANGUO CHENG

CASE

A 58-year-old woman presents with left-sided headache located in the occipital area. She describes the pain as severe with a pulsating or occasionally burning character originating from the left neck, radiating to the left occipital scalp. The pain is intermittent and can occur up to four times a day, lasting from minutes to hours. Episodes of severe pain are generally spontaneous but are sometimes evoked by touching the back of her head, moving her neck, or when she places her head on a pillow. She continues to work full-time. There is no evidence of depression or anxiety, but she feels that the headache is negatively impacting her function and quality of life. Her sleep is mildly affected because of exacerbations in the headaches; she sleeps on her right side. On physical examination, pain is evoked with deep palpation lateral to the occipital condyle on the superior nuchal line. A diagnosis of occipital neuralgia is made after left occipital nerve block, which achieved total pain relief for about 2 weeks.

DEFINITION

Occipital neuralgia (ON) is defined by the International Headache Society (IHS) as "unilateral or bilateral paroxysmal, shooting or stabbing pain in the posterior part of the scalp, in the distribution of the greater, lesser, or third occipital nerves, sometimes accompanied by diminished sensation or dysaesthesia in the affected area and commonly associated with tenderness over the involved nerve(s)."[1] As a primary headache disorder, it is a challenging diagnosis.

There is evident overlap between ON and migraine. Pain in migraine headache by definition is typically severe throbbing or pulsating pain that is often accompanied by episodes of stabbing pain.[2] Allodynia and occipital tenderness are also common in patients with migraine headache.

Furthermore, the response of migraine to occipital nerve blocks is well described.[3-5] Thus, it is important to differentiate ON from other types of headaches, as reflected in the diagnostic criteria. A careful history and physical exam are critical components to accurately identifying ON and distinguishing it from other headache disorders with similar presentations.

PATHOPHYSIOLOGY

Three pairs of nerves can be involved in the pathogenesis of occipital neuralgia. The first is the greater occipital nerve (GON), which is a pure sensory nerve originating from the medial branch of the dorsal ramus of the C2 spinal nerve (Figure 33.1). The GON provides cutaneous sensory innervation to the posterior scalp from the external occipital protuberance to the vertex. It ascends between the inferior oblique capitis muscle and semispinalis capitis and pierces the semispinalis. It then runs rostrolateral deep to the trapezius muscle and pierces the aponeurosis of the trapezius slightly inferior to the superior nuchal ridge, where it becomes subcutaneous and lies medial to the occipital artery.[6] The second is the lesser occipital nerve (LON), which is the lateral branch of dorsal ramus of the C2 spinal nerve. It occasionally originates from the C3 spinal nerve. It is part of the cervical plexus and travels along the posterior border of the sternocleidomastoid muscle and innervates the lateral scalp superior and posterior to the auricle.[7] Finally, the third occipital nerve (TON) is the superficial medial branch of dorsal ramus of the C3 spinal nerve and innervates the C2–C3 zygapophyseal joint as well as the skin in the suboccipital region.

The exact pathophysiology of ON is largely unknown. Most presentations are considered idiopathic. The current belief is that ON occurs because of chronic entrapment or irritation of the GON, LON, or TON. The cause can be

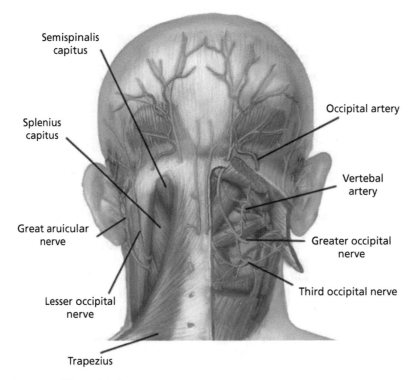

Semispinalis
capitus

Splenius
capitus

Great aruicular
nerve

Lesser occipital
nerve

Trapezius

Occipital artery

Vertebal
artery

Greater occipital
nerve

Third occipital nerve

FIGURE 33.1. Anatomy of the occipital nerves.

vascular (e.g., arteriovenous malformations, arterial compression), neurogenic (Schwannoma, myelitis), or osteogenic (cervical spine spondylosis, fractures, or neoplasms). For example, posterior head trauma and whiplash injuries may result in nerve injury.[8] Myofascial spasm or scarring may cause entrapment or irritation at various locations along the nerve's path, including where the GON branches from C2 between the axis and atlas, between the inferior oblique and semispinalis, as it pierces the belly of the semispinalis, and as it pierces the aponeurosis of the trapezius.[9] Sonography of the GON in a small sample study showed evidence of greater cross-sectional area as it runs between the inferior oblique capitis and semispinalis capitis on the symptomatic as compared to asymptomatic side in individuals with unilateral ON.[10] Case reports have indicated a number of potential structural lesions that cause ON, including a posterior inferior cerebellar artery impinging the dorsal upper cervical roots, dural arteriovenous fistulas, cervical cord cavernous angiomas, neurosyphillis, multiple sclerosis, and myelitis.[11] There are also reported cases of ON after posterior fossa or posterior surgeries in the neck. Neuroimaging, including magnetic resonance imaging (MRI), of the brain and cervical spine can be informative of structural or infiltrative lesions.

EPIDEMIOLOGY

The incidence of ON remains to be determined. A study in the Dutch general population reported a relatively low incidence of 3.2 per 100,000.[12] It accounts for approximately 8% of patients with facial pain. It is more prevalent in the seventh decade of life with a slightly higher prevalence among females. In a sample of 23 cases, ON was more commonly unilateral (85%). Distribution of pain and paresthesia were consistent with GON involvement in 90%, LON in 10%, and both nerves in 9% of the cases.[13]

CLINICAL FEATURES AND DIAGNOSIS

Occipital neuralgia typically has a sudden onset of paroxysmal lancinating pain as its hallmark. It is described as shooting, stabbing, electrical, or shock-like pain in the neck that radiates over the cranium. The pain can be perceived in the retro-orbital area due to the convergence of the C2 dorsal root and the nucleus trigeminus pars caudalis. Given connections with the VIII, IX, and X cranial nerves and the cervical sympathicus, vision impairment or ocular pain, tinnitus, dizziness, and nausea can be present. Patients may describe allodynia or dysesthesia of the scalp in the distribution of the nerve, with sensitivity to touch or pressure on the scalp. Patients may avoid activities that trigger the onset of pain, such as brushing their hair, wearing a hat, or lying on a pillow. Tenderness to palpation along the course of the nerve is common. The International Headache Society has proposed diagnostic criteria for ON (Table 33.1).

Examination may reveal local tenderness and/or hypesthesia in the territory of the affected nerve. Percussion may elicit paresthesia along the distribution of the affected nerve (Tinel's sign). Hyperextension of the neck may reproduce the symptoms (pillow sign).

A careful evaluation of the upper cervical spine and posterior fossa is necessary for patients with suspected occipital neuralgia. For patients with newly diagnosed occipital neuralgia, MRI of the head and cervical spine is recommended to exclude structural or space-occupying lesions. Temporary improvement of these symptoms after treatment with anesthetic blockade of the

GON is diagnostic.[1] However, false positive is a concern as migraine and cluster headache also respond to GON block.[4] Therefore, the latter should be considered in differential diagnosis. In addition, hemicrania continua and tension-type headache should also be ruled out.

There are several other considerations in the differential diagnosis. Temporal arteritis involving the occipital artery may cause occipital headache and scalp tenderness.[14,15] C2 neuralgia due to compressive and inflammatory lesions of the C2 nerve root also presents with lancinating occipital pain. Compared with ON, C2 neuralgia is more likely to involve ipsilateral lacrimation and ciliary injection.[16] Postherpetic neuralgia involving the C2 nerve root or GON should be evaluated with careful inspection of the scalp.

Occipital neuralgia must also be distinguished from referred pain arising from the atlantoaxial, upper facet joints or from myofascial pain in neck muscles. Dull occipital ache as a primary complaint should prompt evaluation for causes of referred occipital pain (cervicogenic headache) from structures innervated by the first three upper cervical spinal nerves, such as the atlantoaxial joints, C2-3 intervertebral disc and zygopophyseal joint, the posterior fossa, and various upper posterior neck muscles.[16] Cervical medial branch blocks can help distinguish if neck pain originates in the upper cervical facet joints. Congenital anomalies such as Chiari malformation and space-occupying lesions also need to be ruled out.

TABLE 33.1. THE INTERNATIONAL HEADACHE SOCIETY DIAGNOSTIC CRITERIA FOR OCCIPITAL NEURALGIA

A. Unilateral or bilateral pain fulfilling criteria B–E

B. Pain is located in the distribution of the greater, lesser, and/or third occipital nerves

C. Pain has two of the following three characteristics:

   1. Recurring in paroxysmal attacks lasting from a few seconds to minutes

   2. Severe intensity

   3. Shooting, stabbing or sharp in quality

D. Pain is associated with both of the following:

   1. Dysesthesia and/or allodynia apparent during innocuous stimulation of the scalp and/or hair

   2. Either or both of the following:

      a. Tenderness over the affected nerve branches

      b. Trigger points at the emergence of the greater occipital nerve or in the area of distribution of C2

E. Pain is eased temporarily by local anesthetic block of the affected nerve

F. Not better accounted for by another ICHD-3 diagnosis.

TREATMENT

Conservative management includes application of local moist heat and posture correction. Carbamazepine, gabapentin, and tricyclic antidepressants all have shown benefit in management of ON. In addition, several interventional approaches may provide pain relief in refractory cases.

Anesthetic block of the GON and LON may confirm the diagnosis and provide temporary pain relief. A couple of studies have demonstrated the efficacy of occipital nerve block with a combination of local anesthetic and corticosteroid in alleviating ON for days to months.[14,17,18]

Injection with botulinum toxin type A was also effective in reducing pain in patients with ON. A reduction of pain on the visual analog scale, from 8 ± 1.8 to 2 ± 2.7, for a mean duration of 16.3 ± 3.2 weeks was reported in a case series.[19] In a prospective pilot study, six patients with

ON treated with botulinum toxin type A were followed for 12 weeks. Improvement in sharp, shooting pain and quality of life measures was observed, but no significant improvement in dull, aching pain or pins and needles–type pain, and no reduction in pain medication usage.[20]

Neuromodulation with pulsed radiofrequency (PRF) and subcutaneous nerve stimulation offer promising treatment options for patients with refractory ON. PRF exposes the nerve to a train of short-duration, high-voltage radiofrequency pulses, which may decrease pain by inducing a low-intensity electrical field around sensory nerves that inhibits long-term potentiation in nociceptive afferents.[21] In contrast to continuous radiofrequency lesioning, PRF is unlikely to cause post-procedure deafferentation pain.[22] A prospective analysis of 19 patients with ON treated with PRF revealed a significant decrease in pain intensity and a significant decrease in medication use. More than half the patients reported substantial improvement at 6-month follow-up.[23] In a retrospective analysis of 102 patients treated with PRF for ON, 51% reported ≥50% pain relief at 3-month follow-up.[24]

Occipital nerve stimulation with percutaneous leads was effective for medically refractory ON.[25] In a series of 13 cases, over 80% of the implanted patients reported good to excellent pain relief at a minimum of 1.5 years of follow-up. In a retrospective analysis of 14 patients who underwent 5- to 7-day trials for medically refractory ON, 10 patients reported a greater than 50% pain reduction and went on to receive a subcutaneous stimulator implant.[26] At a minimum follow-up of 5 months and a mean of 22 months, seven patients continued to have adequate pain relief and a decrease in medication intake. Similar results were reported in other studies.[26,27] Potential complications of occipital nerve stimulation include lead migration, infection, electrode fractures, and hardware erosion.[26]

Finally, surgical removal of the second (C2) or third (C3) cervical sensory dorsal root ganglion is an option to treat intractable ON.[28] Cervical ganglionectomy offers relief to a majority of patients immediately after the procedure, but the effect is short-lived.

GUIDING QUESTIONS
- What are the clinical characteristics of occipital neuralgia (ON)?
- What nerves are involved in ON pathogenesis?

- How do you differentiate ON from other causes of headaches?
- What are the conservative and interventional treatment modalities for ON?

KEY POINTS
- Occipital neuralgia (ON) is unilateral or bilateral paroxysmal, shooting or stabbing pain in the posterior part of the scalp, in the distribution of the greater, lesser, or third occipital nerves.
- Three nerves can be involved in the pathogenesis of ON: (1) the greater occipital nerve (GON), the medial branch of the dorsal ramus of the C2 spinal nerve; (2) the lesser occipital nerve (LON), the lateral branch of dorsal ramus of the C2; and (3) the third occipital nerve (TON), which originates from C3 spinal nerve. The pathogenesis of ON is believed to be entrapment of the occipital nerves.
- Local anesthetic injection is both diagnostic and therapeutic for ON.
- ON should be distinguished from referred pain arising from the atlantoaxial, upper facet joints or from trigger points in neck muscles. Congenital anomalies like Chiari malformation and space-occupying lesions need to be ruled out. In new cases of ON, MRI is recommended to rule out any space-occupying lesion.
- A number of conservative and interventional therapies are options for ON.

REFERENCES

1. The International Classification of Headache Disorders, 3rd edition (beta version). *Cephalalgia.* 2013;33:629–808. doi:10.1177/0333102413485658
2. Kelman L. Pain characteristics of the acute migraine attack. *Headache.* 2006;46:942–953. doi:10.1111/j.1526-4610.2006.00443.x
3. Afridi SK, Shields KG, Bhola R, Goadsby PJ. Greater occipital nerve injection in primary headache syndromes—prolonged effects from a single injection. *Pain.* 2006;122:126–129. doi:10.1016/j.pain.2006.01.016
4. Ashkenazi A, Young WB. The effects of greater occipital nerve block and trigger point injection on brush allodynia and pain in migraine. *Headache.* 2005;45:350–354. doi:10.1111/j.1526-4610.2005.05073.x

5. Caputi CA, Firetto V. Therapeutic blockade of greater occipital and supraorbital nerves in migraine patients. *Headache*. 1997;37:174–179.

6. Guvencer M, Akyer P, Sayhan S, Tetik S. The importance of the greater occipital nerve in the occipital and the suboccipital region for nerve blockade and surgical approaches—an anatomic study on cadavers. *Clin Neurol Neurosurg*. 2011;113:289–294. doi:10.1016/j.clineuro.2010.11.021

7. Lang J. *Clinical Anatomy of the Cervical Spine*. Stuttgart: Thieme Medical Publishers; 1993:127.

8. Magnusson T, Ragnarsson T, Bjornsson A. Occipital nerve release in patients with whiplash trauma and occipital neuralgia. *Headache*. 1996;36:32–36.

9. Loukas M, et al. Identification of greater occipital nerve landmarks for the treatment of occipital neuralgia. *Folia Morphol*. 2006;65:337–342.

10. Cho JC, Haun DW, Kettner NW. Sonographic evaluation of the greater occipital nerve in unilateral occipital neuralgia. *J Ultrasound Med*. 2012;31:37–42.

11. Dougherty C. Occipital neuralgia. *Curr Pain Headache Rep*. 2014;18:411. doi:10.1007/s11916-014-0411-x.

12. Koopman JS, et al. Incidence of facial pain in the general population. *Pain*. 2009;147:122–127. doi:10.1016/j.pain.2009.08.023.

13. Hammond SR, Danta G. Occipital neuralgia. *Clin. Exp Neurol*. 1978;15:258–270.

14. Pfadenhauer K, Weber H. Giant cell arteritis of the occipital arteries—a prospective color coded duplex sonography study in 78 patients. *J Neurol*. 2003;250:844–849. doi:10.1007/s00415-003-1104-2

15. Jundt JW, Mock D. Temporal arteritis with normal erythrocyte sedimentation rates presenting as occipital neuralgia. *Arthritis Rheum*. 1991;34:217–219.

16. Bogduk N. The neck and headaches. *Neurol Clin*. 2004;22:151–171, vii. doi:10.1016/s0733-8619(03)00100-2

17. Newman LC, Levin M. *Headache and Facial Pain*. New York: Oxford University Press; 2008:108–112.

18. Anthony M. Headache and the greater occipital nerve. *Clin Neurol Neurosurg*. 1992;94:297–301.

19. Kapural L, et al. Botulinum toxin occipital nerve block for the treatment of severe occipital neuralgia: a case series. *Pain Pract*. 2007;7:337–340. doi:10.1111/j.1533-2500.2007.00150.x

20. Taylor M, Silva S. Cottrell C. Botulinum toxin type-A (BOTOX) in the treatment of occipital neuralgia: a pilot study. *Headache*. 2008;48:1476–1481. doi:10.1111/j.1526-4610.2008.01089.x.

21. Chua NH, Vissers KC, Sluijter ME. Pulsed radiofrequency treatment in interventional pain management: mechanisms and potential indications—a review. *Acta Neurochirurg*. 2011;153:763–771. doi:10.1007/s00701-010-0881-5

22. Navani A, Mahajan G, Kreis P, Fishman SM. A case of pulsed radiofrequency lesioning for occipital neuralgia. *Pain Med*. 2006;7:453–456. doi:10.1111/j.1526-4637.2006.00217.x

23. Vanelderen P, et al. Pulsed radiofrequency for the treatment of occipital neuralgia: a prospective study with 6 months of follow-up. *Reg Anesth Pain Med*. 2010;35:148–151.

24. Huang JH, et al. Occipital nerve pulsed radiofrequency treatment: a multi-center study evaluating predictors of outcome. *Pain Med*. 2012;13:489–497. doi:10.1111/j.1526-4637.2012.01348.x

25. Weiner RL, Reed KL. Peripheral neurostimulation for control of intractable occipital neuralgia. *Neuromodulation*. 1999;2:217–221. doi:10.1046/j.1525-1403.1999.00217.x

26. Slavin KV, Nersesyan H, Wess C. Peripheral neurostimulation for treatment of intractable occipital neuralgia. *Neurosurgery*. 2006;58:112–119; discussion 112–119.

27. Melvin EA Jr, Jordan FR, Weiner RL, Primm D. Using peripheral stimulation to reduce the pain of C2-mediated occipital headaches: a preliminary report. *Pain Physician*. 2007;10:453–460.

28. Acar F, et al. Pain relief after cervical ganglionectomy (C2 and C3) for the treatment of medically intractable occipital neuralgia. *Stereotact Funct Neurosurg*. 2008;86:106–112, doi:10.1159/000113872

PART VII

Special Forms of Neuropathic Pain

34

Complex Regional Pain Syndrome

BRIAN A. KIM AND TIMOTHY FURNISH

CASE REPORT

A 54-year-old woman presents with a chief complaint of "searing pain" in her right hand and forearm that has been worsening over the past 2 weeks. A month ago she suffered a wrist sprain treated conservatively with NSAIDs, rest, ice, and compression. Over the past 2 weeks she has developed increased swelling, redness, burning sensation, and extreme pain in her hand, wrist, and forearm extending half-way to her elbow beyond the range of her initial wrist injury. She describes her pain as shooting and burning. Movement and light touch exacerbate her pain so much that she has wrapped her right arm in a stocking and has been holding her arm with the elbow flexed against her abdomen, assuming a protective posture. She also reports that her grip strength feels noticeably weak. During the interview she is tearful at times and refuses to have her arm touched or manipulated, but on visual exam reveals a grossly swollen, erythematous right upper extremity. Her right forearm is distinctly warmer than her unaffected limb. Her lab work shows normal WBC, ESR, and CRP and radiographic imaging of her right upper extremity reveals no overt skeletal abnormalities.

DEFINITION

Complex regional pain syndrome (CRPS) is a pain condition of uncertain pathophysiology commonly affecting a single extremity, most frequently after an inciting injury, with the potential for expansion within the affected extremity or migration to a previously unaffected limb. The hallmark of CRPS is pain out of proportion to the initial injury and often described as excruciating and burning in quality. A constellation of sensory, vasomotor, sudomotor, and motor/trophic changes are also observed, and may progress to significant disability and detriment to quality of life. These findings persist beyond the period of normal healing of the injury and may vary greatly over time. CRPS is subdivided into type 1, type 2, and, more recently, not otherwise specified (NOS). The clinical features of both types 1 and 2 are the same, the discriminating factor being the presence of a known nerve injury in type 2. CRPS NOS pertains to a subset of patients who do not completely meet CRPS diagnostic criteria, yet no other diagnosis can be attributed to their presentation. The specific requirements commonly used for the diagnosis of CRPS are discussed later in the Diagnosis section, with emphasis on the International Association for the Study of Pain (IASP) criteria as well as the revised diagnostic criteria, also referred to as "the Budapest criteria."[24–27]

EPIDEMIOLOGY

Internationally, the incidence of CRPS ranges from 5.5 to 26.2 cases per 100,000 individuals.[1,2] It typically occurs after a relatively minor injury, insult, or surgery with time of onset ranging from days to weeks to months. Sprains or strains account for 10%–29%, fractures for 16%, postsurgical for 3%–24%, contusions or crush injuries for 8%, and 6% occur without an identifiable injury.[3,4] In adults the upper extremity is most commonly involved (up to 61%), while pediatric patients typically present with lower extremity lesions (72.6%–85%), ankle sprains being the most common inciting injury.[3,4,15,16] Women are more often affected by the syndrome, accounting for 60%–81% of CRPS patients with peak incidence in the fifth and sixth decades.[1–4]

CLINICAL FEATURES

The most prevalent sensory symptom is intense burning pain presenting as hyperalgesia or allodynia. CRPS pain has also been described as aching, pricking, or shooting in quality, localized in deep somatic tissue often beyond the region of initial injury. Hyperalgesia and allodynia are often evoked and aggravated by mechanical stimuli or joint manipulation. Sensory deficits are also commonplace, with up to 33% of patients revealing hemisensory impairment (decreased temperature and pinprick sensation) ipsilateral to the affected extremity. It has been reported that patients with upper extremity involvement may even present with hypoesthesia or numbness in the trigeminal nerve distribution.[5,6]

Patients often maintain a protective posture to safeguard their affected limb because of the often excruciating allodynia. Sensory abnormalities are generally non-dermatomal, often in a glove-like or stocking-like pattern, and CRPS patients have been noted to wear actual gloves and stockings to prevent further aggravation. Additionally, physical examination and therapy may prove difficult because of the defensive protection of the extremity often seen in these patients.

Autonomic dysfunction in the affected limb is generally manifested as vasomotor and sudomotor instability (see Figure 34.1). These manifestations may be in the form of swelling, color, temperature, and sweating abnormalities. Patients may present with an extremity that is warm, inflamed, and erythematous, or, in contrast, cold, dusky, and mottled. Striking cyanosis may indicate later stages of disease progression and may prove refractory to conventional treatment efforts. Temperature asymmetry of greater than 1°C between the affected and unaffected extremity has also been widely observed, although such changes are dynamic in nature and the affected limb may be warmer or colder than the

unaffected limb.[7,8] Moreover, sweating changes in the affected limb were noted in almost 60% of patients, with most presenting with hyperhidrosis or excessive sweating (94%), hyperhidrosis being a very common early finding in the CRPS disease course.[7]

Motor dysfunction may also be observed in the affected extremity. This can manifest as tremors, dystonia, loss of strength and endurance, as well as muscle spasms. In patients with upper extremity involvement, grip strength was significantly decreased in 78% of CRPS patients.[9] Tremors have been noted in anywhere from 24% to 60% of patients and decreased range of motion is also widely observed.[3,7,10] Causes of decreased range may be due to soft tissue swelling or joint effusions in the early stages and contraction and fibrosis in the later stages.[11] Dystrophic changes are often noted after further disease progression and include increased or decreased nail and hair growth on the affected limb. Skin changes are also common and consist of palmar/plantar fibrosis, hyperkeratosis, and thin, glossy skin.[12] Once disease progression has reached a level of significant muscle atrophy, contracture, and distinct cyanosis, it is more difficult to treat.

CRPS typically affects one extremity at the most distal location (hands and feet); however, there is a 10% incidence of CRPS symptoms spreading to another region (typically more proximally) or to a contralateral previously unaffected limb.[13] A prospective study revealed that contiguous spread, on average, occurred 2.5 months after initial onset, while independent or mirror image migration took significantly longer, about

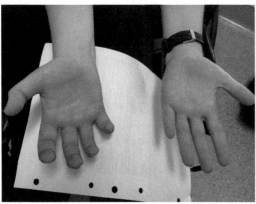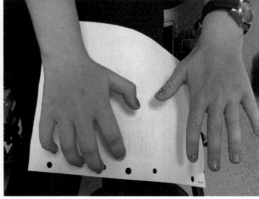

FIGURE 34.1. Left: complex regional pain syndrome (CRPS) diagnosed in the right hand. Right: unilateral CRPS, right hand (left side of the image) displaying swelling, erythema, and dystonic finger positioning in contrast to the unaffected left hand.

2.5 years.[14] Moreover, the recurrence rate once remission is reached has been projected at 1.8% per year.[13]

Although CRPS has been well described in the adult population, emerging evidence demonstrates key differences in the pediatric CRPS population, particularly in terms of remission rates and treatment regimen. Pediatric patients are most commonly females between 8 and 16 years of age, with one case report of a patient as young as 3 years old.[17,18] The diagnosis of CRPS is often delayed by up to 4 months in the pediatric population, and although extension within the affected limb or migration to a previously unaffected limb exists in adults, the incidence of migration in the pediatric population has not been reported.[17]

Most importantly, the reported response in pediatric groups to treatment with conservative measures such as behavioral management and exercise therapy is quite high (88%–93%).[19-21] In his review of CRPS in the pediatric population, Michael Stanton-Hicks attributes this extraordinary and promising remission potential to "plasticity."[17] This is evidenced in children and adolescents by their favorable response to physical therapy and behavioral modifications, with less than 10% requiring any interventional therapies such as epidural catheters, regional blocks, or spinal cord stimulators.[22,23] Although pediatric plasticity may result in a high percentage of patients achieving initial remission, recurrence rates are noticeably higher than in adults (~30%).[19,21] As with adults, pediatric clinicians emphasize the importance of early diagnosis and rehabilitation in CRPS.

PATHOPHYSIOLOGY

The underlying pathophysiology of CRPS is elaborate and incompletely elucidated, with lively debate in the literature. Current evidence reveals an intricate mosaic comprised of many possible disease mechanisms in both the central and peripheral nervous systems, with postulated theories on their interactions. The components of most interest include dysfunction in the autonomic and somatic nervous system, as well the contributions of peripheral inflammation and hypoxia, immunological effects, and psychological mediators, which all may play contributory roles.[30]

Autonomic dysfunction in the form of sympathetically maintained pain has historically been the chief theory to explain many of the significant findings in CRPS, including increased sweating, trophic changes, and vasoconstrictive temperature changes of the affected limb. Traditionally, many of these findings were attributed to sympathetic hyperactivity and sympathetic-afferent coupling—an overexpression of adrenergic receptors on primary afferent nerve endings.[31,32] The classic treatment of CRPS with sympatholytic blocks was directed at uncoupling the hyperalgesia and vasoconstriction associated with sympathetically maintained pain.

The evidence is relatively robust for sympathetic hyperactivity playing at least a partial, although nonobligatory, role in CRPS. Observations reveal increased pain and abnormal vasoconstrictive patterns after central sympathetic arousal.[33,34] Additionally, sympathetic skin reflexes are elevated in CRPS patients and may be attributed to the proliferation of sympathetic innervation centrally in the dorsal horn or peripherally in the upper dermis.[35-37] The triggers for this exaggerated innervation may include inflammatory mechanisms or direct nerve injury. More specifically, studies in humans and primates have shown evidence of $alpha_1$-adrenoreceptor upregulation as a cause of sympathetic afferent–efferent abnormal coupling. In contrast, animal studies point to $alpha_2$-adrenoreceptors as the root cause for excitation and sensitization of nociceptive afferents, potentially via prostaglandin E2.[38-42] Furthermore, the density of alpha-adrenoreceptors is noticeably increased in hyperalgesic skin from CRPS patients, while the sympathetic innervation of sweat glands and vasculature also appear to be abnormal.[43,44]

Adrenergic receptor hypersensitivity may also contribute to the aforementioned findings.[35,45,46] The evidence for this proposed mechanism includes studies that report increased pain levels in CRPS patients after intradermal norepinephrine injection, but not in controls.[47] Serum catecholamine levels from the affected limbs were actually decreased, favoring the proposed role of local adrenergic hypersensitivity as opposed to a pure quantitative increase in adrenergic mediators and receptors.[48] Transiently decreased sympathetic stimulation has been postulated as a potential stimulus for adrenergic receptor upregulation and sensitization.[48] Anecdotally, this is evidenced by a "sympathectomy"-like presentation with vasodilated, erythematous, and edematous limbs frequently observed early on in CRPS.

Hypoxic mechanisms also appear to contribute to sympathetic-mediated pain and sensitization. Studies of CRPS-affected limbs show decreased capillary oxygenation, increased lactate levels, and impaired high-energy phosphate metabolism.[49] Moreover, histopathology of CRPS limbs shows findings consistent with oxidative stress, and induced tissue acidosis has been associated with increased pain rating in these patients.[50,51] The hypoxia in CRPS has been attributed to exaggerated vasoconstriction, which may be sympathetically driven (discussed previously) or due to an imbalance of endothelial mediators. In blister fluid of CRPS-affected limbs, endothelin 1 (ET-1, which promotes vasoconstriction) was found to be elevated in the affected limb, while nitric oxide (NO, a vessel relaxant) was decreased.[52] These findings suggest that endothelial imbalance may contribute to the vasoconstriction and hypoxia evidenced in CRPS extremities.

Of note, murine studies reveal that acute hypoxic insult via tourniquet-induced ischemia (3 hours) resulted in CRPS-like findings in the previously constricted limbs.[56] After rapid reperfusion, neuropathic pain symptoms were observed without microscopic evidence of nerve damage. The authors attributed these results to the triggering of afferent nerves and subsequent exaggerated inflammatory response by free radicals. Furthermore, the involvement of free radicals is supported by randomized clinical trials showing positive outcomes where free radical scavengers were successfully utilized early on in therapy, including dimethylsulfoxide, N-acetylcysteine, and vitamin C.[57,58]

Spinal and supraspinal sensitization also appears to play a role in the generation and maintenance of CRPS and other neuropathic pain disorders. Hyperexcitability and disinhibition states lead to a decreased stimulation threshold contributing to nociceptive dysregulation.[59] Animal-based neuropathic pain models reveal spinal sensitization among postsynaptic receptors, chiefly involving the N-methyl-D-aspartate (NMDA) receptor, the neurokinin-1 (NK-1) receptor, and the alpha-amino-3-hydroxy-5-methyl-4-isoxazoleproprionic acid receptor.[60] Parallel studies in humans prove difficult as they require spinal tissue samples; however, some studies have shown promising benefit after NMDA-receptor antagonism in CRPS.[61]

CRPS commonly exhibits clinical findings suggestive of inflammation, including "dolor, rubor, calor, tumor," often occurring during the early and exacerbation phases of CRPS in affected limbs.[30] Both classic proinflammatory cytokines and neuropeptide-mediated neurogenic inflammation appear to play a role. In artificially produced blisters in the affected extremity of CRPS patients, interleukin-6 (IL-6), tumor necrosis factor alpha (TNF-α), and tryptase were elevated with increased markers for activated monocytes and macrophages.[62-64] Furthermore, there is intensified migration of radiolabeled autologous leukocytes or nonspecific immunoglobulins toward the CRPS affected sites as well.[65,66] Curiously, the classic systemic markers of inflammation such as white blood cell count (WBC), erythrocyte sedimentation rate (ESR), and C-reactive protein (CRP) are normal in most CRPS patients.[53,54]

The neurogenic inflammatory component is mediated by neuropeptides released by nociceptive C-fibers in the extremities, as well as neuropeptide discharge in the dorsal horns, where central sensitization may be mediated. The primary mediators include substance P, calcitonin gene-related protein (CGRP), and bradykinin, all of which are systemically elevated in CRPS patients.[67,68] In murine studies, substance P application induced and/or increased CRPS-like symptoms.[69] In humans with CRPS, intradermal substance P led to abnormal plasma extravasation.[70] Additionally, neuropeptide Y, angiotensin converting enzyme, and vasoactive intestinal protein have been proposed as potential modulators of neuroinflammation but have not been robustly validated.[71]

Interesting evidence supporting immunological mechanisms in CRPS does exist, although the complete nature of its contribution is not well understood. A study by Mailis and Wade revealed elevated levels of both human leukocyte antigen (HLA) class I and II in 80% of treatment-resistant CRPS patients. The authors postulate that CRPS might constitute a neuroimmune disorder.[72] Consistently varying levels, both high and low of heritable antigens, have also been reported in murine studies of neuropathic pain.[73] Additionally, two recent studies revealed autoantibodies against neuronal structures in CRPS patients, although the role of autoantibodies is not completely understood at this time.[74,75] A handful of open-label studies have shown some success using immunomodulating agents such as infliximab, thalidomide, and oral steroids in this patient population.[76-79]

In the past, CRPS was considered by some practitioners to be a manifestation of psychiatric dysfunction, including varying contributions from somatoform disorders and malingering. Experts now view this concept as being outdated.[80] The association of psychological factors and CRPS remains controversial owing to a lack of high-quality studies, with the existing evidence showing no conclusive relationship.[81-83] Some studies have shown debatable association with stressful life events, hypochondria, somatization, depression, and anxiety, although these findings may follow rather than precede the onset of CRPS.[81,82,84] In a small study of the pediatric CRPS population (*n* = 20) Low et al. noted that 55% of pediatric patients were regarded as "high achievers" and common psychosocial themes included family and marital dysfunction, nonverbalization of feelings, pressure for performance at sports or school, and a lack of self-assertiveness.[15]

Moreover, central pain-induced fear appears to affect recovery and prolong disease course due to disuse of the affected extremity. Prolonged immobilization causes decreased range of motion, impaired nutritive perfusion, and trophic alterations.[85] Physical therapy aimed at overcoming movement anxiety is considered to have excellent therapeutic value through desensitization from mechanical and movement allodynia and preventing the buildup of catecholamines, neuropeptides, and other inflammatory mediators.[86,87]

Functional alterations in central processing appear to play a role in the maintenance of CRPS and result in major motor and sensory dysfunction in these patients. This supraspinal dysfunction is evidenced by findings of impaired perceptual learning as well as (secondary) psychological factors such as pain-related fear and movement anxiety.[30] Furthermore, brain imaging studies have associated CRPS with alterations in cerebral perfusion patterns of the amygdala, hippocampus, and prefrontal cortex, with small case studies revealing decreased thalamic activity contralateral to the symptomatic limb.[88,89] Be that as it may, data supporting altered brain function and structure in CRPS have been generally inconsistent and remain a point of contention.[90]

In conclusion, the diverse and often murky pathophysiology of CRPS remains an active and ongoing area of basic science and clinical investigation. The mechanisms described in this chapter

do not differentiate between the subsets of CRPS (types 1, 2, NOS) and continued research may validate clearly defined mechanisms for each in the future.

DIAGNOSIS

The diagnosis of CRPS is one of exclusion and is ultimately determined by the patient's history and physical exam. Prior to 1994, the condition went by a variety of different names, the most common of which was reflex sympathetic dystrophy. There were no widely agreed-upon criteria to diagnose this condition, therefore the International Association for the Study of Pain (IASP) convened a panel to develop the initial diagnostic criteria and renamed the condition complex regional pain syndrome (Table 34.1).[24] In the following years, the IASP criteria were criticized for lacking specificity, resulting in overdiagnosis. A closed panel of international experts again

TABLE 34.1. DIAGNOSTIC CRITERIA OF THE INTERNATIONAL ASSOCIATION FOR THE STUDY OF PAIN (IASP) FOR COMPLEX REGIONAL PAIN SYNDROME (CRPS)

CRPS I (Reflex Sympathetic Dystrophy)
1. Presence of initiating noxious event or cause of immobilization.
2. Continuous pain, allodynia, or hyperalgesia disproportionate to any inciting event.
3. Evidence at some time of edema, skin blood flow changes, or abnormal sudomotor activity in the region of pain.
4. Diagnosis is excluded by existence of conditions that would otherwise account for the degree of pain and dysfunction.
Criteria 2–4 must be satisfied.

CRPS II (Causalgia)
1. Presence of continuing pain, allodynia, or hyperalgesia after a nerve injury, not necessarily limited to nerve distribution.
2. Evidence at some time of edema, skin blood flow changes, or abnormal sudomotor activity in the region of pain.
3. Diagnosis is excluded by existence of conditions that would otherwise account for the degree of pain and dysfunction.
All three criteria must be satisfied.

From Mersky and Bogduk (1994).[24]

convened in Budapest, Hungary in 2003, where the CRPS criteria were refined to address these perceived deficiencies. Aptly, the revised criteria by Harden and Bruehl are commonly referred to as "the Budapest criteria" (see Table 34.2)[25-27] Both sets of criteria have elements that overlap, including alterations in pain, varying sensory, vasomotor, sudomotor, and motor findings, and have been empirically validated to varying degrees. Significantly, the revised "Budapest" criteria include separate sections for the diagnosis of CRPS for clinical versus research purposes. The application of these criteria for

TABLE 34.2. REVISED CLINICAL DIAGNOSTIC CRITERIA (THE BUDAPEST CRITERIA)

For *clinical diagnosis*, the following criteria must be met:

1. Continuous pain, disproportionate to any inciting event.

2. Must report at least one symptom in *three of the four* following categories:
   Sensory: hyperesthesia and/or allodynia
   Vasomotor: temperature asymmetry and/or skin color changes and/or skin color asymmetry
   Sudomotor/Edema: edema and/or sweating changes and/or sweating asymmetry
   Motor/Trophic: decreased range of motion and/or motor dysfunction (weakness, tremor, dystonia) and/or trophic changes (hair, nail, skin)

3. Must display at least one sign at time of evaluation in *two or more* of the following categories:
   Sensory: hyperalgesia (to pinprick) and/or allodynia (to light touch and/or temperature sensation and/or deep somatic pressure and/or joint movement)
   Vasomotor: temperature asymmetry (>1°C) and/or skin color changes and/or asymmetry
   Sudomotor/Edema: edema and/or sweating changes and/or sweating asymmetry
   Motor/Trophic: decreased range of motion and/or motor dysfunction (weakness, tremor, dystonia) and/or trophic changes (hair, nail, skin)

4. There is no other diagnosis that better explains the signs and symptoms.

For *research purposes*, at least one symptom in *all four* symptom categories and at least one sign in two or more sign categories.

From Harden et al. (2007).[27]

clinical diagnosis requires the presence of one symptom in three out of four categories, while the research criteria require one symptom in all four of the diagnostic categories. The more rigorous requirement for research purposes notably increases the specificity of the revised clinical criteria, minimizing false-positive findings.[27]

The differential diagnosis for CRPS is wide-ranging and encompasses neuropathic pain syndromes, vascular diseases, inflammatory conditions, myofascial pain, as well as psychiatric disorders. The criteria require that the definitive diagnosis of CRPS be excluded, if another condition better accounts for the pain and dysfunction.

There is no specific "gold standard" diagnostic test for CRPS. Many tests may be used in creating an overall clinical picture supportive of the diagnosis, but additional studies may be helpful in excluding other potential maladies. Traditional inflammatory markers (WBC, ESR, CRP) are often normal, but may be used to exclude infectious or rheumatological diseases.[53,54] Duplex and ultrasound studies may help rule out peripheral vascular disease, particularly in patients presenting with prominent vasomotor signs and symptoms. Nerve conduction studies may help exclude peripheral neuropathic diseases or in reaffirming specific nerve involvement.

Radiographic studies such as plain radiographs and magnetic resonance imaging (MRI) may be indicated to rule out skeletal or soft tissue pathology. Radiographic imaging may demonstrate osteoporosis, but is of no true diagnostic value by itself.[55] Three-phase bone scintigraphy can reveal increased uptake/hyperperfusion of technetium Tc 99m bisphosphonates in early CRPS due to increased bone metabolism, but is not specific to this diagnosis.[28] In contrast, bone scans in pediatric patients tend to reveal normal or hypoperfused images.[15]

Clinically, thermography may show changes in skin temperature between the affected and nonaffected extremity. A difference of 0.5°C is considered mildly asymmetrical, while a difference of 1.0°C is considered significant.[7,8] The diagnostic value increases if significant differentials are found in multiple sites; however, skin temperature is dynamic in nature and symmetrical thermographic readings do not exclude CRPS.

Other studies may aid in substantiating clinical symptoms and are predominantly used for scientific research purposes. Some of these tests include quantitative sensory testing, resting sweat output, provocative sweat output test by sudomotor axon reflex test, sympathetic skin response, volumetry in edematous extremity, visual analog scales for pain, impairment level sum-score, skills/walking/rising/sitting questionnaires, and limb activity monitoring.[29]

TREATMENT

The treatment modalities for CRPS depend on the degree of severity and disability on presentation. Pain experts emphasize an aggressive, multimodal, multidisciplinary approach for successful treatment and remission. The three main focuses of treatment are rehabilitation, psychological therapy, and pain management. All three components should be part of a well-designed treatment strategy and should be adjusted to patient responsiveness.[91] One interdisciplinary expert panel suggests escalation of treatment modalities every 2 weeks if a favorable response is not achieved and recommends considering invasive or interventional therapies by 12 to 16 weeks if conservative therapies have not proven effective.[91,92] Additionally, comorbidities (depression, anxiety, sleep disturbance, deconditioning, etc.) presenting at the time of clinical diagnosis should be addressed simultaneously.

Physical therapy or rehabilitation historically has been the foundation of CRPS treatment and is one of the few modalities with significant evidence of effectiveness.[19,84,95–98] Physical therapy should proceed in a step-wise, progressive fashion with the ultimate endpoint of achieving functionality of the affected extremity. Initial therapy entails development of a strong therapeutic alliance and desensitization/reactivation exercises. Patients then may move on to isometrics, flexibility exercises, and edema control, as well as treatment of secondary myofascial pain. Next, gentle range of motion, stress loading, and isotonic strengthening may be pursued, followed by aerobic conditioning and postural normalization. Ergonomics, normalization of use, and vocational/functional rehabilitation comprise the final steps. Experts emphasize that this logical step-by-step advancement is paramount to rehabilitation, as the improper or ill-timed application of physical therapy may be detrimental and adversely affect the disease course.[91] Concurrently, psychological and pain control measures should be implemented to optimize patient participation and engagement.

Psychological therapy should be used in the treatment plan of most CRPS patients and includes cognitive-behavioral therapy (CBT),

stress management, coping skills, relaxation techniques, imagery, and self-hypnosis. Biofeedback is also prominently applied and may include electromyography (EMG) feedback, autogenic/limb warming training, progressive muscle relaxation, meditation, and sleep hygiene.[92] Early CRPS (4–6 weeks) patients typically have minimal benefit from full-scale psychological therapy, although education of the syndrome itself as well as its management should be emphasized. Two important concepts that should be conveyed early on in the disease course are that CRPS-related pain does not necessarily indicate tissue damage, and that reactivation of the affected limb will prevent further dysfunction.[91] If the syndrome progresses and persists for more than 6 to 8 weeks, experts strongly recommend clinical psychological assessment, as these factors seem to play a more prominent role in maladaptation and poor coping.[91,99] Additionally, Axis I psychiatric disorders should be ruled out and potential trauma related to any inciting injuries should be addressed. CBT is beneficial in improving quality of life and augmenting physical therapy in chronic pain syndromes, even in individuals without prominent Axis I disorders.[100] Although not specific to CRPS, controlled trials validate the efficacy of psychotherapy in chronic pain management.[100,101]

Pain management is broadly subdivided into pharmacological and interventional therapies. Pharmacological treatment should be directed at the most prominent symptoms and proposed pathophysiology discussed here. It is important to note that few well-designed studies have been performed specifically investigating pharmacological treatments for CRPS. Many of the recommended therapies in guidelines and reviews are based on extrapolation from controlled trials for other neuropathic pain conditions (i.e., diabetic peripheral neuropathy, postherpetic neuralgia).[102]

For patients presenting with pain of neuropathic quality, tricyclic antidepressants (TCAs: amitriptyline, nortriptyline, doxepin) may be beneficial, although there are no specific studies in CRPS. These older antidepressants address neuropathic pain as well as potential sleep impairment and therefore remain a first-line therapy in neuropathic pain conditions.[103–105] A small randomized controlled trial (RCT) of gabapentin found mild improvement in CRPS pain with significant improvement in sensory deficits and serves as a useful adjuvant.[106] The antiepileptic carbamazepine (600 mg/day over 8 days) markedly reduced pain in an RCT of CRPS patients, and may be used if initial conservative measures are ineffective or contraindicated.[110]

Anti-inflammatory agents, particularly free radical scavengers, may have a role in the treatment of CRPS moving forward. Topical dimethyl sulfoxide 50% (DMSO-50%) proved superior to placebo, and oral N-acetylcysteine was almost equally effective as DMSO in RCTs of CRPS groups.[113,114] In two additional RCTs, the corticosteroids prednisone and prednisolone showed evidence of significant CRPS improvement in the early stages of disease, therefore a short-course of steroids may be considered in the acute phase of CRPS with significant inflammatory findings. However, the long-term risk–benefit ratio remains unfavorable, and chronic steroid therapy is not recommended.[111,112] There is no clear evidence for the use of nonsteroidal anti-inflammatory drugs (NSAIDs) and acetaminophen in CRPS, although they are routinely used clinically as opioid-sparing analgesic adjuvants and have been historically used to address the inflammatory findings often observed in CRPS patients.

Opioids remain controversial because of their side-effect profile, abuse potential, and limited evidence in neuropathic pain conditions, but they may be appropriate when conservative therapies have been exhausted. In this scenario, opioids may be employed as part of a pharmacological bridge to allow patient participation in physical therapy or to more aggressive interventional modalities. Of note, sustained-release morphine (90 mg/day) was ineffective in a double-blinded, placebo-controlled trial with neuropathic pain and CRPS patients.[110]

Other medications of interest include the bisphosphonates, alendronate and pamidronate, which reduce the bone turnover often observed in adult CRPS. Both led to promising results, with improvement in spontaneous pain, pressure tolerance, and joint mobility in two separate RCTs, while calcitonin, proposed to have a related mechanism of action to bisphosphonates, proved ineffective in well-designed studies.[112,115,116]

Historically, alpha-adrenergic and antihypertensive medications were commonly used, based on the belief that all CRPS involved sympathetic overactivity. For the subset of patients presenting with cold extremities and hyperactive vasomotor symptoms, alpha-1 adrenergic blockers such as phenoxybenzamine and terazosin have shown some benefit in small case series.[117,118] There are case series that also indicate some benefit to calcium channel blockade with nifedipine, when vasoconstrictive findings are prominent.[118] Furthermore, the alpha-2 adrenoreceptor agonist clonidine has shown some efficacy in transdermal and epidural administrations in CRPS.[119-122] Although case studies have shown some benefit of these agents, there continues to be a lack of robust RCT-supported evidence for the routine use of alpha-adrenergics and antihypertensives at this time.

Topical medications are often prescribed in neuropathic pain conditions but lack significant evidence. These topical agents include capsaicin and transdermal lidocaine. Topical analgesics are generally low risk and may be beneficial in localized CRPS pain, but there is no compelling evidence to support their use.

In patients presenting with severe dystonia, tremors, or myoclonus, muscle relaxants such as oral benzodiazepines, cyclobenzaprine, or baclofen may prove beneficial.[29]

Lastly, NMDA blockade via ketamine in subanesthetic doses has proven effective in both a retrospective case series and randomized double-blinded, controlled trial for CRPS.[107-109] Interestingly, ketamine has recently received growing interest and evidence for treating refractory depression, which may present as a comorbid condition in patients with severe CRPS and chronic pain.[123,124]

Interventional pain therapies are second line if the patient does not respond to initial conservative measures—medication and physical therapy. However, it should be noted that moving on to more invasive therapies should be considered early in the treatment process if conservative therapies are not working. For patients with severe pain, allodynia, or overt sympathetically mediated dysfunction including distinct skin temperature changes, a sympathetic block (stellate ganglion for upper extremity, lumbar sympathetic block for lower extremity) can be considered. If the sympathetic block proves beneficial (at least 50% reduction in pain), the procedure may be repeated, or radiofrequency ablation of the sympathetic ganglion may be offered as an option. Somatic/regional blocks and peripheral nerve stimulation have also been used.[91,125] If symptoms persist without significant improvement, more invasive measures can be undertaken, including spinal cord stimulation (SCS). A randomized trial from the Netherlands comparing SCS and physical therapy versus physical therapy alone in CRPS patients showed significant pain reduction and improved global perceived effect scores for up to 2 years after SCS implantation.[126] However, the pain-alleviating effect appears to progressively diminish over time, beyond the 2- to 3-year mark, and no significant difference was noted in functional status and quality of life.[126] However, at 5-year follow-up, 95% of the patients in the SCS arm of the trial reported high satisfaction ratings and were willing to undergo spinal cord stimulator therapy again.[126] Overall, spinal cord stimulators remain a cost-efficient and efficacious interventional therapy for up to 2 years' duration and potentially beyond in the treatment of CRPS patients warranting interventional therapy. SCS complication rates, however, are high (72%) and include generator failure, lead displacement, infection, and revision of the generator pocket.[126] Intrathecal drug delivery is considered by most to be more invasive than SCS and may be considered in refractory cases. The intrathecal infusion of various analgesics for severe CRPS may include opioids, baclofen, ziconitide, bupivacaine, or clonidine.

Lastly, amputations have been performed but remain a highly controversial intervention and should only be considered in the most severe cases after every other modality has been extensively exhausted. Recent small studies present evidence supporting post-amputation improvements in several metrics (quality of life, quality of sleep, mobility, significant pain reduction, willingness to undergo amputation again), although the occurrence of phantom limb pain was significant (81%).[93,94]

CONCLUSION

CRPS is a challenging pain condition with incompletely elucidated pathophysiology, most often affecting a single extremity after an inciting injury. The most common clinical finding is burning pain out of proportion to any identifiable initiating event with a combination of sensory, vasomotor, sudomotor, and motor/trophic signs and symptoms. The management of CRPS emphasizes early diagnosis and aggressive multimodal treatment based on physical therapy, psychological therapy, and pain management with frequent reassessments of patient progression. In order to prevent permanent life-altering disability, all modalities, including interventional therapies, should be escalated in tandem, based on assessments of patient responsiveness. Clinicians should consider escalating therapy frequently if no improvement is observed, and introducing psychological evaluation if symptoms persist. Lastly, the use of interventional techniques such as sympathetic blocks or SCS should be employed early in refractory cases.[91,125]

GUIDING QUESTIONS

- How do you make a complex regional pain syndrome (CRPS) diagnosis?
- What is the main pathophysiology of CRPS?
- What are the treatment options for CRPS?

KEY POINTS

- The diagnosis of complex regional pain syndrome (CRPS) is one of exclusion and is ultimately determined by the patient's history and physical exam. "The Budapest criteria" emphasize alterations in pain, varying sensory, vasomotor, sudomotor, and motor findings. The criteria include separate sections for the diagnosis of CRPS for clinical versus research purposes. The application of these criteria for clinical diagnosis requires the presence of one symptom in three out of four categories, while the research criteria require one symptom in all four of the diagnostic categories.
- The underlying pathophysiology of CRPS is elaborate and incompletely elucidated. Current evidence reveals an intricate mosaic comprised of many possible disease mechanisms in both the central and peripheral nervous systems, with postulated theories on their interactions. The components of most interest include dysfunction in the autonomic and somatic nervous system, as well the contributions of peripheral inflammation and hypoxia, immunological effects, and psychological mediators, which all may play contributory roles.
- The treatment modalities for CRPS depend on the degree of severity and disability on presentation. An aggressive, multimodal, multidisciplinary approach is required for successful treatment and remission. The three main focuses of treatment are rehabilitation, psychological therapy, and pain management. All three components should be part of a well-designed treatment strategy and should

be adjusted to patient responsiveness.[91] Clinicians should consider invasive or interventional therapies by 12 to 16 weeks if conservative therapies have not proven effective.[91,92] Additionally, comorbidities (depression, anxiety, sleep disturbance, deconditioning, etc.) presenting at the time of clinical diagnosis should be addressed simultaneously.

REFERENCES

1. Sandroni P, Benrud-Larson LM, McClelland RL, Low PA. Complex regional pain syndrome type I: incidence and prevalence in Olmsted county, a population-based study. *Pain*. 2003;103:199–207.

2. de Mos M, de Bruijn AGJ, Huygen FJ et al. The incidence of complex regional pain syndrome: a population-based study. *Pain*. 2007;129:12–20.

3. Harden RN, Bruehl S, Galer BS, et al. Complex regional pain syndrome: are the IASP diagnostic criteria valid and sufficiently comprehensive? *Pain*. 1999;83:211–219.

4. Allen G, Galer BS, Schwartz L. Epidemiology of complex regional pain syndrome: a retrospective chart review of 134 patients. *Pain*. 1999;80:539–544.

5. Rommel O, Gehling M, Dertwinkel R, et al. Hemisensory impairment in patients with complex regional pain syndrome. *Pain*. 1999;80:95–101.

6. Thimineur M, Sood P, Kravitz E, Gudin J, Kitaj M. Central nervous system abnormalities in complex regional pain syndrome: clinical and quantitative evidence of medullary dysfunction. *Clin J Pain*. 1998;14:256–267.

7. Birklein F, Sittl R, Spitzer A, Claus D, Neundorfer B, Handwerker HO. Sudomotor function in sympathetic reflex dystrophy. *Pain*. 1997;69:49–54.

8. Baron R, Blumberg H, Janig W. *Progress in Pain Research and Management*. Seattle, WA: IASP Press; 1996.

9. Zyluk A. The sequelae of reflex sympathetic dystrophy. *J Hand Surg*. 2001;26:151–154.

10. Sieweke N, Birklein F, Riedl B, Neundorfer B, Handwerker HO. Patterns of hyperalgesia in complex regional pain syndrome. *Pain*. 1999;80:171–177.

11. Schwartzman RJ, Kerrigan J. The movement disorder of reflex sympathetic dystrophy. *Neurology*. 1990;40:57–61.

12. Wasner G, Backonja MM, Baron R. Traumatic neuralgias: complex regional pain syndromes; clinical characteristics, pathophysiologic mechanisms and therapy. *Neurol Clin*. 1998;16:851–868.

13. Veldman P, Goris R. Multiple reflex sympathetic dystrophy: which patients are at risk for developing recurrence of reflex sympathetic dystrophy in the same or another limb. *Pain*. 1996;64:463–466.

14. Maleki J, LeBel AA, Bennett GJ, Shwartzman RJ. Patterns of spread in complex regional pain syndrome, type I. *Pain*. 2000;88:259–266.

15. Low AK, Ward K, Wines AP. Pediatric complex regional pain syndrome. *J Pediat Orthop*. 2007;27(5):567–572.

16. Tan EC, Zijlstra B, Essink ML, Goris RJ, Severijnen RS. Complex regional pain syndrome type I in children. *Acta Paediatr*. 2008;97(7):875–879.

17. Stanton-Hicks M. Plasticity of complex regional pain syndrome in children. *Pain Med*. 2010;11:1216–1223.

18. Kozin F, Haughton V, Ryan L. The reflex sympathetic dystrophy syndrome in a child. *J Pediatr*.1977;90(3):417–419.

19. Sherry DD, Wallace CA, Kelley C, Kidder M, Sapp L. Short- and long-term outcomes of children with complex regional pain syndrome type I treated with exercise therapy. *Clin J Pain*. 1999;15(3):218–223.

20. Brooke V, Janselewitz S. Outcomes of children with complex regional pain syndrome after intensive inpatient rehabilitation. *PMR*. 2012;4(5):349–354.

21. Kachko L, Efrat R, Ben Ami S, Mukamel M, Katz J. Complex regional pain syndromes in children and adolescents. *Pediatr Int*. 2008;50(4):523–527.

22. Dadure C, Motais F, Ricard C, et al. Continuous peripheral nerve blocks at home for treatment of recurrent complex regional pain syndrome I in children. *Anesthesiology*. 2005;102(2):387–391.

23. Olsson GL, Meyerson BA, Linderoth B. Spinal cord stimulation in adolescents with complex regional pain syndrome type I. *Eur J Pain*. 2008;12(1):53–59.

24. Mersky H, Bogduk N. *Classification of Chronic Pain: Descriptions of Chronic Pain Syndromes and Definitions of Pain Terms*. Seattle, WA: IASP Press, 1994.

25. Bruehl S, Harden RN, Galer BS, et al. External validation of IASP diagnostic criteria for complex regional pain syndrome and proposed research diagnostic criteria. *Pain*. 1999;81:147–154.

26. Harden RN, Bruehl S, Galer BS, et al. Complex regional pain syndrome: are the IASP diagnostic criteria valid and sufficiently comprehensive? *Pain*. 1999;83:211–219.

27. Harden RN, Bruehl S, Stanton-Hicks M, Wilson PR. Proposed new diagnostic criteria for complex regional pain syndrome. *Pain Med*. 2007;8(4):326–331.

28. Zyluk A. The usefulness of quantitative evaluation of three-phase scintigraphy in the diagnosis

of post-traumatic reflex sympathetic dystrophy. *J Hand Surg Br.* 1999;24:16–21.

29. Perez RS, Zollinger PE, Dijkstra PU, et al. [Clinical practice guideline "Complex regional pain syndrome type I"]. *Ned Tijdschr Geneeskd.* 2007;151:1674–1679.

30. de Mos M, Sturkenboom MC, Huygen FJ. Current understandings on complex regional pain syndrome. *Pain Pract.* 2009;9(2):86–99.

31. Schattschneider J, Binder A, Siebrecht D, Wasner G, Baron R. Complex regional pain syndromes: the influence of cutaneous and deep somatic sympathetic innervation on pain. *Clin J Pain.* 2006;22:240–244.

32. Baron R, Schattschneider J, Binder A, Siebrecht D, Wasner G. Relation between sympathetic vasoconstrictor activity and pain and hyperalgesia in complex regional pain syndromes: a case-control study. *Lancet.* 2002;359:1655–1660.

33. Drummond PD, Finch PM. Persistence of pain induced by startle and forehead cooling after sympathetic blockade in patients with complex regional pain syndrome. *J Neurol Neurosurg Psychiatry.* 2004;75:98–102.

34. Niehof SP, Huygen FJ, van der Weerd RW, Westra M, Zijlstra FJ. Thermography imaging during static and controlled thermoregulation in complex regional pain syndrome type 1: diagnostic value and involvement of the central sympathetic system. *Biomed Eng Online.* 2006;5:30.

35. Bolel K, Hizmetli S, Akyuz A. Sympathetic skin responses in reflex sympathetic dystrophy. *Rheumatol Int.* 2006;26:788–791.

36. Ramer MS, Thompson SW, McMahon SB. Causes and consequences of sympathetic basket formation in dorsal root ganglia. *Pain.* 1999;(Suppl 6):S111–S120.

37. Ruocco I, Cuello AC, Ribeiro-Da-Silva A. Peripheral nerve injury leads to the establishment of a novel pattern of sympathetic fibre innervation in the rat skin. *J Comp Neurol.* 2000;422:287–296.

38. Gonzales R, Sherbourne CD, Goldyne ME, Levine JD. Noradrenaline-induced prostaglandin production by sympathetic postganglionic neurons is mediated by alpha 2-adrenergic receptors. *J Neurochem.* 1991;57:1145–1150.

39. Levine JD, Fields HL, Basbaum AI. Peptides and the primary afferent nociceptor. *J Neurosci.* 1993;13:2273–2286.

40. Stevens DS, Robins VF, Price HM. Treatment of sympathetically maintained pain with terazosin. *Reg Anesth.* 1993;18:318–321.

41. Muizelaar JP, Kleyer M, Hertogs IA, DeLange DC. Complex regional pain syndrome: management with the calcium channel blocker nifedipine and/or the alpha-sympathetic blocker phenoxybenzamine in 59 patients. *Clin Neurol Neurosurg.* 1997;99:26–30.

42. Ghostine SY, Comair YG, Turner DM, Kassell NF, Azar CG. Phenoxybenzamine in the treatment of causalgia: report of 40 cases. *J Neurosurg.* 1984;60:1253–1268.

43. Drummond PD, Skipworth S, Finch PM. Alpha 1 adrenoreceptors in normal and hyperalgesic skin. *Clin Sci.* 1996;91:73–77.

44. Albrecht PJ, Hines S, Eisenberg E, et al. Pathologic alterations of cutaneous innervation and vasculature in affected limbs from patients with complex regional pain syndrome. *Pain.* 2006;120:244–266.

45. Figuerola Mde L, Levin G, Bertotti A, Ferreiro J, Barontini M. Normal sympathetic nervous system response in reflex sympathetic dystrophy. *Funct Neurol.* 2002;17:77–81.

46. Drummond PD, Finch PM, Skipworth S, Blockey P. Pain increases during sympathetic arousal in patients with complex regional pain syndrome. *Neurology.* 2001;57:1296–1303.

47. Ali Z, Raja SN, Wesselmann U, Fuchs PN, Meyer RA, Campbell JN. Intradermal injection of norepinephrine evokes pain in patients with sympathetically maintained pain. *Pain.* 2000;88:161–168.

48. Wasner G, Heckmann K, Maier C, Baron R. Vascular abnormalities in acute reflex sympathetic dystrophy (CRPS I): complete inhibition of sympathetic nerve activity with recovery. *Arch Neurol.* 1999;56:613–620.

49. Heerschap A, den Hollander JA, Reynen H, Goris RJ. Metabolic changes in reflex sympathetic dystrophy: a 31P NMR spectroscopy study. *Muscle Nerve.* 1993;16:367–373.

50. van der Laan L, ter Laak HJ, Gabreels-Festen A, Gabreels F, Goris RJ. Complex regional pain syndrome type I: pathology of skeletal muscle and peripheral nerve. *Neurology.* 1998;51:20–25.

51. Birklein F, Weber M, Ernst M, Riedl B, Neundorfer B, Handwerker HO. Experimental tissue acidosis leads to increased pain in complex regional pain syndrome. *Pain.* 2000;87:227–234.

52. Groeneweg JG, Huygen FJ, Heijmans-Antonissen C, Neihof S, Zijlstra FJ. Increased endothelin-1 and diminished nitric oxide levels in blister fluids of patients with intermediate cold type complex regional pain syndrome type 1. *BMC Musculoskelet Disord.* 2006;7:91.

53. Schinkel C, Gaertner A, Zaspel J, Zedler S, Faist E, Schnermann M. Inflammatory mediators are altered in the acute phase of posttraumatic complex regional pain syndrome. *Clin J Pain.* 2006;22:235–239.

54. Goris RJ, Leixnering M, Huber W, Figl M, Jaindl M, Redl H. Delayed recovery and late development of complex regional pain syndrome in

patients with an isolated fracture of the distal radius: prediction of a regional inflammatory response by early signs. *J Bone Joint Surg Br.* 2007;89:1069–1076.

55. Schurmann M, Zaspel J, Lohr P, et al. Imaging in early posttraumatic complex regional pain syndrome: a comparison of diagnostic methods. *Clin J Pain.* 2007;23:449–457.

56. Coderre TJ, Xanthos DN, Francis L, Bennett GJ. Chronic post-ischemia pain: a novel animal model of complex regional pain syndrome-type I produced by prolonged hindpaw ischemia and reperfusion in the rat. *Pain.* 2004;112:94–105.

57. Perez RS, Zuurmond WW, Bezemer PD, et al. The treatment of complex regional pain syndrome type I with free radical scavengers: a randomized controlled study. *Pain.* 2003;102:297–307.

58. Zollinger PE, Tuinebreijer WE, Breederveld RS, Kreis RW. Can vitamin C prevent complex regional pain syndrome in patients with wrist fractures? A randomized, controlled, multicenter dose-response study. *J Bone Joint Surg Am.* 2007;89:1424–1431.

59. Woolf CJ, Salter MW. Neuronal plasticity: increasing the gain in pain. *Science.* 2000;288:1765–1769.

60. Ji RR, Kohno T, Moore KA, Woolf CJ. Central sensitization and LTP: do pain and memory share similar mechanisms? *Trends Neurosci.* 2003;26:696–705

61. Sinis N, Birbaumer N, Gustin S, et al. Memantine treatment of complex regional pain syndrome: a preliminary report of six cases. *Clin J Pain.* 2007;23:237–243.

62. Huygen FJ, De Bruijn AG, De Bruin MT, Groeneweg JG, Klein J, Zijlstra FJ. Evidence for local inflammation in complex regional pain syndrome type I. *Mediators Inflamm.* 2002;11:47–51.

63. Munnikes RJ, Muis C, Boersma M, Heijmans-Antonissen C, Zijlstra FJ, Huygen FJ. Intermediate stage complex regional pain syndrome type 1 is unrelated to proinflammatory cytokines. *Mediators Inflamm.* 2005;2005:366–372.

64. Heijmans-Antonissen C, Wesseldijk F, Munnikes RJ, et al. Multiplex bead array assay for detection of 25 soluble cytokines in blister fluid of patients with complex regional pain syndrome type 1. *Mediators Inflamm.* 2006;2006:8.

65. Tan EC, Oyen WJ, Goris RJ. Leukocytes in complex regional pain syndrome type 1. *Inflammation.* 2005;29:182–186

66. Okudan B, Celik C. Determination of inflammation of reflex sympathetic dystrophy at early stages with Tc-99m HIG scintigraphy: preliminary results. *Rheumatol Int.* 2006;26:404–408.

67. Birklein F, Schmelz M, Schifter S, Weber M. The important role of neuropeptides in complex regional pain syndrome. *Neurology.* 2001;57:2179–2184.

68. Blair SJ, Chinthagada M, Hoppenstehdt D, Kijowski R, Fareed J. Role of neuropeptides in pathogenesis of reflex sympathetic dystrophy. *Acta Orthop Belg.* 1998;64:448–451.

69. Gradl G, Finke B, Schattner S, Gierer P, Mittlmeier T, Vollmar B. Continuous intra-arterial application of substance P induces signs and symptoms of experimental complex regional pain syndrome such as edema, inflammation, and mechanical pain but no thermal pain. *Neuroscience.* 2007;148:757–765.

70. Leis S, Weber M, Isselmann A, Schmelz M, Birklein F. Substance P-induced protein extravasation is bilaterally increased in complex regional pain syndrome. *Exp Neurol.* 2003;183:197–204.

71. Kramer HH, Schmidt K, Leis S, Schmelz M, Sommer C, Birklein F. Inhibition of neutral endopeptidase facilitates neurogenic inflammation. *Exp Neurol.* 2005;195:179–184.

72. Mailis A, Wade J. Profile of Caucasian women with possible genetic predisposition to reflex sympathetic dystrophy: a pilot study. *Clin J Pain.* 1994;10:210–217.

73. Devor M, Raber P. Heritability of symptoms in an experimental model of neuropathic pain. *Pain.* 1990;42:51–67.

74. Goebel A, Vogel H, Caneris O, et al. Immune responses to Campylobacter and serum autoantibodies in patients with complex regional pain syndrome. *J Neuroimmunol.* 2005;162:184–189.

75. Blaes F, Schmitz K, Tschernatsch M, et al. Autoimmune etiology of complex regional pain syndrome (M. Sudeck). *Neurology.* 2004;63:1734–1736.

76. Huygen FJ, Niehof S, Zijlstra FJ, van Hagen PM, van Daele PL. Successful treatment of CRPS 1 with anti-TNF. *J Pain Symptom Manage.* 2004;27:101–103.

77. Bernateck M, Rolke R, Birklein F, Treede RD, Fink M, Karst M. Successful intravenous regional block with low-dose tumor necrosis factor-alpha antibody infliximab for treatment of complex regional pain syndrome 1. *Anesth Analg.* 2007;105:1148–1151.

78. Schwartzman RJ, Chevlen E, Bengston K. Thalidomide has activity in treating omplex regional pain syndrome. *Arch Intern Med.* 2003;163:1487–1488.

79. Kalita J, Vajpayee A, Misra UK. Comparison of prednisolone with piroxicam in complex regional

pain syndrome following stroke: a randomized controlled trial. *QJM*. 2006;99:89–95.

80. Janig W, Baron R. Is CRPS I a neuropathic pain syndrome? *Pain*. 2006;120:227–229.

81. Geertzen JH, de Bruijn H, de Bruijn-Kofman AT, Arendzen JH. Reflex sympathetic dystrophy: early treatment and psychological aspects. *Arch Phys Med Rehabil*. 1994;75:442–446.

82. Geertzen JH, Dijkstra PU, Groothoff JW, ten Duis HJ, Eisma WH. Reflex sympathetic dystrophy of the upper extremity—a 5.5 year follow-up. Part II. Social life events, general health and changes in occupation. *Acta Orthop Scand*. 1998;279:19–23.

83. Nelson DV, Novy DM. Psychological characteristics of reflex sympathetic dystrophy versus myofascial pain syndromes. *Ref Anesth*. 1996;21:202–208.

84. Birklein F, Riedl B, Sieweke N, Weber M, Neundorfer B. Neurological findings in complex regional pain syndromes—analysis of 145 cases. *Acta Neurol Scand*. 2000;101:262–269.

85. Singh HP, Davis TR. The effect of short-term dependency and immobility on skin temperature and colour in the hand. *J Hand Surg Br*. 2006;31:611–615.

86. Kemler MA, Rijks CP, de Vet HC. Which patients with chronic reflex sympathetic dystrophy are most likely to benefit from physical therapy? *J Manipulative Physiol Ther*. 2001;24:272–278.

87. Bruehl S, Chung OY. Psychological and behavioral aspects of complex regional pain syndrome management. *Clin J Pain*. 2006;22:430–437.

88. Barad MJ, Ueno T, Younger J, Chatterjee N, Mackey S. Complex regional pain syndrome is associated with structural abnormalities in pain-related regions of the human brain. *J Pain*. 2014;15(2):197–203.

89. Iadarola MJ, Max MB, Berman KF, et al. Unilateral decrease in thalamic activity observed with positron emission tomography in patients with chronic neuropathic pain. *Pain*. 1995;63:55–64.

90. van Velzen GA, Rombouts SA, van Buchem MA, Marinus J, van Hilten JJ. Is the brain of complex regional pain syndrome patients truly different? *Eur J Pain*. 2016 May 10. doi: 10.1002/ejp.882.

91. Stanton-Hicks M, Burton A, Bruehl S, et al. An updated interdisciplinary clinical pathway for CRPS: report of an expert panel. *Pain Pract*. 2002;2(1):1–16.

92. Stanton-Hicks M, Baron R, Boas R, et al. Complex regional pain syndromes: guidelines for therapy. *Clin J Pain*. 1999;81:147–154.

93. Midbari A, Suzan E, Adler T, et al. Amputation in patients with complex regional pain syndrome. *Bone Joint J*. 2016;98-B(4);548–554.

94. Krans-Schreuder HK, Bodde MI, Schrier E, et al. Amputation for long-standing, therapy-resistant type-I complex regional pain syndrome. *J Bone Joint Surg [Am]*. 2012;94-A:2263–2268.

95. Watson HK, Carlson L. Treatment of reflex sympathetic dystrophy of the hand with an active "stress loading" program. *J Hand Surg [Am]*. 1987;12:779–785

96. Oerlemans HM, Goris JA, de Boo T, Oostendorp RA. Do physical therapy and occupational therapy reduce the impairment percentage in reflex sympathetic dystrophy? *Am J Phys Med Rehabil*. 1999;8:533–539.

97. Oerlemans HM, Oostendorp RA, de Boo T, Goris RJ. Pain and reduced mobility in complex regional pain syndrome I: outcome of a prospective randomize controlled clinical trial of adjuvant physical therapy versus occupational therapy. *Pain*. 1999;83:77–83.

98. Oerlemans HM, Oostendorp RA, de Boo T, van der Laan L, Severens JL, Goris JA. Adjuvant physical therapy versus occupational therapy in patients with reflex sympathetic dystrophy/complex regional pain syndrome type I. *Arch Phys Med Rehabil*. 2000;81:49–56.

99. Bruehl S, Steger HG, Harden RN. Assessment of complex regional pain syndrome. In: Turk DC, Melzack R, eds. *Handbook of Pain Assessment*. New York: Guilford Press; 2001:549–566.

100. Flor H, Fydrich T, Turk DC. Efficacy of multidisciplinary pain treatment centers: a meta-analytic review. *Pain*. 1992;49:221–230.

101. Carlson CR, Hoyle RH. Efficacy of abbreviated progressive muscle relaxation training: a quantitative review of behavioral medicine research. *J Consult Clin Pasychol*. 1993;61:1059–1067.

102. Kingery WS. A critical review of controlled clinical trials for peripheral neuropathic pain and complex regional pain syndromes. *Pain*. 1997;73:123–139.

103. McQuay HJ, Tramer M, Nye BA, Carroll D, Wiffen PK, Moore RA. A systematic review of antidepressants in neuropathic pain. *Pain*. 1996;68:217–227.

104. Watson CP. The treatment of neuropathic pain: antidepressants and opioids. *Clin J Pain*. 2000;169(2. Suppl):S49–S55.

105. Rowbatham MC. Pharmacologic management of complex regional pain syndrome. *Clin J Pain*. 2006;22:425–429.

106. van de Vusse AC, Stomp-van den Berg SG, Kessels AH, Weber WE. Randomised controlled trial of gabapentin in complex regional pain syndrome type I. *BMC Neurol*. 2004;4:13.

107. Correll GE, Maleki J, Gracely EJ, Muir JJ, Harbut RE. Subanesthetic ketamine infusion therapy: a

retrospective analysis of a novel therapeutic approach to complex regional pain syndrome. *Pain Med.* 2004;5:263–275.

108. Sigtermans MJ, van Hilten JJ, Bauer MC, et al. Ketamine produces effective and long-term pain relief in patients with complex regional pain syndrome type I. *Pain.* 2009;145:304–311.

109. Schwartzman RJ, Alexander GM, Grouthusen JR, Paylor T, Reichenberger E, Perreault M. Outpatient intravenous ketamine for the treatment of complex regional pain syndrome: a double-blind placebo controlled study. *Pain.* 2009;147:107–115.

110. Harke H, Gretenkort P, Ladleif HU, Rahman S, Harke O. The response of neuropathic pain and pain in complex regional pain syndrome I to carbamazepine and sustained-release morphine in patients pretreated with spinal cord stimulation: a double-blinded randomized study. *Anesth Analg.* 2001;92:488–495.

111. Christensen K, Jensen EM, Noer I. The relex dystrophy syndrome response to treatment with systemic corticosteroids. *Acta Chir Scan.* 1982;148:653–655.

112. Kalita J, Vajpayee A, Misra UK. Comparison of prednisolone with piroxicam in complex regional pain syndrome following stroke: a randomized controlled trial. *QJM.* 2006;99:89–95.

113. Zuurmond WW, Langendijk PN, Bezemer PD, Brink HE, de Lange JJ, van Loenen AC. Treatment of acute reflex sympathetic dystrophy with DMSO 50% in a fatty cream. *Acta Anaesthesiol Scan.* 1996;40:364–367.

114. Perez RS, Zuurmond WW, Bezemer PD, et al. The treatment of complex regional pain syndrome type I with free radical scavengers: a randomized controlled study. *Pain.* 2003;102:297–307.

115. Manicourt DH, Brasseur JP, Boutsen Y, Depreseux G, Devogelaer JP. Role of alendronate in therapy for posttraumatic complex regional pain syndrome type I of the lower extremity. *Arthritis Rheum.* 2004;50:3690–3697.

116. Robinson JN, Sandom J, Chapman PT. Efficacy of pamidronate in complex regional pain syndrome type I. *Pain Med.* 2004;5:276–280.

117. Inchiosa MA Jr, Kizelshteyn G. Treatment of complex regional pain syndrome type 1 with oral phenoxybenzamine: rationale and case reports. *Pain Pract.* 2008;8:125–132.

118. Muizelaar JP, Kleyer M, Hertogs IA, DeLange DC. Complex regional pain syndrome: management with the calcium channel blocker nifedipine and/or the alpha-sympathetic blocker phenoxybenzamine in 59 patients. *Clin Neurol Neurosurg.* 1997;99:26–30.

119. Rauck RL, Eisenach JC, Jackson K, Young LD, Southern J. Epidural clonidine treatment for refractory reflex sympathetic dystrophy. *Anesthesiology.* 1993;79:1163–1169.

120. Borg PA, Krijnen HS. Long-term intrathecal administration of midazolam and clonidine. *Clin J Pain.* 1996;12:63–68.

121. Glynn C, O'Sullivan K. A double-blinded randomized comparison of the effects of epidural clonidine, lignocaine, and the combination of clonidine and lignocaine in patients with chronic pain. *Pain.* 1996;64:337–343.

122. Eisenach JC, DuPen S, Dubois M, Miguel R, Allin D. Epidural clonidine analgesia for intractable cancer pain. *Pain.* 1995;61:391–399.

123. Ionescu DF, Swee MB, Pavone KJ, et al. Rapid and sustained reductions in current suicidal ideation following repeated doses of intravenous ketamine: secondary analysis of an open-label study. *J Clin Psychiatry.* 2016;77(6):e719–e725.

124. Zhong X, He H, Zhang C, et al. Mood and neuropsychological effects of different doses of ketamine in electroconvulsive therapy for treatment-resistant depression. *J Affect Disord.* 2016;201:124–130.

125. van Eijs F, Stanton-Hicks M, Van Zundert J, et al. Evidence-based interventional pain medicine according to clinical diagnosis: complex regional pain syndrome. *Pain Pract.* 2011;11(1):70–87.

126. Kemler MA, de Vet HCW, Barendse GAM, van den Wildenberg FAJM, van Kleef M. Effect of spinal cord stimulation for chronic complex regional pain syndrome type I: five-year follow-up of patients in a randomized controlled trial. *J. Neurosurg.* 2008;108:292–298.

INDEX